THE MANAGEMENT OF LABOUR

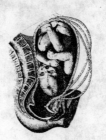

To

Dear Joe & Anne,

With very best wishes

J Warren Regards.

AW

Mr. Joseph Hamlett

—

A great teacher, clinician

friend & Mentor

AW.

THE MANAGEMENT
OF LABOUR

General Editors

S. ARULKUMARAN
MBBS DCH LRCP MRCS FRCS Ed
FRCOG FAMS PhD
Professor and Head
Department of Obstetrics and Gynecology
National University of Singapore
Singapore

S. S. RATNAM
MBBS MD FRCS Ed FRCSG FRCOG FRACOG (Hon)
FWACS (Hon) FACOG (Hon) DSc(Hon)
Director
School of Postgraduate Medical Studies
National University of Singapore
and
Professorial Fellow
Department of Obstetrics and Gynecology
National University of Singapore
Singapore

K. BHASKER RAO
MBBS MD FAMS FRCOG
Formerly
Director, Institute of Obstetrics and Gynecology, Madras
Director-Superintendent,
Government Hospital for Women, Egmore, Madras
and Head of the Department of Obstetrics and Gynecology,
Madras Medical College, Madras, India

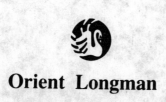

Orient Longman

This book is dedicated to mothers and babies and their caregivers in labour,
all of who have contributed to the understanding of labour
and its optimal management.

Orient Longman Limited

Registered Office
3-6-272 Himayatnagar, Hyderabad 500 029 (A.P.),

Other Offices:
Kamani Marg, Ballard Estate, Bombay 400 038
17 Chittaranjan Avenue, Calcutta 700 072
160 Anna Salai, Madras 600 002
1/24 Asaf Ali Road, New Delhi 110 002

80/1 Mahatma Gandhi Road, Bangalore 560 001
Plot No. 365 Sahid Nagar, Bhubaneswar 751 007
41/316 Gour Mohan, Ambady Lane, Chitoor Road, Cochin 682 011
S.C. Goswami Road, Panbazar, Guwahati 781 001
3-6-272 Himayatnagar, Hyderabad 500 029
House No. 28/31, 15 Ashok Marg, Lucknow 226 001
City Centre Ashok, Govind Mitra Road, Patna 800 004

Laser typeset by
Visvalaya
9 Velders Street
Anna Salai, Madras 600 002

Printed in India at
NPT Offset Pvt. Ltd.
Royapettah
Madras 600 014

Published by
Orient Longman Ltd
160 Anna Salai
Madras 600 002

Foreword

I am pleased to have been asked to write a foreword to this important new text-book 'The Management of Labour' under the editorship of Professors Arulkumaran, Ratnam and Bhasker Rao.

This book will form a significant contribution to the management of labour. The editors and all the contributors are all internationally recognised for their contribution to the management of labour and safe motherhood. All the chapters are well written, readable and the diagrams and charts further simplify the text.

Although most labours are not complicated, all those who provide care for women in labour – midwives, obstetricians and also those who care for the baby – need to know and understand how to manage complications when these arise. This textbook covers all of the aspects. The book makes an important contribution to the management of labour and should become a book that is widely read and used as a reference.

I congratulate the editors and the authors in producing such a comprehensive text.

NAREN PATEL
President
Royal College of Obstetricians
and Gynecologists, UK
Consultant Obstetrician,
Ninewells Hospital and Medical School
Dundee, Scotland, UK

Preface

Passage through the birth canal is the shortest but probably the most hazardous journey made by any individual in his or her life. Hypoxia, trauma and infection are inherent risks. The risks are increased if they are associated with preterm and post-term birth, prelabour rupture of the membranes or antepartum hemorrhage, and when labour is induced as a consequence of medical or obstetric disorders in pregnancy. The mother faces problems of anxiety, pain, infection and if labour is prolonged, the possibility of operative delivery, trauma, postpartum hemorrhage and long term morbidity. At times she runs the risk of losing her life because of complications during childbirth. The women and babies who face these risks every day deserve care to the best of our ability. The art of intrapartum care has evolved and is evidence based. The knowledge of scientific principles should be available to everyone who provides care to the pregnant mother and her unborn child. The end result should be a healthy mother, a healthy baby and emotional satisfaction to those involved including members of the family. These can be achieved by acquiring knowledge, skill and through compassionate team care with attention to details of the needs of the mother, the fetus and the process of labour.

The multi-author volume tries to achieve the goal of providing the knowledge of intrapartum management to the caregiver. It also covers closely related topics which may be of importance just prior to or just after the process of labour. Where possible the book is adequately illustrated. The references cited in each chapter should prove especially useful as they provide recent knowledge in key areas of the field. As editors we have used our vast experience in the subject to fine tune each chapter. We hope that this book will serve the needs of many obstetricians, midwives and trainees who offer valuable care to the pregnant mother in labour.

S. ARULKUMARAN
S. S. RATNAM
K. BHASKER RAO

Contents

List of contributors

C. ANANDAKUMAR
MBBS MMED MRCOG
Associate Professor
Department of Obstetrics and Gynecology
National University of Singapore
Singapore

V. ANNAPOORNA
MBBS MMED
Medical Officer
Department of Obstetrics and Gynecology
National University Hospital
Singapore

S. ARULKUMARAN
MBBS DCH LRCP MRCS FRCS Ed FRCOG FAMS PhD
Professor and Head
Department of Obstetrics and Gynecology
National University of Singapore
Singapore

K. BHASKER RAO
MBBS MD FAMS FRCOG
Consultant Obstetrician and Gynecologist
Formerly
Director, Institute of
Obstetrics and Gynecology, Madras
Director-Superintendent,
Government Hospital for Women
Egmore, Madras and
Head of the Department of Obstetrics and Gynecology
Madras Medical College, Madras, India

A. BISWAS
MBBS MD AIIMSc DIP N B (O & G) MRCOG
Lecturer
Department of Obstetrics and Gynecology
National University of Singapore
Singapore

PAMELA CHAN SIEW LING
MBBS MRCPsych
Lecturer
Department of Psychological Medicine
National University Hospital
Singapore

M. CHOOLANI
MBBS MRCOG MMED MRACOG
Senior Resident/Registrar
Department of Obstetrics and Gynecology
National University Hospital
Singapore

S. CHUA
MBBS MMED MRCOG FAMS
Senior Lecturer and Consultant
Department of Obstetrics and Gynecology
National University Hospital
Singapore

DONALD M. F. GIBB
MBBS MD MRCP FRCOG
Director of Women's Services
Consultant Obstetrician
King's College Hospital
Denmark Hill
London, United Kingdom

R. HATHTHOTUWA
MBBS MRCOG MS (O & G) FRLCOG
Senior Lecturer
Department of Obstetrics and Gynecology
National University Hospital
Singapore

KULDIP SINGH
MBBS MMED (O & G) MRCOG MA in Pop. Research (Exon) FAMS MD
Associate Professor
Department of Obstetrics and Gynecology
National University Hospital
Singapore

LEE TAT LEANG
MBBS MMED (Anaes) FFARACS FAMS
Associate Professor and Head
Department of Anesthesia
National University Hospital
Singapore

K. S. RAGHAVAN
PhD
General Manager
Maternal Health Division
Astra-IDL Ltd
Bangalore

S. S. RATNAM
MBBS MD FRCS Ed
FRCSG FRCOG FRACOG (Hon) FWACS (Hon) FACOG
(Hon), DSc(Hon)
Director
School of Postgraduate Medical Studies
National University of Singapore
and
Professorial Fellow
Department of Obstetrics and Gynecology
National University of Singapore
Singapore

ASHIM C. ROY
Dip Biochem Eng BSc MSc PhD
Senior Research Fellow
Department of Obstetrics and Gynecology
National University of Singapore
Singapore

ROY JOSEPH
MBBS MMed (Ped)
Consultant
Department of Neonatology
National University Hospital
and Associate Professor
Department of Pediatrics
National University of Singapore
Singapore

THAM SUET LAN
MBBS FFARACSI
Senior Registrar
Department of Anesthesia
National University Hospital
Singapore

Y. C. WONG
MBBS MMED FRCOG
Associate Professor
Department of Obstetrics and Gynecology
National University of Singapore
Singapore

1

The Physiopharmacology of Labour

Ashim C Roy
S Arulkumaran

Labour is a multifactorial process which involves myometrial contraction, cervical ripening and dilatation, and the expulsion of the fetus and placenta in an orderly manner. The physiopharmacology of this process has been well documented in various animal species particularly in sheep, but it is not yet fully understood in humans. Biomolecular events that appear to be involved in labour include the formation of gap junctions between the myometrial cells, an increase in the concentration of oxytocin receptors in the uterus and uterine prostaglandin synthesis.

In human parturition, maternal and fetal compartments are interdependent in the regulation of fetal maturation, preparation of the uterus for labour, and initiation of labour. An organ communication system exists between the fetus and mother. This system serves both to maintain pregnancy and to initiate parturition. In the initiation process, the major role is apparently taken by the placental and fetal membranes, while the fetus may modulate the timing of labour.

Both hormonal and paracrine factors have been implicated in the mechanisms of parturition. These include progesterone, oestrogens, oxytocin, prostaglandins, relaxin, second-messengers, corticosteroids, calcium ions and sympathomimetic amines (Roy et al 1985; Roy and Arulkumaran 1991). It is not known whether various tissues involved in the parturition process are under the control of a common factor or are hierarchically organised, one part triggering the action of the other in a chain reaction.

In this review, the current status of some of the prevalent hypotheses of human parturition has been discussed. The emergence of new insights may be useful in the effective management of preterm, term and post-term labour and delivery.

The myometrium and cervix

The uterus is composed of two anatomically distinct but functionally related parts, the myometrium and cervix. They have different functions during gestation and parturition. During pregnancy, the contractility of the myometrium is usually diminished to accommodate and protect the growing products of conception, whereas the cervix forms a tight sphincter to ensure the integrity of pregnancy. Close to term, myometrial activity increases and the cervix undergoes biochemical changes, so called cervical maturation or ripening, by which it becomes soft, distensible and partially dilated. Simultaneously with the initiation of labour contractions, the cervix dilates as a result of the increased compliance and rising intrauterine pressure, and allows birth to occur. The functions of the myometrium and cervix are closely related; they respond in tandem to gestational events, and cooperation between them is essential for normal uterine function. Inappropriate uterine function during pregnancy and labour seriously affects fetal wellbeing and increases perinatal mortality. The myometrial and vascular smooth muscle cells are similar in many respects and share some pharmacological features. This should be taken into account when therapeutic interventions are considered.

Structure and function of the myometrium

The uterus consists of two layers of myometrial smooth muscle. It undergoes a substantial growth in weight (15-fold) and intrauterine volume (500–1,000-fold) during pregnancy. The smooth muscle cells are embedded in an extracellular matrix composed mainly of collagen fibres (Huszar and Walsh 1989). They are linked to one another by gap junctions which are sites of electrical and metabolic coupling in all types of cells. These cells are composed of proteins (connexins) aligned between two cells to form small channels that permit cell-to-cell diffusion of inorganic ions and small molecules such as second-messengers and metabolites (Cole and Garfield 1986). Gap junctions are characterised by low electrical impedance (that is, high conductivity) which allows a rapid spread of the action potentials between neighbouring cells, facilitating the synchronisation of contractile activity.

The development of gap junctions in the myometrium may be one of the necessary steps in the initiation and maintenance of labour. In laboratory animals, the size and density of myometrial gap junctions begin to increase shortly before term, and their number becomes significantly higher during labour and then falls rapidly during postpartum (Garfield et al 1980; Saito et al 1985). Oestrogens and prostaglandins enhance the formation of uterine gap junctions while progesterone partially diminishes this effect (Garfield et al 1980), whereas Ca^{2+} and cyclic adenosine monophosphate (cAMP) exert a regulatory influence over the permeability of gap junction channels (Cole and Garfield 1986, 1988; Garfield et al 1987). Similarly in the human uterus, gap junctions were found to be present between myometrial cells in high numbers in term and preterm patients with frequent uterine contractions, whereas they were present in very low frequencies in women with infrequent uterine contractions and absent in most tissues from nonpregnant women (Garfield and Hayashi 1980, 1981; Balducci et al 1992). Recently, it has been shown that the levels of mRNA encoding the gap junction protein connexin-43 were elevated in the human myometrium towards term and with the onset of labour (Chow and Lye 1994). Therefore if gap junctions are essential for effective labour and delivery, prevention of their formation may be a novel approach for the treatment of preterm labour.

The regulation of myometrial contractility

In pregnant women, uterine activity increases slowly during the second and third trimesters after which a more coordinated pattern of the contractions develops (Braxton-Hicks contractions). The contractions are triggered from various parts of uterus, most commonly near the cornual areas, and they then spread downward towards the lower segment. As term approaches and labour begins, these contractions become stronger, of longer duration and more frequent.

The basic contractile apparatus of the uterus, like that of other smooth muscles, consists of actin and myosin filament (Huszar and Walsh 1989). Myosin is the principal protein of muscle contraction. It is a large molecule made up of two heavy chains and two light-chains. It has three functional sites: the actin combining site where actin interacts with myosin to form actomyosin; the ATPase activity site where ATP is hydrolysed to release energy for contraction; the light-chain site which regulates the actin-myosin interaction. In the myometrium, as in all muscles, the formation of actomyosin constitutes the molecular basis for muscle contraction. Phosphorylation of the light chains by myosin light-chain kinase, an enzyme that requires Ca^{2+} and calmodulin for its activity, promotes contraction, whereas dephosphorylation of the light chains by myosin light-chain phosphatase leads to muscle relaxation. Thus, the muscle contraction is controlled by the concentration of Ca^{2+} in the surrounding cytoplasm. A rise in Ca^{2+} switches it on, and a fall in Ca^{2+} switches it off. However both the normal quiescence of the uterus during pregnancy and the initiation of uterine contractions in labour are results not of a single mechanism but rather of the highly integrated collocation of many different processes.

Peptides   Various peptide hormones and functional peptides participate in the modulation of uterine contractility. The best known and studied is oxytocin which has been traditionally used for the induction and augmentation of labour, and the treatment of uterine inertia (Roy and Arulkumaran 1991). It stimulates myometrial contraction in late pregnancy and this effect is similar to that of spontaneous labour. In early pregnancy, however the uterus remains insensitive even to large doses of oxytocin. An increase in sensitivity which is related to an increase in the myometrial oxytocin receptors occurs around the 20th week of gestation, after which it remains unchanged until just before the beginning of spontaneous labour. The precise mechanism of oxytocin action is not yet clear other than that it increases intracellular calcium levels (Mironneau 1976; Soloff and Sweet 1982). The hormone also promotes myometrial contractility through stimulation of PGE_2 and PGF_2 release (Fuchs and Fuchs 1984). The principal site of stimulation is the decidua or endometrium, and it is associated with increased phosphoinositide turnover (Schrey et al 1986; Silvia and Homanics 1988). Oxytocin induces the synthesis of the second-messenger, IP_3 (Schrey et al 1986) which causes the release of intracellular calcium from the sarcoplasmic reticulum.

Vasopressin has little oxytocic potency in rats, but it has considerable activity in the human. In fact, the nonpregnant human uterus is more sensitive to vasopressin than to oxytocin (Embrey and Moir 1967). In spite of the structural homology, the receptors for oxytocin and vasopressin are of different entities (Guillon et al 1987; Ivanisevic et al 1989). It is also of interest that the density of vasopressin receptors peaks at about 32 weeks of gestation, whereas oxytocin receptors increase throughout pregnancy and labour (Fuchs and Fuchs 1984; Maggi et al 1990).

A peptide hormone known to decrease the myometrial contractility in several animals is relaxin (Roy and Arulkumaran 1991; Roy et al 1984a). The peptide, like isoproterenol, decreases cellular IP_3 and intracellular free calcium concentrations, thereby decreasing myosin light-chain kinase activity (Sanborn et al 1975; Anwer et al 1989). In vivo studies in rats and pigs demonstrated that relaxin inhibited spontaneous myometrial contractility but similar doses had no effect on oxytocin- or prostaglandin-induced contractions (Goldsmith et al 1989; Pupula and MacLennan 1989). Thus relaxin may promote uterine relaxation during pregnancy, but in labour it may bring about cervical maturation without interfering with uterine contractility.

Certain peptide neurotransmitters, such as the vasoactive intestinal polypeptide (VIP), dilate uterine blood vessels and inhibit uterine contractility in a dose-dependent manner (Ottesen et al 1980; Clark et al 1981). The nerves supplying the blood vessels and smooth muscle in the uterus contain VIP (Larsson et al 1977; Ottesen et al 1980). The concentration of VIP in the uterus is modulated by steroid hormones.

Adrenergic stimulation   The human myometrium contains subclasses of both α-adrenoceptors and ß-adrenoceptors; A stimulation of α-adrenoceptors causes uterine contraction, whereas stimulation of ß-adrenoceptors promotes uterine relaxation (Roy and Arulkumaran 1991). Oestrogen and progesterone influence the relative sensitivity of the myometrium to α- and ß-adrenoceptor stimulation. Oestrogen treatment results in reduced myometrial sensitivity to ß-agonist induced relaxation which is antagonised by progesterone. Beta receptors stimulate adenyl cyclase activity (cAMP synthesising enzyme), and $alpha_2$ receptors exert their action by inhibiting adenyl cyclase, whereas $alpha_1$ receptors are coupled to the inositol phosphate pathway. All are regulated by a family of proteins called GTP-binding proteins or G proteins which couple the receptors to their effectors and either stimulate or inhibit second-messenger activity. In late term pregnancy in the rat, α-adrenergic activity appears predominantly in the circular muscle layer of the uterus and ß-adrenergic activity in the longitudinal muscle layer (Kawarabayashi and Osa 1976). Within a few hours after delivery a sharp increase in α_1-adrenoceptors has been observed, whereas the number of ß-adrenoceptors has been seen to drop (Legrand et al 1987). Studies of the human late pregnant uterus have yielded conflicting results. While one group reported decreased ß-adrenoceptor activity at term (Litime et al 1989), another group found no change in the concentrations of ß-receptors or in the efficacy of ß-adrenergic agonists (Dattel et al 1986). Prolonged treatment with ß-agonists results in the down-regulation of ß-adrenoceptors. Administration of ß-agonists in a pulsatile manner has therefore been suggested as a more effective alternative to continuous infusions (Spätling et al 1989).

In late pregnant human myometrial tissue in vitro adrenaline and high concentrations of isoproterenol caused excitatory effects, whereas forskolin, which directly activates cAMP biosynthesis, caused relaxation (Story et al 1989), suggesting a switch to α-receptor dominance from ß-receptor dominance. This indicates that myometrial contraction in response to adrenergic stimuli depends upon the ratio of α- and ß-receptors, independently of the availability of intracellular second-messenger activity. It is possible that individual women vary in the relative α- and ß-receptor dominance, which would explain the woman-to-woman variations in the efficacy of tocolytic therapy.

Cholinergic stimulation   The human uterus is well supplied with both adrenergic and cholinergic nerves (Roy and Arulkumaran 1991). During pregnancy, the uterine adrenergic neurotransmitter is extensively reduced probably leading to functional denervation near term. In contrast, the uterine cholinergic neurotransmitter remains unchanged during pregnancy and labour. Intravenous infusion of acetyl-choline induces labour at term. Although this drug can also produce coordinated uterine contractions, its cardiovascular and other muscarinic side effects are gen-erally considered to preclude its clinical use.

Prostaglandins   Prostaglandins (PGs) are known to play a key role in the physiological activation of the uterus during parturition (Roy and Arulkumaran 1991). Prostaglandins of the E- and F-types stimulate contraction of the human pregnant uterus both in vitro and in vivo. They can stimulate the uterus from the early stages of gestation and terminate pregnancy at all stages, thus differing from the best known oxytocic, oxytocin, which has very little effect in the first and second trimester. Seven different types of prostaglandin receptors have been de-scribed in the human uterus (Coleman et al 1989). The receptors for the contractant prostaglandins are coupled to pathways that increase intracellular Ca^{2+} so that more Ca^{2+} is available to myosin light-chain kinase for its activation to promote contrac-tion through phosphorylation of the myosin light-chains.

   All uterine tissues have the ability to synthesise PGs in vitro. Their uterine synthesis is enhanced by oestradiol, whereas progesterone blocks this increase. Their synthesis is also stimulated by oxytocin whose occurrence may be due to the increased hydrolysis of phosphionosides to diacylglycerol and inositol phos-phates with the subsequent release of arachidonic acid, the precursor of the '2-series' of prostaglandins, from diacylglycerol.

The structure and function of the cervix

In mammals, the cervix represents the terminal portion of the uterus and separates the vagina from the uterine activity. It is a thick-walled, cylindrical structure that tapers at its inferior extremity. The cervix has almost diametrically opposing roles during gestation. It provides an unyielding barrier between the fetus and the outside world for most of the pregnancy. Then, during the very short period of time required for parturition, it gives way and allows the fetus to be born. The dual opposing functions of the cervix have their corresponding physical states. The cervix is rela-tively firm during most of the antepartum course and becomes softer and more compliant as the time for parturition approaches. Finally, during the time of par-turition, the cervix rapidly loses its remaining elasticity, plasticity and viscosity, resulting in complete cervical dilatation (Stys 1986). Even though the most pro-nounced cervical changes occur in late gestation, some changes are evident even quite early in pregnancy (Anthony et al 1982).

   There are three main structural components in the cervix of women. These are smooth muscle, collagen, and the connective tissue 'ground substance' contain-ing glycosaminoglycans. The distribution of smooth muscle in the uterus and cervix varies from segment to segment. About 65–70 per cent of the human myometrium is composed of smooth muscle, whereas smooth muscle content in the cervix is about 25 per cent, 16 per cent and 6 per cent in the upper, middle and lower segments, respectively (Rorie and Newton 1967). In some animal species, smooth muscle has an active role in cervical dilatation. Similar function however has yet to be demonstrated in women. Changes that take place in collagen and in the connective tissue matrix are the primary factors in cervical ripening. During cervical ripening, the ground substance becomes more prominent and the collagen fibrils, previously arranged in an orderly fashion, break up (Harkness and Harkness 1959; Danforth et al 1960, 1974). The cervical distensibility increases, while protein and collagen concentrations decline. The loss of collagen is the result of proteolytic digestion and subsequent elimination of the soluble collagen fragments.

The control of cervical maturation

Cervical ripening by means of which the cervix becomes soft, distensible and partially dilated, is a necessary prerequisite to normal parturition. This is thought to be the result of increasing myometrial contractility in late pregnancy. It takes place slowly but progressively over the last few weeks of pregnancy, and rapidly over a day or two before the spontaneous onset of labour at term. It is accompanied by a similar softening of the connective tissue of the lower segment of the uterine body, leading to the thinning of this area in response to Braxton-Hicks contractions of the myometrium (Roy and Arulkumaran 1991).

The biochemical mechanisms of cervical softening are poorly understood in the human. It is known that cervical collagen breakdown is influenced by various connective tissue hormones. It is widely accepted that prostaglandins have discrete softening and effacement effects on the cervix that are not possessed by oxytocin. Intracervical administration of PGE_2 or $F_{2\alpha}$ produces cervical changes in women without uterine contraction (Hillier and Wallis 1981; Goeschen et al 1985). Prostaglandins have the capacity to increase the production of glycosaminoglycans from fibroblasts in culture (Roy and Arulkumaran 1991). Cervical tissues have the ability to generate prostaglandins (Ellwood et al 1980), and thus endogenous PGs may participate in the cervical ripening process. The clinical value of prostaglandins for preoperative cervical dilatation and pre-induction cervical ripening has now been well established.

Oestrogens may also play a physiological role in cervical ripening. They have been used clinically to soften the cervix, but the results are equivocal. Some researchers reported the softening of an unfavourable cervix with oestradiol, whereas others have reported negligible effects. The administration of the progesterone receptor antagonist, RU486 (mifepristone) to pregnant animals and women for the induction of abortion was associated with cervical ripening (Wolf et al 1989; Elger et al 1990; Silvestre et al 1990). Progesterone may therefore be essential for the maintenance of firmness of the cervix. However since RU486 blocks not only progesterone but also glucocorticoid receptors (Editorial 1990), whether cervical ripening resulted from progesterone withdrawal or other action of the antagonist is not known. It is unlikely to have caused prostaglandin release in cervical tissues because there is evidence to suggest that RU486 treatment suppresses prostaglandin release (Elger et al 1990). The action of RU486 may be indirect and due to oestrogen receptor replenishment following the blockade of progesterone action. Human cervical tissue possesses oestrogen receptors (Honnebier et al 1989), and oestrogens including DHEAS (dehydroepiandrosterone sulphate) have been shown to be accumulated in the ripening cervix (Ishikawa and Shimizu 1989). DHEA has recently been used widely in Japan for the induction of cervical ripening (Ishikawa and Shimizu 1989).

Some strong evidence suggests that relaxin may have a role in human gestation and cervical maturation similar to that in rodents. The level of this ovarian polypeptide hormone increases significantly in the human cervical tissue towards the end of pregnancy (Von Maillot et al 1979). It is also present in the decidua and chorion laeve at term, and has a paracrine effect on the amnion, inhibiting PGE production during gestation but favouring PGE production during spontaneous labour (Lopez-Bernal et al 1980). Fetal membranes and the decidua also express the relaxin gene (Sakburn et al 1990). Specific receptors for relaxin have been identified in the amnion, and in this tissue relaxin increases the production and secretion of collagenase activity (Koay et al 1983). Double-blind randomised trials in pregnant women showed that the vaginal application of preparations of purified relaxin, made from porcine ovaries before surgical or oxytocic induction of labour, was associated with cervical ripening in most cases (MacLennan et al 1980, 1981; Evans et al 1983). Relaxin was as effective as prostaglandins when administered in this way, but there was no additive effect when these hormones were used in combination (MacLennan et al 1981).

The initiation of labour

The role of steroid hormones

The hypothesis postulating a uterine-stimulating action of oestrogen and a uterine-relaxing effect of progesterone has long been promulgated. Oestrogen causes the development and growth of uterine muscle accompanied by increased activity and contractility, whereas progesterone elicits relaxation of the myometrial cells. Progesterone is necessary for the maintenance of a relatively quiescent uterus during pregnancy in most mammals (Thorburn and Challis 1979). In non-primate species, labour is preceded by an increase in the oestrogen : progesterone ratio. It has previously been held that removal of the progesterone block to uterine activity was necessary for labour to occur in women (Csapo 1977). However in the human and in the rhesus monkey, peripheral plasma concentrations of progesterone and oestrogens do not change significantly immediately preceding labour at term or preterm (Thorburn and Challis 1979). This applies to both free and protein-bound, and conjugated as well as unconjugated placental steroids. The levels of oestrogens and progesterone in uterine arterial and venous blood also remain constant (Davidson et al 1987). A recent study in which salivary oestriol and progesterone levels were measured in women before, during and after spontaneous labour also found no significant change in the concentration of either steroid immediately preceding or during labour (Lewis et al 1987).

Neither measurements of uterine tissue levels of oestradiol and progesterone, nor the levels of their myometrial receptors at term and after the onset of labour revealed any significant labour related changes in pregnant women (Giannopoulos et al 1979, 1980). At term, the myometrial receptor levels of both oestradiol and progesterone were found to be as low or lower than in nonpregnant women. The percentage of occupied receptors was considerably higher in pregnant than in nonpregnant women, indicating an active progestational state with no changes at the onset of labour. The low levels of unoccupied oestrogen and progesterone receptors reflect the ability of progesterone to suppress the replenishment of both oestrogen and progesterone receptors in uterine tissues (Leavitt and Takeda 1986; Okulicz 1986, 1989).

On the other hand, RU486 (mifepristone), an antagonist to progesterone activity, induces abortion in women during the first trimester and oestradiol increases uterine activity in pregnant women (Pinto et al 1964; Ulmann et al 1987). These observations suggest that changes in the oestrogen : progesterone ratio may play a role in controlling uterine activity. It has been found, however, that the rhesus monkey treated in late gestation with RU486 had only temporary induction of uterine activity and did not go into labour unless oxytocin was administered (Wolf et al 1989; Elger et al 1990; Haluska et al 1990). Such treatment induced cervical changes and increased uterine oestrogen receptor levels but these changes were not observed in animals with spontaneous labour (Haluska et al 1990).

It has been suggested that modulation of progesterone and oestrogen biosynthesis in human fetal membranes could occur at term, resulting in the local withdrawal of progesterone and increased oestradiol synthesis which is not detectable by measurements of concentrations in the maternal peripheral circulation (Mitchell and Challis 1988). The human amnion, chorion, and decidua are steroidogenic tissues, producing oestrogens and progesterone primarily from sulfated precursors (Mitchell and Challis 1988; Gibb et al 1988). It has been found that the steroid synthesising enzyme, steroid sulfohydrase activity is increased in the chorion after spontaneous labour (Mitchell and Challis 1988). Another enzyme, 17ß, 20α-hydroxysteroid dehydrogenase (17ß, 20α-HSD) which catalyses the conversion of oestrone to the more biologically active oestradiol and progesterone to the inactive progestin 20α-dihydroprogesterone is also found to be present in fetal membranes, the decidua and placenta (Strickler et al 1981; Mitchell and Challis 1988). There is some evidence that placental 17ß, 20α-HSD activity is increased towards term, but data regarding 17ß, 20α-HSD in fetal membranes is not available. Mitchell and Challis (1988) contend that regulation of substrate supply and enzymatic activity could determine local oestrogen and progesterone levels in the fetal membranes. In turn, the alterations in the local levels of oestrogens and progesterone effect the onset of labour via their influence on local prostaglandin production.

Progesterone appears to inhibit prostaglandin $F_{2\alpha}$ production in human endometrial tissues, which suggests that it may also regulate decidual prostaglandin production (Abel and Baird 1980). Oestrogens stimulate prostaglandin production in the human amnion, decidua and endometrial tissues, and may thus favour the onset of labour (Abel and Baird 1980; Olson et al 1983). In recent studies on chorion laeve cells however it was glucocorticoids, not progesterone, which inhibited prostaglandin production, and oestrogens failed to stimulate prostaglandin production (Gibb et al 1988). Further studies are needed to define more clearly the role of steroids in the control of intrauterine prostaglandin production, as there may be differences in the responses of tissues taken before and after labour.

Further evidence is needed to support the hypothesis of a local withdrawal of progesterone and an increase in oestrogen production at term by human fetal membranes and the decidua. Under the circumstances, it may be assumed that uterine activity is initiated by uterine stimulating hormones such as oxytocin, vasopressin and/or prostaglandins.

The role of oxytocin

Historically oxytocin was considered to be the primary factor responsible for the onset of labour. It is one of the most potent and specific uterine contractile agents known. Exogenously administered oxytocin induces contractions resembling those of spontaneous labour, and when given at term, is effective in inducing parturition in all mammalian species studied. However the role of endogenous oxytocin in the initiation of human parturition remains suspect because increased maternal plasma levels do not appear until the second stage of labour (Soloff 1988).

Recently Fuchs et al (1991) reexamined the secretory pattern of oxytocin in pregnant and parturient women using a more sensitive and specific antibody to oxytocin than previously used. Blood samples were taken at 1-min interval of 30 min at three stages: prior to the onset of labour, in the first stage of labour, and in the second stage of labour. A pulsatile pattern of oxytocin secretion was evident in all patients, the frequency of pulses was found to vary significantly in the three groups of patients. The lowest frequency was observed in women not in labour, and the highest frequency was noted in the second and third stages of labour. The pulses were similar to those produced by bolus injections of oxytocin administered intravenously. These results provide clear evidence of increased oxytocin secretion during all stages of human labour in quantities sufficient to induce uterine contractions. The pulsatile secretion pattern explains the failure of some investigators who collected samples at infrequent intervals, to detect a rise in plasma oxytocin during labour (Sellers et al 1981), or only during the expulsive phase (Leake et al 1981). Moreover, oxytocin originates not only in the hypothalamus-posterior pituitary, but also in the decidua, amnion, chorion and placenta (Lefebvre et al 1992; Chibbar et al 1993), and hormone released from the latter sources may not necessarily be reflected in an increased plasma level.

Fetal pituitary oxytocin may also play a role in the initiation of labour. The human fetal pituitary gland is able to secrete oxytocin at birth, and the fetus releases large amounts of oxytocin during spontaneous labour and parturition (Roy et al 1985). There are relatively high levels of oxytocin found in the umbilical cord blood (artery > vein) after normal labour and delivery (Sellers et al 1981). Labour has been induced by intramuscular administration of oxytocin into anencephalic fetuses (Honnebier and Swaab 1974), thus providing clear evidence of the transport of oxytocin from the fetus to the mother. Substantial amounts of biologically active oxytocin have been found in the human placenta after spontaneous vaginal delivery (Fields et al 1983), indicating that the placenta does not degrade oxytocin as rapidly as is commonly believed.

It has been postulated that the increasing sensitivity of the myometrium to basal levels of oxytocin receptors at term is the key to the onset of labour (Soloff 1988). The changes in uterine sensitivity to oxytocin during the stages of pregnancy correlate well with the uterine oxytocin receptor levels which increase in parallel, reaching the maximum at the time of labour (Fuchs and Fuchs 1984). Oestrogen increases and progesterone decreases the formation of oxytocin receptors during gestation. The rise in oxytocin receptor levels is thought to be the biological basis for the increased oxytocin response. The rise in receptor levels lowers the threshold for stimulation so that the low amplitude pulses of oxytocin become sufficient to elicit contractions in late gestation. The fact that administration of ethanol which inhibits oxytocin and vasopressin release, or atosiban which is an oxytocin receptor antagonist abolishes Braxton-Hicks contractions of late pregnancy and early labour, adds strong support to the notion that endogenous oxytocin plays an important role in the initiation of human labour (Landesman and Fuchs 1973; Akerlund et al 1987). Moreover the lower concentration of oxytocin receptors found in advanced labour than at the onset of labour also suggests that oxytocin is a less important uterine stimulator in advanced labour than in the early stages of the delivery process (Fuchs 1990; Maggi et al 1990). The decrease in receptor concentration may be related to the down-regulating effect of oxytocin on its own receptor. An increase in maternal circulating oxytocin during labour may be related, but a more substantial release of oxytocin from uterine and fetoplacental sources (Lefebvre et al 1992; Chibbar et al 1993) may be the cause of lowered oxytocin receptor concentration as delivery progresses. A further confirmation of the existence of such a mechanism of down-regulation is the recent finding of a tendency for reduced oxytocin receptor concentration in women who had received oxytocin infusion for ≥ 3 hours or of a total dose > 5 nmol in comparison with those who had shorter treatment or lower total dose (Bossmar et al 1994).

The role of vasopressin

Vasopressin has little oxytocic potency in rats, but has considerable activity in the human. In fact the nonpregnant human uterus is more sensitive to vasopressin than to oxytocin (Embrey and Moir 1967). During pregnancy, the uterine sensitivity to vasopressin rises proportionately but less than to oxytocin, and at term the oxytocin sensitivity is higher than the vasopressin sensitivity (Embrey and Moir 1967). Maternal plasma levels of vasopressin remain low during pregnancy and labour, but considerable amounts of vasopressin can be demonstrated in the cord blood with a remarkable arteriovenous difference, indicating the fetal origin of the hormone (Pohjavuori and Fyhrquist 1980; Parboosingh et al 1982). Umbilical arterial vasopressin levels are particularly high during fetal distress and fetal hypoxia has been shown to be a powerful stimulus for vasopressin release in sheep (Alexander et al 1972; Stark et al 1982). The great arteriovenous difference in umbilical cord vasopressin concentrations means that large amounts of fetal vasopressin enter the placenta and possibly the maternal circulation as well, which may add considerable stimulating activity to the circulating oxytocin. A significant fraction of fetal vasopressin appears in the amniotic fluid (Stark et al 1982) in which little degradation occurs because oxytocinase (aminopeptidase) activity, which is also known to inactivate vasopressin, decreases to minimal levels at term (Roy et al 1984b, 1986). Vasopressin receptor levels in the myometrium and decidua also rise during pregnancy and are about 50 per cent lower than oxytocin receptor levels at term (Ivanisevic et al 1989). Both the neuropeptide hormones show considerable affinity to each other's binding sites and may share a common receptor. Oxytocin antagonists effectively block both oxytocin and vasopressin receptors (Ivanisevic et al 1989; Bossmar et al 1994). Interestingly, myometrial oxytocin effect is mediated only by oxytocin receptors, whereas vasopressin acts on both oxytocin and vasopressin receptors and thus may play a role in the regulation of labour (Bossmar et al 1994).

The role of prostaglandins

All the uterine tissues have the capacity to synthesise prostaglandins in vitro, although the spectrum of PGs produced varies somewhat from tissue to tissue (Fuchs and Fuchs 1984). An increase in intrauterine PG production occurs during labour in all mammals studied, including the human. Prostaglandins are potent myometrial contractile agents, and they induce labour and interrupt pregnancy at any time during gestation. Prostaglandin synthetase inhibitors can delay the onset of parturition and suppress uterine contractions during preterm labour. Amniotic fluid prostaglandin levels increase during term labour but not before term, and circulating prostaglandin metabolites increase during advanced labour. The urinary excretion of prostaglandins markedly rises on the day following delivery which attests to their increased production during labour. These facts strongly suggest a key role for prostaglandins in the mechanism of labour.

No difference has been found in the uterine arterial and venous concentrations of PGE and PGF, or in their metabolites in samples obtained at caesarean section prior to the onset of labour. However in samples obtained during active labour, increased concentrations of the prostaglandins were found in the uterine veins (Fuchs and Fuchs 1984; Davidson et al 1987). These findings indicate that uterine PG production increases during labour in women, and that PGs probably do not initiate human labour.

The endogenous capacity to form prostaglandins by uterine tissues is present throughout pregnancy, and no marked changes in this capacity occur at the onset of labour (Fuchs and Fuchs 1984). It is not yet clear whether under in vivo conditions uterine PG synthesis is suppressed during pregnancy by endogenous inhibitors that are withdrawn during parturition, or alternatively whether stimulatory factors increase the rate of production of prostaglandins during labour. A total withdrawal of inhibitory action may not be necessary; a shift in the balance of inhibiting and stimulating factors in favour of simulators may suffice.

An endogenous inhibitor of prostaglandin synthesis (EIPS) has been shown to be present in the human amniotic fluid. This amniotic fluid EIPS activity decreases towards term and particularly in labour (Saeed et al 1982). The source of EIPS in human amniotic fluid is as yet uncertain. EIPS-like activity has been suggested to be present in the amnion at term before the onset of labour (Mortimer et al 1985). This activity was reported to be completely absent in the amnion obtained after labour. Antiphospholipase proteins have been detected in the amniotic fluid and intrauterine tissues. These could presumably decrease the availability of the substrate for conversion to prostaglandins (Wilson et al 1985; Liggins and Wilson, 1986). Decidual prolactin has also been shown to inhibit the amnion PGE_2 production (Tyson et al 1985). Disruption of the contact between the decidua and the fetal membranes results in increased prostaglandin formation by the membranes. It has been suggested that disruption of contact in vivo could serve as a trigger for labour. Romero et al (1987) have found that a decidual conditioned medium inhibits amnion cell PGE_2 synthesis, suggesting that the decidua secretes a substance which suppresses amnion prostaglandin production.

Oxytocin was the first endogenous compound shown to stimulate prostaglandin formation in uterine tissues at term (Fuchs and Fuchs 1984). Vasopressin, which stimulates prostaglandin synthesis in the adult kidney as well, may also affect the amniotic fluid prostaglandin levels by stimulating the fetal kidney to produce PGE which is then secreted with fetal urine. Histamine and bradykinin also have the capacity to stimulate prostaglandin release from various tissues including the decidua and amnion. It is possible that activation of the uterine mast cells or kininogens of fetal origin might lead to their release and subsequently to prostaglandin release. Other fetal excretory products recently found in the amniotic fluid which stimulate prostaglandin formation in the amnion cell include the platelet-activating factor (PAF) (Bleasdale and Johnston 1985), the epidermal growth factor (EGF) (Casey et al 1987), the transforming growth factor alpha (TGFα) (Mitchell 1988), and some of the interleukins (Mitchell et al 1993; Dudley et al 1994). The levels of these substances increase in the amniotic fluid during late pregnancy or labour. These substances may provide a link between fetal development and the onset of labour. Another family of small proteins found in the amniotic fluid are endothelins (Mitchell et al 1991). Their concentrations are elevated in the amniotic fluid in women with infections of the amniotic fluid who are delivered preterm. Infections also cause the production of cytokines which stimulate prostaglandins production. This probably does not take place in normal and uncomplicated labour. Cytokines also stimulate the production of endothelins by the amnion (Mitchell et al 1991). Endothelins have been shown to be potent both in elevating cytoplasmic calcium concentrations and in increasing myosin phosphorylation in the human myometrium (Word et al 1990). Hence, if endothelins secreted by the amnion were to reach the myometrium, it could have a significant effect on contractile function.

The interaction between oxytocin and prostaglandins

An interaction of oxytocin with prostaglandins in the uterus may be very important for the mechanism of labour (Roy and Karim 1983a and b). Oxytocin plays a dual role in the mechanism of parturition: it stimulates myometrial contractions by activating myometrial oxytocin receptors, and it stimulates prostaglandin production in the decidual tissue which also has oxytocin receptors (Fuchs and Fuchs 1984). However stimulation of myometrial contractions by oxytocin is not mediated by intracellular prostaglandin generation. Its mechanism of contractile action involves an increase in the level of free Ca^{2+} in the cells mediated by the second-messenger, inositol 1,4,5-triphosphate (IP_3) system (Fuchs 1990).

The prostaglandins also have a dual action: they promote cervical softening and potentiate oxytocin-induced myometrial contractions (Fuchs and Fuchs 1984; Coleman and Parkington 1988). Induction of labour with oxytocin in women at term succeeds in dilating the cervix only when the infusion is associated with increased maternal prostaglandin F production. The linking of oxytocin receptors to the prostaglandin synthase system in the decidua is therefore of crucial importance in the mechanism of labour. The determination of the temporal relationship of plasma oxytocin and prostaglandin F metabolite levels during spontaneous labour supports this view. The concentrations of plasma oxytocin were significantly increased over prelabour values in early as well as late labour, whereas the concentrations of the metabolite were increased only in the later stages (Fuchs and Fuchs 1984).

The released prostaglandins in the decidua may diffuse into the adjacent myometrium and potentiate oxytocin induced contraction. Amniotic fluid levels of prostaglandins and their metabolites remain low throughout oxytocin-induced labour and delivery (Padayachi et al 1986). Moreover, it has been shown that the PGF metabolite appearing in the maternal circulation during oxytocin-induced labour is of decidual origin (Fuchs and Fuchs 1984). This indicates that prostaglandin production by the fetal membranes is not essential for the progress of labour or cervical dilatation. Atosiban, the oxytocin antagonist which also binds to decidual receptors (Ivanisevic et al 1989) is likely to block both direct contractile effects of oxytocin on the myometrium and the oxytocin induced decidual prostaglandin synthesis.

Fuchs and collaborators have suggested that oxytocin rather than $PGF_{2\alpha}$ may be the major stimulus that initiates labour, whereas $PGF_{2\alpha}$ may be responsible for the progress of labour (Fuchs and Fuchs 1984). Support for this hypothesis is provided by the observation that the administration of ethanol, which inhibits oxytocin and vasopressin release, abolishes the Braxton-Hicks uterine contractions and prevents early but not advanced labour (Fuchs and Fuchs 1984). Similarly, the finding that the myometrial oxytocin receptor concentration was lower in advanced labour than at the beginning of labour (Fuchs 1990; Bossmar et al 1994) suggests that oxytocin is less important as a uterine stimulator in advanced labour than in the early stages of labour.

Decidual activation

Decidual activation may be a contributing factor to the onset of labour. Casey and MacDonald (1988) suggested that the maintenance of pregnancy and the initiation of parturition are closely aligned by way of the timely regulation of decidual function. Human decidua parietalis contains a number of different cell types besides the large decidualised stromal cells. Small numbers of epithelial cells, mast cells, lymphocytes, and macrophages are present throughout gestation (Nehemiah et al 1981). All of these cell types are potential sources of prostaglandins and other compounds such as histamine, cytokines and endothelin that may serve in a paracrine fashion to modulate the function of decidual cells (Salamonsen and Findlay 1990). Significant amounts of these compounds are accumulated in the amniotic fluid during labour. Human decidua has also an endocrine function: it possesses several enzymes involved in the steroid metabolism (Lopez-Bernal et al 1980; Gibb et al 1988; Mitchell and Challis 1988).

Decidual function is regulated by a fetal-decidual paracrine system, whereby the fetus contributes to the maintenance of pregnancy (Casey and MacDonald 1988). The withdrawal of fetal support of this paracrine system results in the activation of the decidua. The stromal and epithelial cells are the main sites of prostaglandin synthesis. The activated mast cells release histamine and the activated macrophages release cytokines, which in turn can stimulate the stromal cells to release prostaglandins. This may be an important factor in the pathogenesis of infection related preterm labour. It is not known, however, whether decidual macrophages and mast cells are activated at the onset of labour in normal pregnant women. Whatever triggers the synthesis of decidual prostaglandins, they immediately and directly diffuse into the adjacent myometrium without entering the vascular system, thereby avoiding degradation in the lungs and other organs. Decidual secretory products may also diffuse through the adjacent chorioamnion and influence fetal functions.

Immune function

One of the most intriguing concepts of pregnancy is the fetus as allograft. In the absence of immunotolerance, the fetus will be rejected by the maternal host and it is thought that this is the cause of recurrent abortion in some women (Mowbray and Underwood 1985). The exact mechanism of this rejection and subsequent labour is unknown. Whether normal parturition is due to the timely rejection of a previously tolerated allograft is still open to speculation.

Several hypotheses have been developed in an effort to understand why the immunocompetent mother does not reject the fetoplacental allograft. These include: a lack of transplantation antigens on the trophoblast; the placenta as an immunological barrier; local suppression of the maternal immune system. Recent studies reveal a novel regulation of major histocompatibility complex (MHC) antigens by placental cells in such a way that a complete lack of or only partial expression of MHC antigens occur on some cell types (Fisher and Lawler 1984; Sutton et al 1986; Bulmer et al 1988; Hunt et al 1988). Antibody formation to MHC antigens occurs in a large percentage of multiparous (36–64%) and primiparous (nearly 25%) women (Burke and Johansen 1974; Beard et al 1983). Trophoblast antigens other than those of the MHC antigens have also been described. Some of these antigens are immunogenic (McIntyre et al 1983). Yet, in normal pregnancies, antibodies formed to MHC or non-MHC antigens fail to damage the placenta or fetus. In fact, many consider maternal antibody formation to fetal antigens a normal and necessary response to pregnancy (Mowbray and Underwood 1985).

The maternal antibodies formed to fetal antigens rarely gain access to the fetus. This may be largely because the placenta serves as an immunological barrier. In addition to the physical barrier between the maternal and fetal circulations provided by the placenta, extravillous trophoblast cells have the capacity to bind, internalise, and inactivate the maternal antibodies produced by fetal antigens (Beer and Sio 1982).

Immunosuppression may be another mechanism by which the fetal allograft is tolerated. There are factors in the maternal serum which block cell-mediated immune function (Daya et al 1985, 1987). Many investigators have suggested that fetoplacental hormones play a role in immunosuppression. Progesterone, chorionic gonadotropin (CG) and chorionic somatomammotropin (CS) are all produced in high concentrations by the fetoplacental unit. While experiments fail to show a clear immunosuppressive role for either CG or CS, progesterone has definite immunosuppressive properties as shown by its ability to block lymphocyte responses in in vitro tests and its ability to impair graft rejection in laboratory animals (Siiteri and Stites 1982).

It has been reported that lymphocyte cytotoxicity is increased at the time of term and preterm labour in women (Szekeres-Bortho et al 1986). A local withdrawal of immunosuppressive factors such as progesterone, or decidual immunosuppressive factors could result in an increase in the cytotoxicity of maternal lymphocytes. It is possible that when maternal immunotolerance is lost, graft rejection could occur, and that this may involve macrophage, T lymphocyte, and B lymphocyte infiltration into the graft region, the maternal-fetal interface. Activated macrophages produce a tissue necrosis factor (TNF) and interleukin (IL)-1. TNF is important for cell lysis while IL-1 causes T cell proliferation. Stimulated T cells produce IL-2 which is necessary for the clonal proliferation of T-helper and cytotoxic-T cells. In addition to mediating the complex interactions of macrophages and lymphocytes, cytokines are known to increase the prostaglandin production by intrauterine tissues; thus the mechanism of graft rejection may precipitate uterine contractions, leading to labour.

The onset of labour is a complex biological phenomenon controlled by multiple regulatory mechanisms which remain largely unknown in humans. Gap junctions are a necessary component of the human myometrium during term and preterm labour for coordinated contractions of the uterine smooth muscle. The increase in the number of uterine oxytocin receptors before or during the onset of labour is an important marker of the preparational events for parturition. Many hormonal and paracrine factors involved in parturition may regulate the formation of gap junctions and oxytocin receptors.

The steroid hormones, progesterone and oestrogens, may play only a facilitatory role in the initiation of labour. Oestrogens or rising oestrogens/progesterone ratios are important both in increased uterine sensitivity to oxytocic agents and in cervical ripening in pregnant animals. In women, the evidence is less clear, but oestrogens would appear to promote cervical softening, possibly by stimulating prostaglandin synthesis within the cervix, and progesterone could have the opposite effect and favour maintenance of pregnancy by inhibiting prostaglandin release and collagenase activity. A definite role for fetal adrenal steroids in the parturition process has also to be established.

Oxytocin and prostaglandins E and F are powerful stimulants of uterine contraction. The prostaglandins stimulate the pregnant uterus from early gestation unlike oxytocin which has little effect in the first and second trimesters. Their effects are modulated by other hormones and substances. The effect of oxytocin on the myometrium and decidua is mediated by oxytocin receptors, and oxytocin receptor antagonists block the effect of the peptide hormone. Oxytocin from maternal and fetal sources reaches all parts of the myometrium simultaneously and therefore induces synchronised uterine contractions. In contrast, prostaglandin $F_{2\alpha}$ reaches the inner layers of the myometrium particularly from the decidua through the paracrine route and causes local contractions. Formation of the prostaglandin by the decidua may be controlled by a balance of endogenous inhibitors and stimulators of prostaglandin synthesis produced intracellularly in the decidua or chorioamnion. Prostaglandins E and F are also produced by cervical tissue and have an effect on the remodelling of the cervical collagenase framework required for cervical dilatation and therefore for successful parturition. Thus, oxytocin may be important for the initial phase of labour, whereas increased synthesis of prostaglandins may be essential for the progress of labour. It is becoming increasingly evident that vasopressin may also be involved in the mechanism of labour.

Relaxin may also have a direct role in the initiation of labour through the participation of steroid hormones, prostaglandins and oxytocin. It has strong effects on the cervical tissue of pregnant animals and women. The mechanism of graft rejection may have a role in the uterine contractions leading to labour, and this may be one of the causes of recurrent abortion. However, whether normal parturition is due to the timely rejection of a previously tolerated allograft is still open to speculation.

References

Abel MH, Baird DT 1980. The effect of 17ß-estradiol and progesterone on prostaglandin production by human endometrium maintained in organ culture. *Endocrinology* 106: 1599-1606.

Akerlund M, Stromberg P, Hauksso A, et al 1987. Inhibition of uterine contractions of premature labor with an oxtyocin analogue. Results from a pilot study. *Br J Obstet Gynecol* 94: 1040-1044.

Alexander DP, Forslig ML, Martin MJ 1972. The effect of maternal hypoxia on fetal pitui- tary hormone release. *Biol Neonate* 21:219-228.

Anthony GS, DeGrood RM, Compton AA 1982. Forces required for surgical dilatation of the pregnant and non-pregnant human cervix. *Br J Obstet Gynecol* 89: 913-916.

Anwer K, Hovington JA, Sanborn BM 1989. Antagonism of contractants and relaxants at the level of intracellular calcium and phosphoinositide turnover in the rat uterus. *Endocrinology* 124:2995-3002.

Balducci J, Risek B, Gilula NB et al 1992. Gap junction formation in human myometrium: A key to preterm labor? *Am J Obstet Gynecol* 168: 1609-1615.

Beard RW, Braude P, Mowbray JF, Underwood JL 1983. Protective antibodies and spontaneous abortion. *Lancet* 2: 1090.

Beer AE, Sio JO 1982. Placenta as an immunological barrier. *Biol Reprod* 26: 15-27.

Bleasdale JE, Johnston JM 1985. Prostaglandins and human parturition: regulation of arachidonic acid mobilization. *Rev Perinatol Med* 5: 151-160.

Bossmar T, Akerlund M, Fantoni G, Szamatowicz J, Melin P, Maggi M 1994. Receptors for and myometrial responses to oxytocin and vasopressin in preterm and term human pregnancy: Effects of the oxytocin antagonist atosiban. *Am J Obstet Gynecol* 171: 1634-1642.

Bulmer JN, Smith J, Morrison L, Wells M 1988. Maternal and fetal cellular relationships in the human placental basal plate. *Placenta* 9: 237-246.

Burke J, Johansen K 1974. The formation of HLA antibodies in pregnancy: the antigenicity of aborted and term fetuses. *J Obstet Gynecol Br Cwlth* 81: 222-228.

Casey ML, MacDonald PC 1988. Biomolecular process in the initiation of parturition: Decidual activation. *Clin Obstet Gynecol* 31: 533-552.

Casey ML, Mitchell MD, MacDonald PG 1987. Epidermal growth factor stimulates PGE2 production in human amnion cells specifically, and nonarachidonic acid dependency. *Mol Cell Endocrinol* 53:169-176.

Chibbar R, Miller FD, Mitchell BF 1993. Synthesis of oxytocin in amnion, chorion and decidua may influence the timing of human parturition. *J Clin Invest* 91: 185-192.

Chow L, Lye SJ 1994. Expression of the gap junction protein connexion - 43 is increased in the human myometrium toward term and with the onset of labour. *Am J Obstet Gynecol* 170: 788-795.

Clark KE, Mills EG, Stys SJ, Seeds AE 1981. Effects of vasoactive polypeptides on the uterine vasculature. *Am J Obstet Gynecol* 139:182-188.

Cole WC, Garfield RE 1986. Evidence for physiological regulation of myometrial gap junction permeability. *Am J Physiol* 251:C411-C420.

Cole WC, Garfield RE 1988. Effects of calcium ionophore, A23187 and calmodulin inhibitors on intercellular communication in the rat myometrium. *Biol Reprod* 38:55-62.

Coleman RA, Kennedy I, Humphrey PPA, Bunce K, Lumley P 1989. Prostanoids and their receptors. In: Hansch C, Sammes PG, Tayler JB, eds. Comprehensive Medicinal Chemistry. Elmsford, NY: Pergamon Press, 3: 643-714.

Coleman HA, Parkington H 1988. Induction of prolonged excitability in myometrium of pregnant guinea pig prostaglandin $F_{2\alpha}$. *J Physiol* (Lond) 399: 33-47.

Csapo AI 1977. The 'See-Saw' theory of parturition. In: Knight J, O'Conner M, (eds.) The Fetus and Birth. Amsterdam: Elsevier/Excerpta Medica, p 159.

Danforth DN, Buckingham JC, Roddick JW 1960. Connective tissue changes incident to cervical effacement. *Am J Obstet Gynecol* 80:939-945.

Danforth DN, Veis A, Breen M, et al 1974. The effects of pregnancy and labor on the human cervix: changes in collagen, glycoprotein and glycosaminoglycans. *Am J Obstet Gynecol* 120:641-651.

Dattel BJ, Lam F, Roberts JM 1986. Failure to demonstrate decreased ß-adrenergic receptor concentration or decrease agonist efficacy in term or preterm human parturition. *Am J Obstet Gynecol* 154:450-456.

Davidson BJ, Murray RD, Challis JRC, Valenzuela GJ 1987. Estrogen, progesterone, prolactin, PGE_2, $PGF_{2\alpha}$, PGFM and 6-keto-$PGF_{1\alpha}$ gradients across the uterus in women in labor and not in labor. *Am J Obstet Gynecol* 157:754-758.

Daya S, Clark DA, Delvin C, Jarrell J 1985. Preliminary characterisation of two types of suppressor cells in the human uterus. *Fertil Steril* 44: 778-785.

Daya S, Rosenthal KL, Clark DA 1987. Immunosuppressor factor(s) produced by decidua-associated suppressor cells: a mechanism for fetal allograft survival. *Am J Obstet Gynecol* 156: 344-350.

Dudley DJ, Hunter C, Mitchell MD, Varner MW 1994. Clinical value of amniotic fluid interleukin-6 determinations in the management of preterm labour. *Br J Obstet Gynecol* 101: 592-597.

Editorial 1990. Mifepristone (RU486). *New Engl J Med* 322: 691-693.

Elger W, Chwalicz K, Fahnrich M, et al 1990. Studies on labor conditioning and labor inducing effects of antiprogestins in animal models, In: Garfield RE, ed. Uterine Contractility. Norwell, Mass: Serono Symposia USA, p 153.

Ellwood DA, Mitchell MD, Anderson ABM, Turnbull AC 1980. The in vitro production of prostanoids by the human cervix during pregnancy: preliminary observations. *J Obstet Gynecol* 87:210-214.

Embrey MP, Moir JC 1967. A comparison of the oxytocic effects of synthetic vasopressin and oxytocin. *J Obstet Gynecol Br Cwlth* 74: 648-652.

Evans MI, Dougan M-B, Moawad AH, Evans WJ, Bryant-Greenwood GD, Greenwood FC 1983. Ripening of the human cervix with porcine ovarian relaxin. *Am J Obstet Gynecol* 147:410-414.

Fields PA, Eldridge RK, Fuchs A-R, et al 1983. Human placental and bovine luteal oxytocin. *Endocrinology* 112:1544-1546.

Fisher RA, Lawler SD 1984. The expression of major histocompatibility antigens in the chorionic villi of molar placentae. *Placenta* 5: 237-242.

Fuchs A-R 1990. Oxytocin and oxytocin-receptors: maternal signals for parturition. In: Garfield RE (ed). Uterine Contractility. Norwell, Mass: Serono Symposia USA, p 177.

Fuchs A-R, Fuchs F 1984. Endrocrinology of human parturition: a review. *Br J Obstet Gynecol* 91: 948-967.

Fuchs A-R, Romero R, Keefe D, et al 1991. Pulsatile oxytocin secretion increases during labor in women. *Am J Obstet Gynecol* 167:1515-1523.

Garfield RE, Hayashi RH 1980. Presence of gap junctions in the myometrium of women during various stages of menstruation. *Am J Obstet Gynecol* 138: 569-574.

Garfield RE, Hayashi RH 1981. Appearance of gap junctions in the myometrium of women during labor. *Am J Obstet Gynecol* 140:254-260.

Garfield RE, Hayashi RH, Harper MJK 1987. In vitro studies on the control of human myometrial gap junctions. *Int J Gynaecol Obstet* 25:241-248.

Garfield RE, Kannon MS, Daniel EE 1980. Gap junction formation in myometrium: Control by estrogens, progesterone and prostaglandins. *Am J Physiol* 238:C81-C89.

Giannopoulos G, Goldberg P, Shea TB, Tulchinsky D 1980. Unoccupied and occupied estrogen receptors in myometrial cytosol and nuclei from nonpregnant and pregnant women. *J Clin Endocrinol Metab* 51: 702-710.

Giannopoulos G, Tulchinsky D 1979. Cytoplasmic and nuclear progestin receptors in human myometrium during the menstrual cycle and in pregnancy at term. *J Clin Endocrinol Metab* 49:100-106.

Gibb W, Riopel L, Collu R, Ducharme JR, Mitchell MD. Lavoie JC 1988. Cyclooxygenase products formed by primary cultures of cells from human chorion laeve: influence of steroids. *Can J Physiol Pharmacol* 66: 788-793.

Goeschen K, Fuchs A-R, Fuchs F, et al 1985. Effect of beta-mimetic tocolysis on cervical ripening and plasma prostaglandin F metabolite level with PGE2 gel. *Obstet Gynecol* 65:166-177.

Goldsmith LT, Skurnick JH, Wojtczuk AS, et al 1989. The antagonistic effect of oxytocin and relaxin on rat uterine segment contractility. *Am J Obstet Gynecol* 161:1644-1649.

Guillon G, Balestre MN, Roberts JM, Bottari SP 1987. Oxytocin and vasopressin: distinct receptors in myometrium. *J Clin Endocrinol Metab* 64:1129-1135.

Haluska GJ, West NB, Novy MJ, Brener RM 1990. Uterine estrogen receptors are increased by RU486 in late pregnant macaques but not after spontaneous labor. *J Clin Endocrinol Metab* 70:181-186.

Harkness MLR, Harkness RD 1959. Changes in the physical properties of the uterine cervix of the rat during pregnancy. *J Physiol* 148:524-547.

Hillier K, Wallis P 1981. Prostaglandins, steroids and the human cervix. In: Ellwood DA, Anderson AM, eds. The Cervix in Pregnancy and Labor. Clinical and Biochemical Investigations. Edinburgh: Churchill Livingstone, pp 34-40.

Honnebier MBOM, Figueroa JP, Rivier JP, et al 1989. Studies on the role of oxytocin in late pregnancy in the pregnant rhesus monkey: plasma concentrations of oxytocin in the maternal circulation throughout the 24h day and the effect of the synthetic oxytocin antagonist [1B-Mpa^{1}B(Ch$_2$)$_5$-5 (OMe)Tyr-8 Orn]OT on spontaneous nocturnal myometrial contractions. *J Dev Physiol* 12:225-232.

Honnebier WJ, Swaab DF 1974. The effect of hypophysial hormones and human chorionic gonadotropin on the anencephalic fetal adrenal cortex and parturition in the human. *J Obstet Gynecol Br Cwlth* 81:423-438.

Hunt JS, Fishback JL, Andrews GK, Wood GW 1988. Expression of class I HLA genes by trophoblast cell. *J Immunol* 140: 1293-1299.

Huszar G, Walsh MP 1989. Biochemistry of the myometrium and cervix. In: Wynn R, Jollie W, eds. Biology of the Uterus, 2nd ed. New York: Plenum Medical, pp 355-402.

Ishikawa M, Shimizu T 1989. Dehydroepiandrosterone sulfate and induction of labor. *Am J Perinatol* 6:173-175.

Ivanisevic M, Behren O, Helmer H, Fuchs A-R 1989. Vasopressin receptors in human pregnant myometrium and decidua: interaction with oxytocin and vasopressin agonists and antagonists. *Am J Obstet Gynecol* 161:1637-1643.

Kawarabayashi T, Osa T 1976. Comparative investigations of α- and ß-effects on the longitudinal and circular muscles of the pregnant rat myometrium. *Jpn J Physiol* 26:403-406.

Koay ESC, Too CKL, Greenwood FC, Bryant-Greenwood GD 1983. Relaxin stimulates collagenase and plasminogen activator secretion by dispersed human amnion and chorion cells in vitro. *J Clin Endocrinol Metab* 56: 1332-1334.

Landesman R, Fuchs F 1973. Control of uterine activity and prevention of premature birth. In: Cutinho E, Fuchs F, eds. Physiology and Genetics of Reproduction. *Basic Life Sciences*, vol IV, part B. New York: Plenum; p 219.

Larsson L-I, Fahrenkrug J, Schaffalitzky de Muckadell OB 1977. Vasoactive intestinal polypeptide occurs in nerves of the female genitourinary tract. *Science* 197:1374-1375.

Leake RD, Weitzman RE, Glatz TH, Fisher DA 1981. Plasma oxytocin concentration in men, nonpregnant women and pregnant women before and during spontaneous labor. *J Clin Endocrinol Metab* 53: 730-733.

Leavitt WW, Takeda A 1986. Hormonal regulation of estrogen and progesterone

receptors in decidual cells. *Biol Reprod* 35:475-484.

Lefebvre DL, Giaid A, Bennett H et al 1992. Oxytocin gene expression in rat uterus. *Science* 256: 1533-1555.

Legrand C, Maltier JP, Benghan-Eyene Y 1987. Rat myometrial adrenergic receptors in late pregnancy. *Biol Reprod* 37:641-650.

Lewis PR, Galvin PM, Short RV 1987. Salivary oestriol and progesterone concentrations in women during late pregnancy, parturition, and the puerperium. *J Endocrinol* 115: 177-181.

Liggins GC, Wilson T 1986. Isolation of an inhibitior of phospholipase A2 from human chorion. Abstract #40 presented at the Meeting of the International Union of Physiological Sciences, Vancouver Island, Canada.

Litime MH, Pointis G, Breuiller M, et al 1989. Disappearance of ß-adrenergic response of human myometrial adenylate cyclase at the end of pregnancy. *J Clin Endocrinol Metab* 69:1-6.

Lopez-Bernal A, Flint APF, Anderson ABM, Turnbull AC 1980. 11-beta-hyroxysteroid dehydrogenase activity in human placenta and decidua. *J Steroid Biochem* 13:1081-1087.

MacLennan AH, Green FR, Bryant-Greenwood GD, Greenwood FC 1981. Cervical ripening with combinations of vaginal prostaglandin F2α, estradiol and relaxin. *Obstet Gynecol* 58: 601-604.

MacLennan AH, Green RC, Bryant-Greenwood GD, Greenwood FC, Seamark RF 1980. Ripening of the human cervix and induction of labour with purified porcine relaxin. *Lancet* 1:220-223.

Maggi M, Del-Carlo P, Fantoni G, et al 1990. Human myometrium during pregnancy contains and responds to V1 VP receptors as well as oxytocin receptors. *J Clin Endocrinol Metab* 70: 1142-1154.

McIntyre JA, Faulk WP, Verhulst SJ, Colliver JA 1983. Human trophoblast-lymphocyte cross-reactive (TLX) antigens define a new alloantigen system. *Science* 222: 1135-1137.

Mironneau J 1976. Effect of oxytocin on ionic currents underlying rhythmic activity and contraction in uterine smooth muscle. *Pflügers Arch* 3363:113-118.

Mitchell MD 1988. Action of transfroming growth factors on amnion cell prostaglandin bio-synthesis. *Prostaglandins, Leukotrienes, Ess Fatty Acids*, 33:157-158.

Mitchell BF, Challis JRG 1988. Estrogen and progesterone metabolism in human fetal membranes. In: Mitchell BF, ed. The Physiology and Biochemistry of Human Fetal Membranes. Ithaca, New York: Perinatology Press, p 5.

Mitchell MD, Edwin SS, Lundin-Schiller S, Silver RM, Smotkin D, Trautman AD 1993. Mechanism of interleukin-1 beta stimulation of human amnion prostaglandin biosynthesis: mediation via a novel inducible cyclo-oxygenase. *Placenta* 14: 615-625.

Mitchell MD, Lundin-Schiller S, Edwin SS 1991. Endothelin production by amnion and its regulation by cytokines. *Am J Obstet Gynecol.* 165: 120-124.

Mortimer G, Hunter IC, Stimson WH, Govan ADT 1985. A role for amniotic epithelium in control of human parturition. *Lancet* 1: 1074-1075.

Mowbray JF, Underwood JL 1985. Immunology of abortion. *Clin Exp Immunol* 60: 1-7.

Nehemiah JL, Schwitzer JA, Schulman H, Novikoff AB 1981. Human-chorionic trophoblasts, decidual cells, and macrophages: a histochemical and electron microscopy analysis. *Am J Obstet Gynecol* 140:261-268.

Okulicz WC 1986. Progesterone receptor replenishment during sustained progesterone treatment in the hamster uterus. *Endocrinology* 118: 2488-2494.

Okulicz WC 1989. Temporal effects of progesterone inhibition of occupied nuclear estrogen receptor retention in the rat uterus. *J Endocriol* 121:101-107.

Olson DM, Skinner K, Challis JRG 1983. Estradiol-17ß and 2-hydroxyestradiol-17ß-induces differential production of prostaglandins by cells dispersed from human intrauterine tissues at parturition. *Prostaglandins* 25(5): 639-651.

Ottesen B, Wagner G, Fahrenkrug J 1980. Vasoactive intestinal polypeptide (VIP) inhibits prostaglandin-F_2-induced activity of the rabbit myometrium. *Prostaglandins* 19:427-435.

Padayachi T, Norman RJ, Reddi K, et al 1986. Changes in amniotic fluid prostaglandin with oxytocin induced labor. *Obstet Gynecol* 68:610-613.

Parboosingh J, Lederis K, Singh N 1982. Vasopressin concentration in cord blood: Correlation with method of delivery and cord pH. *Obstet Gynecol* 60: 179-183.

Pinto RM, Votta RA, Montuori E, Baleiron H 1964. Action of estradiol-17ß on the activity of the pregnant human uterus. *Am J Obstet Gynecol* 88: 759-769.

Pohjavuori M, Fyhrquist F 1980. Hemodynamic significance of vasopressin in the newborn infant. *J Pediatr* 97: 462-465.

Pupula M, MacLennan AH 1989. Effect of porcine relaxin on spontaneous, oxytocin-driven and prostaglandin-driven pig myometrial activity in vitro. *J Reprod Med* 34:819-823.

Romero R, Lafreniere D, Hobbins JC, Mitchell MD 1987. A product from human decidua inhibits prostaglandin production by human amnion. *Prostaglandins, Leukotrienes. Med* 30: 29-35.

Rorie DK, Newton M 1967. Histologic and chemical studies of the smooth muscle in the human cervix and uterus. *Am J Obstet Gynecol* 99:466-469.

Roy AC, Arulkumaran, S 1991. Pharmacology of parturition. *Ann Acad Med Singapore* 20: 71-77.

Roy AC, Karim SMM 1983a. Interaction between oxytocin and prostaglandins in reproduction. *Sing J Obstet Gynecol* 14: 5-15.

Roy AC, Karim SMM 1983b. Review. Significance of the inhibition by prostaglandins and cyclic GMP of oxytocinase activity in human pregnancy and labour. *Prostaglandins* 25: 55-70.

Roy AC, Kottegoda SR, Ratnam SS. 1984a. Relaxin and reproduction. Review. *Sing J Obstet Gynecol.* 15: 65-69.

Roy AC, Kottegoda SR, Ratnam SS 1985. Another look at initiation of human parturition. *Aust NZ J Obstet Gynecol* 25: 94-100.

Roy AC, Kottegoda SR, Ratnam SS 1986. Oxytocinase activity in human amniotic fluid and its relationship to gestational age. *Obstet Gynecol* 68: 614-617.

Roy AC, Yang M, Tan SM, Kottegoda SR, Ratnam SS 1984b. Oxytocinase activity in human amniotic fluid. *IRCS Med Sci* 12: 856-857.

Saeed SA, Stricklan DM, Young DC, Dang A, Mitchell MD 1982. Inhibition of prostaglandin synthase by human amniotic fluid: acute reduction in inhibitory activity of amniotic fluid obtained during labor. *J Clin Endocrinol Metab* 55: 801-803.

Saito Y, Sakamoto H, MacLusky NJ, Naftolin F 1985. Correlation between gap junctions and steroid hormone receptors in myometrial tissue of pregnant and postpartum rats. *Am J Obstet Gynecol* 151:805-812.

Sakburn V, Ali SM, Greenwood FC, Bryant-Greenwood GD 1990. Human relaxin in the amnion, chorion, decidua parietalis and placental trophoblast by immunocytochemistry and Northern blot. *J Clin Endocrinol Metab* 70:508-514.

Salamonsen LA, Findlay JK 1990. Regulation of endometrial prostaglandins during the menstrual cycle and in early pregnancy. *Reprod Fertil Dev* 2: 443-457.

Sanborn BM, Held B, Kuo HS 1975. Specific estrogen binding proteins in human cervix. *J Steroid Biochem* 6:1107-1112.

Schrey MP, Read AM, Steer PJ 1986. Oxytocin and vasopressin stimulate inositol phosphate production in human gestational myometrium and decidual cells. *Biosci Rep* 6:613-619.

Sellers SM, Hodgson HT, Mountford LA, Mitchell MD, Anderson ABM, Turnbull AC 1981. Is oxytocin involved in parturition? *Br J Obstet Gynecol* 88: 725-729.

Siiteri PK, Stites DP 1982. Immunologic and endocrine interrelationship in pregnancy. *Biol Reprod* 26: 1-4.

Silvestre L, Dubois C, Renault M, et al 1990. Voluntary interruption of pregnancy with mifepristone (RU486) and a prostaglandin analogue. *N Engl J Med* 322:645-648.

Silvia WJ, Homanics GE 1988. Role of phospholipase C in mediating oxytocin-induced release of prostaglandin $F_{2\alpha}$ from ovine endometrial tissue. *Prostaglandins* 35:535-548.

Soloff MS 1988. The role of oxytocin in the initiation of labor, and oxytocin-prostaglandin interactions. In: McNellis D, Challis JRG, MacDonald PC, Nathanielsz PW, Roberts JM, eds. The Onset of Labor: Cellular and Integrative Mechanisms. Ithaca, New York: Perinatology Press, p 87.

Soloff MS, Sweet P 1982. Oxytocin inhibition of (Calcium-Magnesium)-ATPase activity in rat myometrial plasma membranes. *J Biol Chem* 257:10687-10693.

Spätling L, Fallenstein F, Schneider H, Dancis J 1989. Bolus tocolysis: treatment of preterm labor with pulsatile administration of a ß-adrenergic agonist. *Am J Obstet Gynecol* 160:713-717.

Stark RI, Wardlaw SL, Daniel SS, et al 1982. Vasopressin secretion induced by hypoxia in sheep: developmental changes and relationship to beta-endorphin release. *Am J Obstet Gynecol* 143:204-215.

Story ME, Hall S, Ziccone SP, Pauli JD 1989. Effects of adrenaline, isoprenaline and forskolin on pregnant human myometrium. *Clin Exp Pharmacol Physiol* 15:707-713.

Strickler RC, Tobias B, Covey DF 1981. Human placental 17ß-estradiol dehydrogenase and 20α-hydroxysteroid dehydrogenase: two activites at a single site. *J Biol Chem* 256: 316-321.

Stys S 1986. Endocrine regulation of cervical function during pregnancy and labor. In: Huszar G, ed. Physiology and Biochemistry of the Uterus in Pregnancy and Labor. Boca Raton, Fla: CRC Press, pp 281-295.

Sutton L, Gadd M, Mason DY, Redman CWG 1986. Cells bearing class II MHC antigens in the human placenta and amniochorion. *Immunology* 58: 23-29.

Szekeres-Bortho J, Varga P, Pacsa AS 1986. Immunologic factors contributing to the initiation of labor - lymphocyte reactivity in term labor and threatened preterm delivery. *Am J Obstet Gynecol* 155: 108-112.

Thorburn GD, Challis JRG 1979. Endocrine control of parturition. *Physiol Rev* 59: 863-917.

Tyson JE, McCoshen JA, Dubin NH 1985. Inhibition of fetal membrane prostaglandin production by prolactin: relative importance in the initiation of labor. *Am J Obstet Gynecol* 151: 1032-1038.

Ulmann A, Dubois C, Philibert D 1987. Fertility control with RU486. *Hormone Res* 28: 274-278.

Von Maillot K, Stuhlsatz HW, Mohanaradha-krishnan V, Greiling H 1979. Changes in the glycosaminoglycans distribution pattern in the human cervix during pregnancy and labor. *Am J Obstet Gynecol* 135:503-506.

Wilson T, Liggins GC, Aimer GP, Skinner SJM 1985. Partial purification and characterisation of two compounds from amniotic fluid which inhibit phospholipase activity in human endometrial cells. *Biochem Biophys Comm* 131: 22-29.

Wolf JP, Sinosich M, Anderson TL, et al 1989. Progesterone antagonist (RU 486) for cervical dilatation, labor induction, and delivery in monkeys: effectiveness in combination with oxytocin. *Am J Obstet Gynecol* 160:45-47.

Word RA, Kamm KE, Stull JT, Casey ML 1990. Endothelin increases cytoplasmic calcium and myosin phosphorylation in human myometrium. *Am J Obstet Gynecol.* 162: 1103-1108.

2

Management of the First Stage of Labour

S Arulkumaran
S Chua

The management of spontaneous labour has become an important issue both in the developing and the developed world. In the developing world, prolonged labour associated with high levels of morbidity and mortality is still common because of a lack of adequate health care, in particular antibiotics and the surgical facilities necessary for caesarean section. The causes of death and morbidity include obstructed labour, sepsis, rupture of the uterus and postpartum hemorrhage (Rao 1992). In the developed world, the increasing caesarean section (CS) rate for dystocia or difficult labour contributes at least a third to the overall CS rate, and repeat CS following primary CS contributes up to another third (NIH 1981). CS leads to increased maternal morbidity as well as mortality, especially when it is performed as an emergency procedure (Hall 1990). Maternal and fetal morbidity and mortality due to prolonged labour and the CS rate for dystocia can be reduced by the proper management of poor progress in labour.

Normal labour

Normal labour is difficult to define precisely but the archetype can be described as spontaneous painful uterine contractions associated with the effacement and dilatation of the cervix and the descent of the presenting part. The process culminates in the birth of a healthy fetus followed by the expulsion of the placenta. In most cases, the outcome can be predicted prospectively by observing the progress of cervical dilatation. Although labour is a continuous process, it is divided into three functional stages for the purpose of management: the first, second and third stage of labour.

The basis for the scientific study of the progress of labour was developed by Friedman (1954), who described it graphically by plotting the rate of cervical dilatation against time. The resulting graph of cervical dilatation forms the basis of the modern partogram, which now incorporates many relevant parameters related to labour, like the condition of the mother and the fetus in relation to each other chronologically on one page. These parameters include cervical effacement and dilatation, the descent of the presenting part (in fifths of the head palpable above the pelvic brim rather than the station in cm above or below the ischial spines), fetal heart rate (FHR), the frequency and duration of uterine contractions, the colour and quantity of amniotic fluid passed per vaginum, maternal parameters such as temperature, pulse and blood pressure, and drugs used. The pictorial documentation of labour facilitates the early recognition of poor progress. Plotting of cervical dilatation also enables prediction of the time of onset of the second stage of labour.

Nomograms of cervical dilatation

The rate of cervical dilatation in labour has been studied in various ethnic groups in different countries (Philpott 1972; O'Driscoll et al 1973; Studd 1973; Ilancheran et al 1977). The nomograms derived show similar rates of cervical dilatation in different ethnic groups and comparative studies have confirmed that differences in ethnicity have little influence on the rate of cervical dilatation (Duignan et al 1975) or uterine activity in spontaneous normal labour (Arulkumaran et al 1989a). Observations during the first stage of labour (defined as from the time of admission to the labour ward to full dilatation of the cervix) show that the rate of cervical dilatation has two phases: a slow 'latent phase' of labour during which the cervix shortens from about 3 cm long to less than 0.5 cm long (effacement) and dilates to 3 cm; and a faster 'active phase', when the cervix dilates from 3 cm to full dilatation (taken by convention to be 10 cm because of the presenting diameters of the well flexed vertex presentation of 9.5 × 9.5 cm, although in reality it refers to a situation when the cervix is not palpable). In order to identify parturients at the risk of prolonged labour, a line of acceptable progress is drawn on the partogram. If the rate of cervical dilatation in any particular case crosses to the right of the line, progress is deemed unsatisfactory. The line of acceptable progress can be based on the mean, median or slowest tenth percentile rate of cervical dilatation observed in women who progress without intervention and deliver normally, or it can be a line parallel and 1–4 h to the right of these. Accordingly, the proportion of labours deemed to have unsatisfactory progress can vary from 5 to 50%. In the presence of good contractions (at least > 2/10 min, each lasting > 40 sec), the latent phase may last for up to 8 h in nulliparas and up to 6 h in multiparas. During the peak of the active phase of labour, the cervix dilates at a rate of approximately 1 cm/h in both nulliparas and multiparas. Multiparas appear to dilate faster because they have shorter labours overall; not only do they have a shorter latent phase resulting in a more advanced cervical dilatation on admission, they have an increased rate of progress approaching full dilatation. Construction of nomograms of expected normal progress or alert lines, with the addition of acceptable progress or action lines, prevents prolongation of labour being overlooked and is of considerable diagnostic and educational value (Fig 2.1).

Diagnosis of labour

The correct diagnosis of established labour may be difficult.   If the contractions are painful and regular and if the cervix is dilated to > 3 cm (that is, in the active phase) there is little difficulty in diagnosing labour. On the other hand if the patient is in the latent phase of labour, two examinations at least two hours apart may be necessary to observe cervical effacement and dilatation and to conclude that she is in labour.

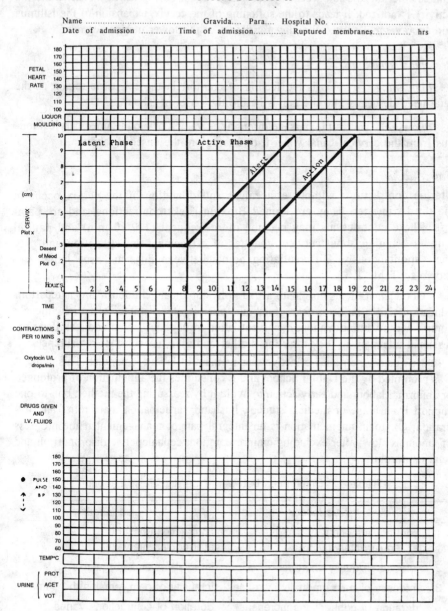

Fig 2.1   WHO partograph showing alert and action lines in the latent and active phase of labour. Cervical dilatation, descent of head, fetal parameters (FHR, colour of liquor, caput and moulding), maternal parameters (pulse, blood pressure, results of urine tests and drugs used) can be entered.

Prelabour

This is a period of a few weeks before active labour during which increased uterine activity is noticed. It leads to the softening of the cervix, expansion of the isthmus and supravaginal cervix allowing formation of the lower uterine segment.

Prelabour symptoms

a. *Lightening*   This is the feeling of comfort in the epigastric region as the fetal head descends into the pelvis before the onset of labour.

b. *Show*   This is the passage through the vagina of bloodstained cervical mucus from the cervical canal when it dilates before the onset of labour.

False labour

Uterine contractions without effacement and dilatation of the cervix occur in the third trimester. They are termed Braxton-Hicks contractions, and are painless. These contractions may become more frequent (1–2/10 min) and painful without bringing about cervical changes of effacement and dilatation and may abate spontaneously. Differentiating points between false and true labour are shown in Table 1.

Good antecedents for 'natural' or 'physiological' childbirth are antepartum education that eliminates fear of labour; exercise to promote relaxation, muscle control and breathing without hyperventilation throughout labour and a skilled professional attendant to look after the mother and give her constant reassurance.

Nowadays the policy of active management of labour is popular. This concept was promoted by the Dublin School and it constitutes the anticipation of prolonged or abnormal labour and early action to avoid it by reassuring the mother, one-to-one support by a nurse or medical student, husband participation, pain relief and hydration. Oxytocin augmentation is an integral part of management if the progress of labour is slow, after excluding malpresentation, cephalopelvic disproportion and fetal compromise.

Table 1:   Differences between True and False Labour

	True labour	False labour
1.	contractions occur at regular intervals	contractions occur at irregular intervals
2.	interval gradually shortens	interval remains irregular
3.	intensity of pain gradually increases	intensity of pain remains the same
4.	duration of contractions increases	duration of contractions varies and tends to become less
5.	There is progressive cervical effacement and dilatation.	There is no progress in cervical effacement and dilatation.
6.	progress of labour not stopped by sedation	Usually painful contractions are relieved by sedation and there is no progress in labour.

Management of the first stage of labour

The general principles of management are

1. initial assessment
2. observation and intervention if labour becomes abnormal
3. close monitoring of the fetal and maternal condition
4. pain relief
5. emotional support and
6. adequate hydration.

Initial assessment

At the time of arrival initial assessment should be done by eliciting a detailed history, by clinical examination and basic investigations. The aim is to identify high risk pregnancies; a proportion being identified as high risk before the onset of labour and others being identified as at risk only during labour.

History

Detailed history should include the time of onset of contractions and their frequency and duration. It should be verified whether the membranes are ruptured, and if they have, the colour and quantity of amniotic fluid should be noted. Present and previous obstetrical history and any significant medical or drug history should be noted.

General examination

This should include the general condition of the woman: whether she has pallor or jaundice, the state of hydration, her blood pressure, pulse, temperature and breathing should be checked, the condition of her breasts, heart and chest and whether she has edema.

Abdominal examination

Uterine contractions should be assessed with relevance to their frequency and duration over a 10 min period (Fig 2.2). The fundal height should be measured. Fetal presentation and the level of the presenting part should be determined. The head level should be measured in 'fifths' (Fig 2.3) because it excludes variability due to caput and moulding and also variability produced by different depths of pelvis. It is easily reproducible. The fetal heart rate should be auscultated for a period of one minute, preferably soon after a contraction, and should be repeated ideally every 15 min in the first stage of labour and after every 5 min in the second stage of labour.

Vaginal examination

The following points should be noted during vaginal examination: any discharge from the vagina; evidence of rupture of the membranes, the colour and quantity of amniotic fluid and whether it is clear, bloodstained or meconium stained; the consistency, position, effacement and dilatation of the cervix; the level of the presenting part in relation to the ischial spine and caput or moulding of the head. Finally, a bony pelvis should be assessed with regard to its adequacy for childbirth.

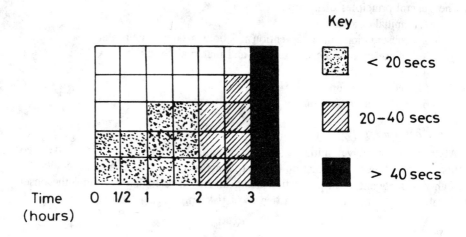

Fig 2.2   Quantification of uterine contractions by clinical palpation. Frequency per 10 min is recorded by shading the equivalent number of boxes. The type of shading indicates the duration of each contraction.

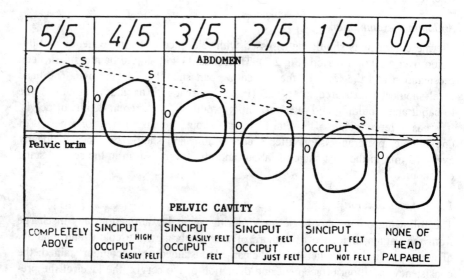

Fig 2.3   Clinical estimation of descent of head in fifths palpable above the pelvic brim

Investigations

Blood should be tested for hemoglobin (if there is no recent estimation), and grouped and typed (if it has not been done) and urine examination for albumin, ketones and sugar should be performed. This enables additional steps to be taken should there be abnormal results.

It is advisable to give the woman a small enema if the bowels are loaded with hard stools to enable the head to descend and for efficient uterine action. In addition it prevents soiling of the vulva and perineum, offering a clean environment for the baby at delivery. An intravenous line may be inserted if there is need for hydration. This will also allow quick access should the need arise for any immediate medication. In developing countries many women come in an advanced stage of or with obstructed labour. They need to be hydrated and intravenous antibiotics may be necessary. Five per cent dextrose is used commonly but it is best to give dextrose in saline, or normal saline, to maintain the fluid and electrolyte balance. This will also help to avoid water intoxication if oxytocin is used over a long period in large doses. During labour solid food should be restricted in order to avoid vomiting and aspiration, should the mother need general anesthesia. Sips of water, ice chips or hard candies may be allowed. It is preferable not to confine the mother to bed in early labour. She may prefer ambulation or sitting in a chair which may give psychological and perhaps physiological benefit. In bed she may be allowed to assume the position she finds most comfortable; sitting, reclining or the lateral recumbent position. The latter position is advantageous as it promotes more venous return and thus a better uterine perfusion.

Use of analgesia and anesthesia

Analgesia or anesthesia is initiated on the basis of discomfort and pain. The kind of analgesia to be used and the dose and frequency of administration are based to a considerable degree on the anticipated interval of time to delivery, the woman's preference, availability of the different modalities and the experience of the medical attendants. A brief description of some analgesic and anesthetic agents is given below. Details are given in the chapter relating to pain relief in labour.

1. Systemic analgesia These include (a) sedatives and hypnotics: butobarbitone and phenobarbitone. (b) Tranquillizers: phenothiazines (promazine, chlorpromazine, promethazine), diazepam and meprobamate. (c) Narcotic analgesia: these are pethidine, hydrochloride, pentazocine or morphine. New drugs include salbuphine and butarphanol. The usual duration of action of narcotic drugs is 2–4 hours. If the baby has respiratory depression (because the drugs are administered too soon before delivery) it should be given naloxone, 0.02 mg i/m, immediately after birth.

2. Inhalational analgesia The commonly used agent is entonox which is a mixture of nitrous oxide and oxygen. Other agents are methane flurane and trichloroethylene.

3. Local analgesia   These drugs produce a temporary block of pain impulses along the nerve. The commonly used drugs are lignocaine and bupivacain. The following blocks are used in obstetrics:
  a.   perineal infiltration prior to performing an episiotomy
  b.   a para cervical block (rarely used in current obstetric practice)
  c.   a pudendal block prior to outlet instrumental deliveries
  d.   a caudal block prior to instrumental deliveries
  e.   a lumbar epidural block prior to an instrumental or breech delivery and in multiple pregnancies. Caesarean sections' or manual removal of the placenta can also be performed.

     The anesthetic technique that provides the greatest pain relief in labour is the epidural block. It produces segmental anesthesia, which works in all stages of labour, but skilled and trained personnel are required to administer it.

Analgesia during the first stage of labour

Early labour   This is managed with minimal analgesia. Sedatives may be given.

Late labour   It is preferable to provide an epidural block if a centre has the facility. The other option is i/m narcotics every 3–4 hours. Commonly, pethidine is used in 75–100 mg doses.

Diagnosis of poor progress of labour

Labour is monitored by observing the progressive effacement and dilatation of the cervix and the descent of the presenting part against time in a chronological manner. The frequency and duration of uterine contractions is also noted as indicated before. The maternal condition is monitored by observing the pulse, blood pressure, temperature and hydration. In addition, the use of anesthetic and oxytocic drugs can be recorded.

     Fetal monitoring is by observation of the fetal heart rate at regular intervals. A gradual increase in the basal FHR or prolonged bradycardia indicates the possibility of fetal distress. The colour of the amniotic fluid if heavily stained with meconium (thick or grade 3), with scanty fluid or fresh passage of meconium, or the absence of amniotic fluid at the time of the rupture of membranes is suggestive of possible hypoxia.

     The use of a partogram for the management of labour has been shown to be beneficial in that it clearly differentiates normal from abnormal progress in labour and identifies women likely to require intervention (WHO 1994). This can be used at all levels of obstetric care by basic care providers who are trained to assess cervical dilatation. When used properly, it helps to detect cases of abnormal labour without delay, thus allowing timely intervention. In a WHO multicentre trial (WHO 1994) in southeast Asia involving 35,484 women, introduction of the partograph with an agreed labour management protocol reduced both prolonged labour (from 6.4 to 3.4% of labours) and the proportion of labours requiring augmentation (from 20.7 to 9.1%). Emergency caesarean sections fell from 9.9 to 8.3%, and intrapartum stillbirths from 0.5 to 0.3%. Improvements in maternal and fetal mortality and morbidity took place among both nulliparous and multiparous women.

The term dystocia or difficult labour refers to poor progress of labour and is diagnosed when the rate of cervical dilatation in the active phase is slower than the mean, median or slowest tenth centile, according to the policy of the obstetrician. When a woman is admitted in the active phase of labour with regular painful contractions, her cervical dilatation can be plotted on the partogram and an expected progress line or alert line can be constructed. Another line, the action line, can be constructed 1–4 h parallel and to the right of the alert line. Alternatively, an action line can be added by the use of a stencil (Studd et al 1975) in which an individualised alert line is constructed from the cervical dilatation on admission. If the progress of labour is to the right of the action line, it is considered to be poor, needing augmentation. The outcome of such labours has been studied and various abnormal labour patterns have been described (Studd et al 1975; Cardozo et al 1982; Gibb et al 1982). The latent phase is usually considered prolonged if it is greater than 8 h in a nullipara and 6 h in a multipara, although to some extent this will depend on the Bishop score on admission: the slowest 20 per cent of labours will improve the Bishop score by at least one point per hour in the latent phase (Beazley and Alderman 1976). If the progress of labour is slow in the active phase of labour and is to the right of the nomogram, it is termed 'primary dysfunctional labour'. If labour progresses normally in the early active phase but the cervix subsequently fails to dilate or dilates slowly, prior to full dilatation, it is termed 'secondary arrest' of labour (Fig 2.4). The same patient may exhibit both a prolonged latent phase and primary dysfunctional labour (Fig 2.4).

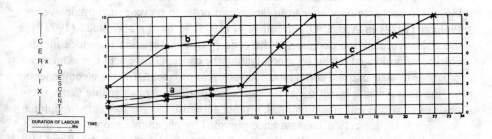

Fig 2.4   Abnormal labour patterns

(a) prolonged latent phase, (b) secondary arrest, (c) prolonged latent phase and primary dysfunctional labour

The use of a partogram with the expected progress line constructed for an individual patient allows easy recognition of an unsatisfactory rate of cervical dilatation. The descent of the presenting part as the number of fifths palpable abdominally is also plotted at each review and a poor rate of descent also indicates potentially problematic labour. Poor progress may be related to inadequate uterine contractions and/or to an increased resistance of the birth canal to the passage of the fetus. This latter can be due to disproportion between the presenting part and the birth canal, or to an unfavourable cervix. Poor progress in labour does not identify the specific cause (that is, a fault with the powers, passage or passenger).

Secondary arrest of labour need not indicate cephalopelvic disproportion, as some-times in these patients inadequate uterine contractions can be corrected by oxytocin and result in spontaneous vaginal delivery (Arulkumaran et al 1987a). When there is failure to progress, obvious problems in the passenger (for example, hydrocepha-lus, brow presentation, undiagnosed shoulder presentation, large/macrosomic baby) and passage (for example, a congenitally small pelvis, a deformed pelvis due to an accident or disease or masses in the pelvis) should be excluded. Commonly, there is no recognisable compromise in the cephalopelvic relationship. Unfavour-able pelvic diameters may result in cephalopelvic disproportion. However the fetus is more commonly the cause of relative disproportion by presenting a larger di-ameter of the vertex due to malposition or deflexion attitudes. In such cases, dystocia may be overcome by further flexion, rotation of the head to the occipito-anterior position and moulding, and efficient uterine contractions. Inefficient uterine contractions have been recognised as the most common cause for poor progress of labour and in these cases, the appropriate use of oxytocin will usually produce efficient contractions and bring about vaginal delivery (Steer et al 1985a; Arulku-maran et al 1991).

Management options for poor progress of the first stage of labour

Augmentation

Indications   Prolonged labour has been known to be associated with maternal infection, obstructed labour, uterine rupture and postpartum hemorrhage which at times may end with maternal mortality. It has been a common axiom 'not to allow the sun to set twice on a woman in labour', in order to prevent such tragic events. Philpott (1972) in Africa, O'Driscoll et al (1973) in Dublin and Studd (1973) in the UK advocated and popularised the concept of augmentation to reduce the in-cidence of prolonged labour by promulgating the concept of the active management of labour to diagnose and correct the poor progress of labour. The main components of 'the active management of labour' are regular assessment to enable early diag-nosis of slow cervical dilatation rates, prompt administration of oxytocin (to correct 'inefficient uterine action'), reassurance provided by one-to-one support by a nurse or a medical student, the husband's or partner's participation, pain relief and hy-dration. The use of active management as practised in the National Maternity Hospital, Dublin, has been associated with reduction in the incidence of prolonged labour, fetal and maternal infection, operative deliveries and poor maternal and fetal outcome (O'Driscoll et al 1970, 1973).

The decision to augment labour should be governed primarily by the rate of cervical dilatation after the exclusion of gross disproportion or malpresentation. Minor degrees of disproportion due to malposition and poor flexion of the head may be overcome by oxytocin infusion. Forceful uterine contraction causes flexion at the atlanto-occipital joint and reduces the presenting diameter. This allows ro-tation of the occiput from a posterior or lateral to an anterior position. The increased force of contractions would also help in further moulding and reduce the presenting diameter of the head as well as effect an increase in pelvic dimensions due to the descending head and widening of the sacroiliac and symphysis pubic joints. Mould-ing is a process whereby the parietal, occipital and frontal bones of the skull first come together (moulding +). This is followed by one parietal bone going under the other and the occipital and frontal bones going below the parietal bones. Gentle digital pressure is adequate to reduce the overlapping of the bones (moulding ++). If the moulding is severe (+++), gentle digital pressure will not restore the overlapping bones to their original position. Caput is the soft tissue swelling caused by the edema of the scalp which develops as the fetal head descends in the pelvis. The degree of caput increases, the tighter the fit and the longer the labour.

When to augment labour   The 'efficiency' of uterine contractions should be defined in terms of how much they have achieved, that is, the progress of cervical dilatation and descent of the head, and not in relation to the magnitude of uterine contractions, because the normal progress of labour is observed with a wide range of uterine activity in nulliparas and multiparas (O'Driscoll and Meagher 1980; Gibb et al 1984; Arulkumaran et al 1984). The more rapid the rate of progress for a

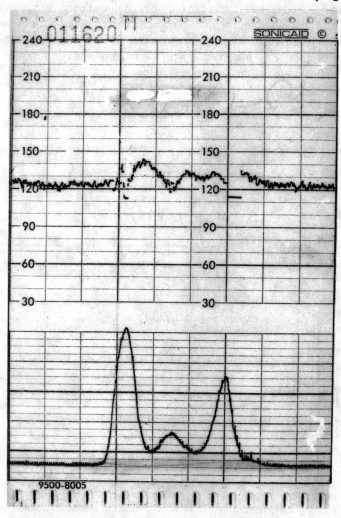

Fig 2.5   Mild degree of incoordination of uterine contractions

given level of uterine activity, the more 'efficient' the contractions. It is also important to recognise the difference between the concept of inefficient uterine activity and that of 'incoordinate' uterine contractions. Inefficiency is the failure of the uterus to work in such a way that the progress of labour is not normal. It can be demonstrated only when the end-point of such activity has been observed to be deficient. This clinical situation is one of poor cervimetric progress in the absence of cephalopelvic disproportion or malposition (although both of these may coexist with inefficient uterine action). Incoordinate uterine action is a descriptive term for a tocographic tracing (Figs 2.5 and 2.6). Most records of uterine contractions show some degree of irregularity. Quantification of irregularity is difficult, but there appears to be an intrinsic pattern of uterine contractile rhythm, which each individual patient assumes once labour is established. This pattern does not change substantially during active labour. Regular uterine contractions are often associated with the normal progress of labour. While incoordinate patterns may be inefficient (Ferreira and Odendaal 1994), this can only be concluded once vaginal examination has confirmed that labour has failed to progress. Therefore the decision to augment labour should be governed primarily by the rate of cervical dilatation after exclusion of gross disproportion or malpresentation. The issue of whether oxytocin augmentation is appropriate in the presence of slow progress but apparently normal

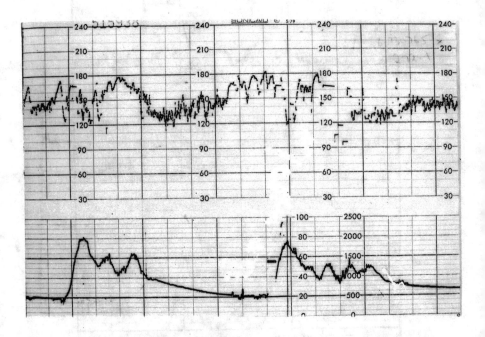

Fig 2.6   Severe degree of incoordination of uterine contraction

contractions as demonstrated by intrauterine pressure measurement needs further elucidation.

Practical aspects of labour management

A variety of techniques is used for the detection of slow progress in labour. However it is universally agreed that the diagnosis of active labour depends fundamentally on a careful assessment of the cervical state (dilatation, effacement, consistency, position and descent of the head) and not on soft indicators such as regular painful contractions, a show, or even rupture of the amniotic membranes. On admission, the cervical dilatation should be plotted on a partogram. In our unit, an alert line is drawn at 1 cm/h once the active phase of labour is reached and an action line is drawn parallel to it and 2 h to the right. If the observed progress is slow and is to the right of the action line, augmentation is considered. There is no consensus as to the placement of the action line, whether it should be 1, 2, 3 or 4 h to the right of the alert line. Various centres use different intervals. Modifying factors include the level of nursing and medical care available for the supervision of labour (because oxytocin is likely to be used once the cervical dilatation rate crosses the action line), the risk of complications associated with prolonged labour (which is likely to be higher in disadvantaged communities) and the social milieu of the clients (in many Western settings there is a consumer demand for 'natural childbirth', which generally means avoiding intervention unless it becomes inescapable). The fact that there is a line drawn to indicate that action is necessary at some point (preferably 1-4 h) is more important than the time interval between the alert and action lines. When action is needed, amniotomy alone may be adequate to correct slow progress, although oxytocin will be needed in most cases if the progress after amniotomy is poor in the next 2 or 3 hours.

Augmentation in the latent phase of labour

The duration of the latent phase of labour varies widely and is a period when the diagnosis of labour is difficult. An appreciable proportion of women have painful contractions for long periods in the latent phase of labour with little cervical change. These contractions may subside and labour may not get established. Due to the variation in the duration of the latent phase and the uncertainty regarding the establishment of labour, the management of the latent phase should usually be conservative and consist of reassurance, hydration, nutrition and ambulation. The decision to augment labour in the latent phase should be based on medical or obstetric indications. In women with 'spurious labour' who have been managed conservatively, there is a slightly higher risk of fetal distress in subsequent labour (Arulkumaran et al 1987b). Hence it may be useful to confirm fetal wellbeing by cardiotocography before deciding to manage the latent phase conservatively. Augmentation of labour in the latent phase with a poor cervical score may be associated with a higher risk of caesarean section and therefore a clear indication is a prerequisite for intervention. However when the woman has contractions for a long time some action has to be taken. There is limited literature available in relation to the management of a prolonged latent phase, but the results of a large WHO multicentre study using a partogram with a cut-off at 8 h in the latent phase appear to be satisfactory for the management of the prolonged latent phase (WHO 1994).

Augmentation in the active phase of labour

The decision to augment in the active phase of labour is based on the observed progress in relation to the expected (alert) and satisfactory (action) progress line drawn from the first cervical dilatation observed in the active phase. Most patients are admitted in the active phase with the cervical dilatation > 3 cm. The expected progress line or the 'alert line' can be drawn using a stencil (Studd et al 1975) or can be a line drawn at a rate of 1 cm/h (Arulkumaran and Ingemarsson 1985). O'Driscoll et al (1970, 1973) augment labour when the progress of labour is to the right of the alert line, whereas others are less stringent and advocate augmentation when the progress has deviated to the right of the 'action line' drawn 2, 3, or 4 h parallel to the alert line. By allowing a 2 h 'period of grace', fewer patients will be augmented: 55% of nulliparas with no period of grace (O'Driscoll et al 1973) compared to 19% with a 2 h period of grace (Arulkumaran et al 1987a). Both methods of management yield comparable results, although prompt intervention does decrease the duration of labour and therefore may be most appropriate when labour ward staffing is adequate and/or the bed strength is limited. Alternatively, if women are more in favour of 'natural childbirth', preference should be given to a protocol with lower intervention rates (by drawing the action line 3 or 4 hours to the right of the alert line) if obstetric outcomes are not very different. The WHO study with the action line drawn 3 h to the right of the alert line in the active phase in order to reduce the number of patients needing oxytocin has shown a reduction in prolonged labour and caesarean section rates (WHO 1994).

The role of artificial rupture of membranes (ARM)

The artificial rupture of membranes need not be performed as a routine. Once the active phase has started, that is, when the cervix is more than 3 cm, the membranes may be ruptured. This procedure is popular in centres which believe in the active management of labour. When it is not done routinely, there are some occasions when the rupture of the membranes is indicated

    a.   to increase the frequency, duration and strength of uterine contractions when the progress of labour is abnormal;

    b.   to exclude the presence or absence of meconium stained amniotic fluid in a high risk labour especially if the fetal heart rate pattern is abnormal;

    c.   to facilitate the insertion of intrauterine pressure catheters or internal scalp electrodes when the FHR or uterine contraction recordings are poor with external transducers.

ARM has a few drawbacks. When the presenting part is high there is a chance of cord prolapse and if the labour becomes prolonged there is an increased chance of intrauterine infection.

Oxytocin dosage and time increment schedules

The uterus of a patient in labour is sensitive to oxytocin and may be hypersensitive even to small doses (Sica Blanco and Sala 1961). The drug is best titrated in an arithmetical or geometric manner starting from a low dose. Oxytocin is often administered by gravity fed drips, which are not reliable. Overdosage may lead to fetal distress, while a suboptimal dose may lead to failure to progress, resulting in unnecessary intervention. The dangers to the fetus (Kubli and Ruttgers 1961; Liston and Campbell 1974; Gibb and Arulkumaran 1982) and to the mother (Daw 1973) of uncontrolled infusion are well documented. Ideally, for precise control, a peristaltic infusion pump should be utilised.

Published protocols variously recommend a starting dose of 2–6 mµ/min of oxytocin and geometric increases every 15–30 min for the induction of labour (Turnbull and Anderson 1968; Steer et al 1985a and b; Knutzen et al 1977). They have been adapted for the augmentation of labour in many centres. The recommendations were based on earlier in vitro pharmacological studies in which the half-life of oxytocin was thought to be 3–4 min (Fuchs and Fuchs 1984; Saameli 1963). However recent in vivo studies (Seitchik et al 1984) have suggested that the half-life of oxytocin is in fact 10–15 min. Continuous intravenous infusion of oxytocin has also shown first-order kinetics, with a progressive stepwise increase. With every increase in infusion rate, a steady plasma concentration is reached 40–60 min after the alteration of an infusion. A shorter increment interval results in the dose being increased before maximum plasma levels are reached. These findings, along with a number of litigation cases due to the misuse of oxytocin (Fuchs 1985), have prompted a closer look at intervals between dose increments. Seitchik et al (1984) recommend an incremental interval of 30 min as a reasonable compromise to avoid overdosage and the danger of uterine hyperstimulation leading to fetal distress on the one hand, and undue delay in delivery on the other. Retrospective studies (Foster et al 1988) and prospective studies (Blakemore et al 1990; Chua et al 1991) on the optimal interval between dose increments suggest that a 30 min increment interval is likely to be associated with less incidence of hyperstimulation, fetal heart rate changes and a lower total dose of oxytocin infusion without increasing the length of labour compared with shorter incremental intervals. These studies lend weight to the recommendations on oxytocin regimes made by the American College of Obstetricians and Gynecologists (1987). Recent radioimmunoassays of oxytocin in vivo and retrospective studies on contraction patterns in augmented labour support these recommendations (Brindley and Sokol 1988).

Achievement of optimal uterine activity

The literature is limited regarding the level of uterine activity that should be produced by oxytocin titration to effect a good obstetric outcome. It has been suggested that the use of pre- and post-augmentation uterine activity measurements with the use of an intrauterine catheter may identify those who are likely to need caesarean section for failure to progress (Reddi et al 1988). It is known that active contraction area measurements using an intrauterine catheter correlate better with the rate of cervical dilatation than the individual variables of frequency or amplitude of contractions (Steer 1977). Hence if there is no progress with optimal uterine activity, it may suggest disproportion. Despite this possible theoretical advantage, the measurement of uterine activity using an intrauterine catheter or oxytocin titration to achieve preset active contraction area profiles has not been shown to produce a better obstetric outcome in augmented labour, compared with oxytocin titration to achieve a preset frequency of contractions (Arulkumaran et al 1989b).

The question is what the frequency should be if oxytocin titration to achieve a preset frequency offers a good obstetric outcome? Steer et al (1985b) suggest that when facilities are not available for computation of uterine activity measurements, the dose of oxytocin should not be increased beyond 8 mμ/min and the target frequency of contractions should not exceed one in 3 min. He postulates, that practice contrary to this may lead to more babies with poor Apgar scores. In most centres facilities for quantification of uterine activity in labour are not available. In a prospective study, two-thirds of women who showed failure to progress despite no evidence of cephalopelvic disproportion had two or fewer contractions in 10 min, while one-third had an 'optimal' contraction frequency of one in 3 min over a period of 4 h. In the latter group, oxytocin titration to achieve a contraction frequency of 4 in 10 min with each contraction duration lasting > 40 s was associated with the vaginal delivery of babies in good condition in 96% (24/25) (Arulkumaran et al 1991). It may therefore be that three contractions in 10 min should be the target uterine activity with oxytocin titration, but if there is no progress with this frequency of contractions, the oxytocin dose should be increased to achieve a contraction frequency of four or five in 10 min provided the FHR pattern is normal.

The measurement of uterine contractions

The frequency of contractions can be assessed by either external or internal tocography. Some centres use intrauterine catheters when oxytocin is administered because they feel that hyperstimulation of the uterus can be identified early and that oxytocin infusion rates can be adjusted accordingly, resulting in a reduction in fetal hypoxic episodes and a better neonatal outcome. In most instances, prior to hyperstimulation there is an increase in frequency followed by an increase in the amplitude of contractions, which precedes elevation of the baseline tone. However excessively frequent contractions can also be identified by external tocography. A prospective randomised study did not show a better obstetric outcome when an intrauterine catheter was used, compared with the use of external tocography in augmented labour (Chua et al 1990). In a busy clinical practice, it may be easier, less invasive and cheaper to assess uterine contractions using external tocography. On the other hand, in high risk cases (such as pregnancies complicated by intrauterine fetal growth deficiency, or in practices where medicolegal concerns are important), there are theoretical advantages to the use of intrauterine pressure measurement. In addition, the use of intrauterine catheters may be of value in restless or obese parturients where external tocography does not record well. There are circumstances where the contraction frequency is three or four in 10 min with each contraction lasting > 40 s but progress of labour is poor. In these situations and in cases where high doses of oxytocin (> 15mμ/min) are used, quantification of uterine activity by the use of an intrauterine catheter may prevent hyperstimulation with consequent fetal hypoxia. The use of intrauterine pressure measurement has also been recommended in cases with a previous caesarean scar which are augmented with oxytocin, as a sudden decline in uterine activity may be the first and only sign of scar dehiscence in a proportion of cases (Beckley et al 1991; Arulkumaran et al 1992).

Duration of augmentation

It is generally agreed that the use of the partogram and oxytocic augmentation for the management of poor progress of labour are valuable. There is, however, a debate as to how long one should augment labour prior to deciding on caesarean section for failure to progress. A prospective study of 2,803 patients admitted in spontaneous labour evaluated the mode of delivery and neonatal outcome when augmentation was continued in those who had unsatisfactory progress (< 1 cm/h) in the first 4 h of augmentation (Arulkumaran et al 1987a). Of the 19.0% of nulliparas and 7.3% of multiparas who had poor progress, 65.5% of nulliparas and 83.8% of multiparas showed good response to oxytocic augmentation and dilated at a rate >1 cm/h in the first 4 h of augmentation. In those who showed such good progress, only 1.4% of nulliparas and 1.2% of multiparas needed caesarean section and these were for reasons other than poor progress. In those who had poor progress in the first 4 h (35.5% of nulliparas and 16.2% of multiparas), a further 4 h of augmentation was allowed. This resulted in vaginal delivery for 50.7% of nulliparas with primary dysfunctional labour and 33.3% for those with secondary arrest in labour. The corresponding figures for multiparas were 41.7% and 25.0% respectively. The neonatal outcome was uniformly good. These data suggest that augmentation of slow labours (< 1 cm in 3 h) benefits both nulliparas and multiparas. A period of 8 h of augmentation with adequate monitoring in the absence of gross disproportion should result in the majority of nulliparas and multiparas delivering vaginally with little risk of intrauterine or birth asphyxia or injury. It is doubtful whether more than 8 h of augmentation in the presence of poor progress will result in a significantly greater number of patients delivering vaginally without compromise to the fetus.

Augmentation in special circumstances

Multiparas   Caution has to be exercised in augmenting multiparas, especially grand multiparas, where the cause of the poor progress may be unrecognised disproportion. Augmentation in such situations might lead to rupture of the uterus. In these women, if there is no progress despite adequate spontaneous uterine contractions, it may be better to observe them for a few hours than to use oxytocin. One has also to be careful when augmentation is undertaken for failure to progress in the late first stage of labour (> 7 cm cervical dilatation). A prolonged period of augmentation should be avoided. Failure to progress despite augmentation may be due to disproportion and an early decision should be made as to the mode of delivery.

Previous caesarean section   Opinion regarding augmentation if there is poor progress in cases of previous caesarean section or breech presentation varies widely. When there is failure to progress in cases of previous caesarean section, and major disproportion seems unlikely (there is no history of pelvic injury, clinical pelvimetry is normal and the head is no more than three-fifths palpable per abdomen), if contractions are not optimal (frequency less than three in 10 min and duration less than 40 sec) it may be justified to augment labour. The role of intrauterine pressure measurement in this situation is disputed. There are no prospective studies which show a high incidence of scar rupture with careful oxytocin augmentation and yet some clinicians refuse to use oxytocin in the trial of scars for fear that rupture will occur. On purely logical grounds, it would seem reasonable to augment contractions at least to the average level for spontaneous labour. In practice, augmentation may lead to higher levels of uterine activity than spontaneous normal labour (Arulkumaran et al 1989c, d). Since a substantial proportion of those who fail to make adequate progress in the first 4 h of augmentation need operative delivery (Arulkumaran et al 1989d), and since, with further prolongation of labour they become more susceptible to scar rupture (Beckley et al 1991; Arulkumaran et al 1992), the period of augmentation should probably be limited to 4 h unless adequate cervical dilatation rates resume themselves. Those who show satisfactory progress can be allowed a further period of augmentation. This concept is discussed further in the chapter on management of previous caesarean section.

Breech   Dysfunctional labour is more common in breech presentation than in cephalic presentation. If augmentation is carried out in the presence of breech presentation, it should be performed cautiously. It is probably wise to estimate fetal weight clinically and preferably by ultrasound before augmentation, as fetal weights greater than 3.8 kg are associated with a significantly higher rate of obstructed labour. X-ray pelvimetry can be used to exclude gross disproportion (Arulkumaran et al 1988a), although it is becoming increasingly appreciated that pelvimetry is a poor indicator of the likely mode of delivery (Krishnamurthy et al, 1991). Knowledge of the adequacy of uterine activity may also be useful before a decision is made about augmentation (Arulkumaran et al 1988b). Good results have been reported provided there is ready resort to caesarean section if there is no progress in the first 4 h of augmentation (Arulkumaran et al 1989e; Ingemarsson et al 1989).

Genuine cephalopelvic disproportion and disproportion due to malposition

If the progress of labour is unsatisfactory despite adequate augmentation, mechanical factors that might contribute to disproportion have to be considered. Disproportion may be diagnosed when two-fifths or more of the head is palpable abdominally. Vaginal examination may reveal a loosely applied presenting part, an edematous cervix, gross moulding and caput. Furthermore, deflexion or malposition of the head may be identified with the maximal diameter of the head still high in the pelvis. A cardiotocographic tracing may show either early or variable decelerations suggestive of head compression. Meconium-stained amniotic fluid sometimes appears. These signs indicate an absolute cephalopelvic disproportion if the occiput is anterior with a well-flexed vertex presentation, and relative disproportion due to malposition if the head is deflexed with the occiput felt laterally or posteriorly. Diagnosis of disproportion at full dilatation becomes a difficult issue. Fetal weight estimation, the proportion of the head palpable abdominally, the degree of caput and moulding, the station of the bony part and the position of the presentation have to be carefully evaluated. The descent of the head with contraction and bearing down effort and the possibility of palpating the fetal ear give additional clues.

In relative cephalopelvic disproportion due to malposition, the degree of flexion is unsatisfactory and a larger anteroposterior occipitofrontal (11 cm) diameter is presented instead of the smaller suboccipito bregmatic (9.5 cm) diameter in a well-flexed occipito-anterior position. The subtle distinction between 'absolute' cephalopelvic disproportion and 'relative' cephalopelvic disproportion due to malposition may be useful in deciding on trial of labour or a repeat elective caesarean section in the next pregnancy. A patient who has a caesarean section for disproportion due to malposition and deflexed head in her first pregnancy may well have a normal delivery in her subsequent labour if the head flexes and presents in an occipito-anterior position with a smaller diameter. Thus two-thirds of patients allowed a trial of labour despite a previous caesarean section for failure to progress due to 'disproportion', deliver vaginally in their subsequent pregnancy without a significant increase in maternal or fetal morbidity (Clark et al 1984; Phelan et al 1987; Chua et al 1989).

X-ray pelvimetry

In the majority of cases that fail to progress in labour, the relative contribution by the passenger and the passage is difficult to evaluate. The dynamic nature of labour continuously alters the dimensions of the pelvis and of the presenting part by flexion, rotation and moulding. Static measurements are probably of little value in such situations. Prospective studies of prenatal and intrapartum x-ray pelvimetry have been shown not to alter planned management policies (Hanna 1965; Laube et al 1981; Jagani et al 1981). In a woman with a cephalic presentation, unless there is evidence of gross disproportion, a well-conducted trial of labour is the best test for the adequacy of the pelvis.

Labour is a natural phenomenon leading to childbirth. Many women have the rewarding experience of a safe vaginal delivery, while a small proportion die of the consequences of prolonged labour and its sequelae. In an attempt to reduce adverse events, obstetric interventions have become popular. However public suspicion about unnecessary interventions have often threatened to bring the medical profession into disrepute (Sir Anthony Carlisle first voiced these concerns in the British Parliament as long ago as 1834 when speaking to the Select Committee on Medical Education, concerns echoed in the most recent report on childbirth produced by the Select Committee on Health 11 in 1992). These concerns, widely expressed by the general public in recent years, are perfectly valid and will increase if practice is not continually scrutinised and subjected to appropriate clinical trials whenever possible. Interventions in labour should not only be made in good faith but should be based on sound knowledge of normal labour and its variations. Perhaps in obstetrics more than in other fields of medicine, opinions differ as to management policies especially when an intervention is needed. The physician is in a dilemma when he intervenes because, on the one hand, if complications ensue the decision to intervene may be questioned and, on the other, if fetal or maternal morbidity or mortality follow non-intervention, the consequences may be even more difficult to face. During the last four decades, research concerning the management of labour has been directed to formulating guidelines based on scientific data. Further research is needed to improve current practice. Some areas of current interest related to poor progress of labour concern the usefulness of drugs like prostaglandins (Keirse 1989), and technology related research like the use of catheter-mounted transducers to quantify intrauterine pressure and head-to-cervix force (Gough et al

1990). But the conclusions of research have to be tailored to an appropriate use of technology to cut down cost without compromising the health of the mother and her baby.

References

Arieff AI, Guisado R 1967. Effects on CNS of hyponatraemic states. *Kidney International* 10:104-109.

American College of Obstetricians and Gynecologists 1987. Induction and Augmentation of Labour, *Tech Bull* No. 110, November.

Arulkumaran S, Gibb DMF, Lun KC, Heng SH, Ratnam SS 1984. The effect of parity on uterine activity in labour. *Br J Obstet Gynecol* 91:843-848.

Arulkumaran S, Ingemarsson I 1985. New concepts in the management of spontaneous labour. *Sing J Obstet Gynecol* 16:163-172

Arulkumaran S, Koh CH, Ingemarsson I, Ratnam SS 1987a. Augmentation of labour. Mode of delivery related to cervimetric progress. *Aust NZ J Obstet Gynecol* 27:304-308.

Arulkumaran S, Michelson J, Ingemarsson I, Ratnam SS 1987b. Obstetric outcome of patients with a previous episode of spurious labour. *Am J Obstet Gynecol* 157:17-20.

Arulkumaran S, Tariq K, Ingemarsson I 1988a. Management of the term breech presentation in labour. *Sing J Obstet Gynecol* 19:44-52.

Arulkumaran S, Ingemarsson I, Gibb DMF, Ratnam SS 1988b. Uterine activity in spontaneous labour with breech presentation. *Aust NZ J Obstet Gynecol* 28:275-278.

Arulkumaran S, Gibb DMF, Chua S, Piara Singh, Ratnam SS 1989a. Ethnic influences on uterine activity in spontaneous normal labour. *Br J Obstet Gynecol* 96:1203-1206.

Arulkumaran S, Yang M, Ingemarsson I, Piara S, Ratnam SS 1989b. Augmentation of labour. Does oxytocin titration to achieve preset active contraction area values produce better obstetric outcome? *Asia Oceania J Obstet Gynecol* 15:333-337.

Arulkumaran S, Gibb DMF, Ingemarsson I, Kitchener CH, Ratnam SS 1989c. Uterine activity during spontaneous normal labour after previous caesarean section. *Br J Obstet Gynecol* 96:933-938.

Arulkumaran S, Ingemarsson I, Ratnam SS 1989d. Oxytocin augmentation in dysfunctional labour after previous caesarean section. *Br J Obstet Gynecol* 96:939-941.

Arulkumaran S, Thavarasah AS, Ingemarsson I, Ratnam SS 1989e. An alternative approach to assisted vaginal breech delivery. *Asia Oceania J Obstet Gynecol* 15:47-51.

Arulkumaran S, Chua S, Chua TM, Yang M, Piara S, Ratnam SS 1991. Uterine activity in dysfunctional labour and target uterine activity to be aimed at with oxytocin titration. *Asia Oceania J Obstet Gynecol* 17:101-106.

Arulkumaran S, Chua S, Ratnam SS 1992. Symptoms and signs with scar rupture: Value of uterine activity measurements. *Aust NZ J Obstet Gynecol*, 32:208-212.

Arulkumaran S 1994. Poor progress in labour including augmentation, malpositions and malpresentations. In: James DK, Steer PJ, Gonig S, Weiner C, eds. High Risk Pregnancy Management Options. London: WB. Saunders Co Ltd, pp 1061-1075.

Beazley JM, Alderman S 1976. The 'inductograph', a graph describing the limits of the latent phase of induced labour in low risk situations. *Br J Obstet Gynecol* 83:513-517.

Beckley S, Gee H, Newton JR 1991. Scar rupture in labour after previous lower segment caesarean section: The role of uterine activity measurement. *Br J Obstet Gynecol* 98:265-269.

Blakemore KJ, Qin NG, Petrie RH, Paine LL 1990. A prospective comparison of hourly and quarter hourly oxytocin dose increase intervals for the induction of labour at term. *Obstet Gynecol* 75:757-761.

Borten M 1983. Breech presentation. In Friedman EA, Cohen WR, eds. Management of Labour. Baltimore, MD: University Park Press, pp. 253-256.

Brindley BA, Sokol RJ 1988. Induction and augmentation of labour. Basis and methods for current practice. *Obstet Gynecol Surv* 43:730-743.

Caldeyro Barcia R, Sica Blanco Y, Poseiro J et al 1957. A quantitative study of the action of synthetic oxytocin on the pregnant human uterus. *J Pharmacol* 121:18-26.

Cardozo LD, Gibb DMF, Studd JWW, VaSant RV, Cooper DJ 1982. Predictive value of cervimetric labour patterns in primigravidae. *Br J Obstet Gynecol* 89:33-38.

Caesarean child birth 1981. Summary of a National Institutes of Health Consensus Statement. *Br Med J* 282:1600-1604.

Chua S, Arulkumaran S, Piara S, Ratnam SS 1989. Trial of labour after previous caesarean section: Obstetric outcome. *Aust NZ J Obstet Gynecol* 29:12-17

Chua S, Kurup A, Arulkumaran S, Ratnam SS 1990. Augmentation of labour. Does internal tocography result in better obstetric outcome than external tocography? *Obstet Gynecol* 76:164-167.

Chua S, Arulkumaran S, Kurup A, Tay D, Ratnam SS 1991. Oxytocin titration for induction of labour: A prospective randomised study of IS versus 30 minute dose increment schedules. *Aust NZ J Obstet Gynecol* 31:134-137.

Clark SL, Eglinton GS, Beall M, Phelan JP 1984. Effect of the indication for previous caesarean section on subsequent delivery outcome in patients undergoing a trial of labour. *J Reprod Med* 29:22-25.

Clinch J 1989. Abnormal fetal presentations and positions. In: Turnbull A, Chamberlain G, eds. Obstetrics, London: Churchill Livingstone, pp 793-812.

Cruikshank DP, Cruikshank JE 1981. Face and brow presentation: A review. *Clin Obstet Gynecol* 24:33-351.

Dahlenburgh GW, Burnell RH, Braybrook R 1980. The relation between cord serum sodium levels in newborn infants and maternal intravenous therapy during labour. *Br J Obstet Gynecol* 87:519-524.

Daw E 1973. Oxytocin induced rupture of the primigravid uterus. *J Obstet Gynecol Br Cwlth* 80:374-375.

Duignan NM, Studd JWW, Hughes AO 1975. Characteristics of labour in different racial groups. *Br J Obstet Gynecol* 82:593-601.

Ferguson JKW 1941. A study of the motility of the intact uterus at term. *Surg, Gynecol and Obstet* 73:359-366.

Ferreira CJ, Odendaal HJ 1994. Does coupling of uterine contractions reflect uterine dysfunction? *S Afr Med J* 84:20-3.

Foster TCS, Jacobson JD, Valenzuela GJ 1988. Oxytocin augmentation of labour A comparison of 15 and 30 minute dose increment intervals. *Obstet Gynecol* 71:147-149.

Friedman EA 1954. The graphic analysis of labour. *Am J Obstet Gynecol* 68: 1568-1571.

Fuchs AR, Fuchs F 1984. Endocrinology of human parturition: A review. *Br J Obstet Gynecol* 91:948:967

Fuchs F 1985. Caution on using oxytocin for inductions. *Contemp Obstet Gynecol* 25: 13-16.

Gibb DMF, Arulkumaran S 1982. Oxytocin: A reappraisal. *Sing J Obstet Gynecol* 13:152-158.

Gibb DMF, Cardozo LD, Studd JWW, Magos AL, Cooper DJ 1982. Outcome of spontaneous labour in multigravidae. *Br J Obstet Gynecol* 89:708-711.

Gibb DMF, Arulkumaran S, Lun KC, Heng SH, Ratnam SS 1984. Characteristics of uterine activity in nulliparous labour. *Br J Obstet Gynecol* 91:220-227.

Goodfellow CF, Studd C 1979. The reduction of forceps in primigravidae with epidural analgesia: A controlled trial. *Br J Clin Pract* 33:287-288.

Gough GW, Randall NJ, Genevier ES, Sutherland IA, Steer PJ 1990. Head to cervix pressure and their relationship to the outcome of labour. *Obstet Gynecol* 75:613-618.

Hall MH 1990. Confidential enquiry into maternal death. *Br J Obstet Gynecol* 97:752-753.

Hanna WJ 1965. X-ray pelvimetry: Critical appraisal. *Am J Obstet Gynecol* 91:333-341.

Holmberg NG, Lilieqvist B, Magnusson S, Segerbrand E 1977. The influence of the bony pelvis in persistent occiput posterior position. *Acta Obstet Gynecol Scand (Suppl)* 66:49-54.

Ilancheran A, Lim SM, Ratnam SS 1977. Nomograms of cervical dilatation in labour. *Sing J Obstet Gynecol* 8:69-73.

Ingemarsson I, Arulkumaran S, Westgren M 1989. Breech delivery: Management and long term outcome. In: Tejani N, ed. Obstetrical events and developmental sequelae. Boca Raton, FL: CRC Press, pp. 143-159.

Jagani N, Schulman H, Chandra P, Gonzalez P, Fleischer A 1981. The predictability of labour outcome from a comparison of birth weight and x-ray pelvimetry. *Am J Obstet Gynecol* 139:501-511

Keirse WNC 1989. Augmentation of labour. In: Chalmers 1, Enkin M, Keirse MJNC, eds. Effective Care in Pregnancy and Childbirth, Oxford: Oxford University Press, pp. 951-968.

Kenepp NB, Shelley WC, Kumar S, Stanley CA, Gutsche BB 1980. Effects on newborn of hydration with glucose in patients undergoing caesarean section with regional anesthesia. *Lancet* i:645.

Kenepp NB, Shelley WC, Gabbe SG, Kumar S, Stanley CA, Gutsche BB 1982. Fetal and neonatal hazards of maternal hydration with 5% dextrose before caesarean section. *Lancet* i:1150-1152.

Knutzen VK, Tanneberger U, Davey DA 1977. Complications and outcome of induced labour. *S Afr Med J* 52:482-485.

Krishnamurthy S, Fairlie F, Cameron AD, Walker JJ, MacKenzie JR 1991. The role of postnatal pelvimetry after caesarean section in the management of subsequent delivery. *Br J Obstet Gynecol* 98:716-718.

Kubli F, Ruttgers H 1961. Iatrogenic fetal hypoxia. In: Gevers RH, Ruys JH, eds. Physiology and Pathology in the Perinatal Periods, Leiden: Leiden University Press, pp. 55-75.

Laube WD, Vamer MW, Cruikshank DP 1981. A prospective evaluation of x-ray pelvimetry. *JAMA* 246:2187-2190.

Liston WA, Campbell AJ 1974. Dangers of oxytocin induced labour to the fetus. *Br Med J* 3:606-607.

Morton KE, Jackson MC, Gillmer MDG 1985. A comparison of the effects of four intravenous solutions for treatment of ketonuria during labour. *Br J Obstet Gynecol* 92:473-479.

Myerscough P 1989. Cephalopelvic disproportion. In: Turnbull A, Chamberlain G, eds. Obstetrics, London: Churchill Livingstone, pp. 813-821.

O'Driscoll K, Stronge JM, Minogue M 1973. Active management of labour. *Br Med J* iii: 135-138.

O'Driscoll K, Jackson RJA, Gallagher JT 1970. Active management of labour and cephalopelvic disproportion. *J Obstet Gynecol Br Cwlth* 77:385-389.

O'Driscoll K, Meagher D 1980. Active Management of Labour: *Clin Obstet Gynecol.* Philadelphia, PA: W B Saunders. p 317.

Paintin DB, Vincent F 1980. Forceps delivery: Obstetric outcome. In: Beard RW, Paintin DB, eds. Outcome of Obstetric Intervention in Britain, London: Royal College of Obstetricians and Gynecologists, pp. 17-32.

Phelan JP, Clark SL, Diaz F, Paul RH 1987. Vaginal birth after caesarean. *Am J Obstet Gynecol* 157:1510-1515.

Philpott RH 1972. Graphic records in labour. *Br Med J* iv: 163-165.

Rao KB 1992. Obstructed labour. In: Ratnam SS, Bhasker Rao K, Arulkumaran S, eds. Obstetrics and Gynecology for Postgraduates, Vol. 1, Madras:Orient Longman., pp. 127-133.

Reddi K, Kambaran SR, Philpott PA 1988. Intrauterine pressure studies in multigravid patients in spontaneous labour. Effect of oxytocin augmentation in delayed first stage. *Br J Obstet Gynecol* 95:771-777.

Richardson JA, Sutherland IA, Allen DW 1978. A cervimeter for continuous measurement of cervical dilatation in labour: Preliminary results. *Br J Obstet Gynecol* 85:178-184.

Saameli K 1963. An indirect method for the estimation of oxytocin blood concentration and half-life in pregnant women near term. *Am J Obstet Gynecol* 85:186-192.

Seeds JW, Cefalo R C 1982. Malpresentations. *Clin Obstet Gynecol* 25:145-156.

Seitchik J, Amico J, Robinson AG et al 1984. Oxytocin augmentation of dysfunctional labour. iv. Oxytocin pharmacokinetics. *Am J Obstet Gynecol* 150:225-232.

Sica Blanco Y, Sala NL 1961. Oxytocin: Proceedings of an International Symposium, London: Pergamon Press, pp. 127-134.

Spencer SA, Mann NP, Smith ML, Woolfson AMJ, Benson S 1981. The effects of intravenous therapy during labour on maternal and cord serum sodium levels. *Br J Obstet Gynecol* 88:488-492.

Steer PI 1977. The measurement and control of uterine contractions. In: Beard RW, Campbell S, eds. The Current Status of Fetal Heart Rate Monitoring and Ultrasound in Obstetrics, London: Royal College of Obstetricians and Gynecologists, pp 48-70.

Steer PJ, Carter MC, Beard RW 1985a. The effect of oxytocin infusion on uterine activity levels in slow labour. *Br J Obstet Gynecol* 92: 1120-1126.

Steer PJ, Carter MC, Choong K et al 1985b. A multicentre prospective randomised controlled trial of induction of labour with an automatic closed-loop feedback controlled oxytocin infusion system. *Br J Obstet Gynecol* 92:1127-1133.

Stewart DB 1984. The pelvis as a passageway. 11. The modem human pelvis. *Br J Obstet Gynecol* 91:618-623.

Studd JWW 1973. Partograms and nomograms in the management of primigravid labour. *Br Med J* iv:451-455.

Studd J, Clegg DR, Saunders RR, Hughes AO 1975. Identification of high risk labours by labour nomogram. *Br Med J* ii:545-547.

Thavarasah AS, Arulkumaran S 1988. Administration of intravenous fluids in labour - a critical evaluation. *Int J Feto-Mat Med* 1:42-50.

Turnbull AC, Anderson AB 1968 Induction of labour. *J Obstet Gynecol Br Cwlth* 75:32-41.

Vasika A, Kumaresan P, Han GS Kumaresan M 1978. Plasma oxytocin in initiation in labour. *Am J Obstet Gynecol* 130:263-273.

World Health Organization 1988. The Partograph. Sections 1, 11, 111 and IV. WHO/MCH/88.4. Geneva: WHO/Maternal and Child Health Unit, Division of Family Health.

World Health Orgainization Maternal Health and Safe Motherhood Programme 1994. World Health Orgainization partograph in management of labour. *Lancet* 343:1399-1404.

3

Pain Relief in Labour

Tham Suet Lan
Lee Tat Leang

The most important consideration in pregnancy is that there are in fact two individuals receiving treatment : mother and baby.

Anesthetic requirements in the peripartum period include long periods of constant pain relief, and an increased depth of analgesia might be needed as labour progresses and pain increases. Instrumental delivery might necessitate even deeper levels of sensory blockade, and any analgesic technique used will have to accommodate a sudden need for expeditious delivery.

Changes in maternal physiology are marked during pregnancy and labour, and will require modifications in anesthetic technique. A detailed discussion on this topic has been presented in Chapter 1 of this book, hence only a brief outline will be mentioned where appropriate.

Labour and delivery cause pain in most patients. Nulliparous women are more likely to experience severe pain than multiparous women (Melzack 1984).

Pain may be aggravated by anxiety, fear, maternal expectations and the mother's state of preparation for delivery. It increases maternal oxygen consumption, cardiac output and circulating catecholamine levels (Schnider et al 1983). The rise in serum catecholamines may cause fetal tachycardia, bradycardia or dysfunctional uterine contractions.

An ideal analgesic technique should therefore take into consideration maternal wishes and preferences, available expertise, support staff and facilities. Practices in various countries may vary from culture to culture. The technique used should be cheap, easy to administer, produce good and reliable relief from pain, but not impair consciousness or cooperation. It should be nontoxic to mother and fetus and not produce cardiorespiratory depression in the fetus. The technique must have no tocolytic action and not delay labour.

Methods of pain relief

Table 1:   Non-pharmacological methods

Non-Pharmacological Methods available for Relief of Obstetric Pain		
Natural childbirth	**Acupuncture**	**Touch and massage**
emotional support	transcutaneous electrical nerve stimulation	hydrotherapy
hot and cold compresses		biofeedback
vertical position	psychoprophylaxis	hypnosis

Attempts to minimise the pain of labour non-pharmacologically first began in the early twentieth century.

Natural childbirth was pioneered by Grantly Dick-Read in 1932. He suggested that the pain of childbirth was brought about by fear and tension and recommended passive muscle relaxation to reduce the pain (Dick-Read 1933, 1944).

Psychoprophylaxis is a technique which involves educating the mother about the functioning of her body and the physiology of labour. It originated in Russia and was later popularised in France by Lamaze (Lamaze 1958). The aims of psychoprophylaxis were similar to those of natural childbirth but directed at blocking pain impulses from the uterus and perineum by conditioned reflexes. The establishment of conditioned reflexes involved an intensive training period. Unlike Dick-Read, Lamaze did not rule out the use of analgesics in labour. Leboyer (1975) advocated a modification of natural childbirth and advised delivery in a dark and quiet place, with massage of the newborn and a warm bath for the baby shortly after delivery. He claimed that this technique produced a happier and healthier neonate.

Studies on these methods have shown mixed results, with some researchers finding that they resulted in decreased analgesic requirements, shorter labours and lower instrumentation rates. Others however found no differences from control groups (Minnich 1994).

Other techniques include simple emotional support from the patient's partner or another labour companion, touch and massage, the application of hot or cold compresses, hydrotherapy and adoption of the vertical position. This last technique includes ambulation during early labour, use of the squatting position or a birthing chair, and may aid maternal comfort (Minnich 1994).

Some techniques require fairly extensive preparation and antenatal training. These include biofeedback, acupuncture, hypnosis and transcutaneous electrical nerve stimulation (TENS).

Transcutaneous electrical nerve stimulation (TENS) involves applying an intermittently pulsed electrical current to the back over the lower thoracic and upper lumbar spine. Sensory fibres are stimulated, and synapse with interneurones in the substantia gelatinosa. These feed back to inhibit the release of a neurotransmitter in the sensory fibres themselves. Studies show that TENS shortens the overall duration of labour and gives great maternal satisfaction (Vincenti et al 1982). Another trial has shown (Chia et al 1990) that TENS is effective in labour up to 4 cm cervical dilation.

The advantages of all these techniques include quick discontinuation, non-invasiveness and lack of any demonstrable ill effects on the fetus.

Table 2: Pharmacological methods in pain relief

Systemic drugs	Inhalational agents	
opiates	Peripheral nerve blockade	Central nervous blockade
benzodiazepines	paracervical	spinal
barbiturates	local infiltration	lumbar epidural
ketamine	pudendal	caudal epidural
phenothiazines		combined spinal
non-steroidal		and epidural
anti-inflammatory agents		

Systemic drugs: sedatives and analgesics

All drugs given systemically will cross the placenta to some extent. Drugs which may reach the fetus in larger amounts are those with higher lipid solubilities and low degrees of ionisation (Ginsburg 1971). In some cases placental metabolism may help to lower fetal drug levels.

Opiates   Opiates help the patient to tolerate pain better, but do not provide total analgesia. They can be given orally, intramuscularly, intravenously or subcutaneously, either as intermittent boluses or continuously as an infusion or via a patient-controlled analgesia pump. This last technique generally provides good analgesia at lower analgesic dosages, and gives great patient satisfaction (Wakefield 1994).

Maternal side effects include nausea, vomiting, drowsiness, decreased gastric emptying, respiratory depression and dysphoria. Fetal effects include respiratory depression at birth, and decreased baseline variability in the fetal heart rate. The most commonly used opiates will be discussed briefly.

Pethidine (meperidine in the U.S.) is the most commonly used opiate in obstetric practice. It is a weak base, and a phenomenon known as 'ion-trapping' can occur. Weak bases like lignocaine and pethidine have high pKa values (pethidine has a pKa of 8) and are thus more ionised than un-ionised at the normal maternal pH of 7.4. The fetus is more acidotic (pH of 7.0) than the mother, so at this lower pH more of the weak base will be ionised. The ionised drug cannot diffuse back through the placenta and so tends to accumulate in the fetus. Furthermore, the ionised form of the drug is cleared more slowly than the un-ionised form from the fetal circulation, and this situation will be worsened by any increase in fetal acidosis (for example, due to hypoxia).

Pethidine is a synthetic opioid and the usual dose is 50 to 100 mg intramuscularly. Levels peak in the fetus between 2 and 3 hours after intramuscular administration, therefore delivery should be timed to occur outside this period. An active breakdown product of pethidine is norpethidine, which has a half-life of 60 hours in the neonate (Caldwell et al 1978). Norpethidine is thought to be responsible for poor neonatal neurobehavioural scores.

Pethidine has been used in combination with phenothiazines or hyoscine, which provide antiemesis and sedation. However the somnolence and amnesia caused by these drugs are no longer thought to be desirable.

Pethidine may also be given epidurally (Baraka et al 1982) and intrathecally. Pethidine is unique among opioids in that it possesses weak local anesthetic properties and has been used as a sole intrathecal anesthetic for surgery. It might thus provide effective analgesia in labour when given intrathecally. Doses used have been in the range of 10 to 20 mg (Swayze et al 1991). When given with bupivacaine, epidural pethidine provides effective analgesia while preventing the shivering that sometimes occurs during labour and with epidurals (Brownridge et al 1992).

Morphine has been infrequently used in obstetrics in doses of 5 to 10 mg intramuscularly. Levels peak in maternal blood at 20 to 40 minutes after intramuscular administration. It was part of the original 'twilight sleep' cocktail of drugs (Gauss 1905). Morphine has been shown to produce greater respiratory depression in neonates than pethidine, and the neonatal brain is thought to be more permeable to morphine than the adult brain (Way et al 1965).

Intrathecal morphine produces fairly reliable analgesia in the latent stage of labour but is less effective for the late first and second stages. Epidural morphine appears to be effective only in doses that produce significant side effects in both mother and baby.

Fentanyl has the benefit of rapid onset and lack of active metabolites but its very short duration of action (15–30 minutes) means that it has to be given intravenously either by very frequent boluses or by a continuous infusion.

Fentanyl is the most popular opioid given epidurally in combination with bupivacaine. It allows better analgesia with the use of more dilute local anesthetic solutions, thus reducing the risks of high spinal block and local anesthetic toxicity. Maternal motor blockade is less, which may help to reduce prolongation of the second stage of labour (Chestnut et al 1987).

Mixed agonist-antagonist opioids have the advantage of having a ceiling effect on respiratory depression. Butorphanol (Maduska et al 1978) has been found to provide similar analgesia to pethidine with fewer maternal side effects like nausea, vomiting and dizziness (Hodgkinson et al 1979). Trials with nalbuphine and pentazocine have been less successful and maternal sedation, dysphoria and psychomimetic effects were greater than with pethidine (Wilson et al 1986; Refstad and Lindbaek 1980).

Sufentanil and alfentanil are new opioid agents which are very short acting and have to be given by infusion. They have shown promise when given extradurally along with bupivacaine (Phillips 1987; Huckaby et al 1989). Sufentanil has been approved by the FDA for epidural administration but alfenatil awaits further evaluation as it appears to cause neurobehavioural changes in the fetus (Golub et al 1986).

Phenothiazines   Phenothiazines are still used occasionally in obstetric practice. Desired effects include sedation, antiemesis and lack of fetal respiratory depression. Most phenothiazines do however depress the baseline variability of the fetal heart rate. Drugs in use include chlorpromazine, propiomazine, prochlorperazine and promethazine.

Benzodiazepines   Benzodiazepines are used for maternal sedation. Diazepam has an active metabolite, desmethyldiazepam, which has a very long half-life. Fetal side effects include hypotonicity, decreased activity, respiratory depression, impaired temperature regulation and decreased response to metabolic stress (McAllister 1980). Lorazepam is relatively long acting (half-life 12 hours) but has no active metabolites. It provides good anterograde amnesia, which may not however be desirable during the birth experience. Midazolam has the advantage of being water-soluble and causes less pain when injected intravenously. It has a shorter duration of action than lorazepam, has inactive metabolites and provides good amnesia.

Other drugs   Non-steroidal anti-inflammatory drugs are not used much in obstetric practice because of deleterious side effects like tocolysis and premature closure of the patent ductus arteriosus. Ketorolac has been tried, but per se has not been found to be as effective as an opiate (Walker et al 1988).

Barbiturates like pentobarbital and secobarbital have been tried to allay maternal anxiety. However, fetal respiratory depression occurs with repeated doses, and this category of drugs can be antanalgesic if not given with opioids (Wakefield 1994).

Ketamine is a phencyclidine derivative which is used mainly in anesthetic practice. In small doses (0.3–0.5 mg/kg) it is a good analgesic. It is a bronchodilator and is useful in asthmatic patients. Ketamine also produces sympathetic stimulation, which is useful in hypovolemic patients. It should therefore not be used in patients with pregnancy-induced hypertension. Other undesirable side effects include a 40% rise in uterine tone, when ketamine is used in larger doses (1.5–2 mg/kg). It has been shown to produce neonates with lower Apgar scores, respiratory depression and hypotonia (Akamatsu et al 1974). Another problem is that it produces maternal hallucinations during emergence.

Inhalational agents

The use of inhalational analgesics necessitates specialised equipment, such as vaporisers and blenders. Pollution of the environment and the possible ill effects of trace concentrations on personnel are matters of concern. Analgesia is not complete, drowsiness and maternal amnesia and the potential for loss of airway reflexes are other problems associated with inhalational agents.

Ether, the halogenated anesthetics and trichloroethylene have all been tried over the years. However by far the most popular agent has been and remains nitrous oxide.

The advantages of nitrous oxide include lack of tocolysis, lack of accumulation of the agent in either mother or baby and minimal effect on the fetus. Either pre-mixed cylinders of nitrous oxide and oxygen in a 50-50 ratio (Entonox) must be used, or else blenders mixing oxygen and nitrous oxide should be available. The blender should limit the amount of nitrous oxide obtainable to 50%. If pre-mixed Entonox cylinders are used, care must be taken in cold weather to prevent the liquid nitrous oxide from settling in the tank and producing unintentional delivery of high concentrations of nitrous oxide. Other problems with nitrous oxide include the possibility of maternal diffusion hypoxia when administration is terminated. Good timing is also needed, as the mother must start inhalation of nitrous oxide when the contraction begins and continue it until the contraction ends.

With regard to halogenated anesthetics, a major disadvantage has been dose-related relaxation of the uterine smooth muscle (Munson et al 1977). Other problems include drowsiness and the risk of aspiration pneumonitis. Methoxyflurane, once popular, has fallen into disuse because of nephrotoxicity. Other inhalational agents : isoflurane, enflurane and recently, desflurane (Swart et al 1991) have all been used successfully.

Peripheral nerve blockade

Mechanisms of pain

There are two types of pain transmitted from the female reproductive tract, visceral and somatic.

Visceral pain is caused by the distention of the cervix and the lower uterine segment. Sympathetic visceral afferents transmit sensation to various plexuses and then to the lumbar sympathetic chain. From the sympathetic chain, impulses pass into the spinal cord through the tenth, eleventh, and twelfth thoracic and the first lumbar nerves (Bonica 1975). These must be blocked to gain relief from pain during the first stage of labour. Sensation from the cervix is also transmitted via parasympathetic afferents along the second, third and fourth sacral nerves.

Somatic afferents transmit sensation from the vagina and the perineum in the later stages of labour. Impulses pass to the spinal cord via the pudendal nerve to the second, third and fourth sacral nerves.

Local anesthetics

Local anesthetics block sodium channels in nerve fibres reversibly and can thus block the transmission of painful impulses at several points along the pain pathway. Painful impulses can be blocked along the peripheral nerves, at the paracervical ganglia or centrally. The trend in the west in the last few decades has been increasingly towards central neural blockade.

In overdose or with inadvertent intravenous injection, local anesthetics also have cardiovascular, respiratory and central nervous system side effects in addition to their effects on nerve fibres. Central nervous system effects include anxiety, agitation and fits, and these are followed by first respiratory and then by myocardial depression.

Bupivacaine

Bupivacaine is used in obstetrics in concentrations ranging from 0.05% to 0.5%. The maximum dose recommended by the manufacturers (Astra, Sweden) is 2 mg/kg every 4 hours. The duration of action of the 0.5% solution without adrenaline is approximately 2–3 hours. Bupivacaine has been shown to provide a very good sensory block without much motor block. It is also effective in very low concentrations. However it has been shown to be more cardiotoxic than lignocaine if given intravascularly by accident (Kotelko et al 1984), and this effect may be enhanced by acidosis and hypoxia. The use of 0.75% bupivacaine has been associated with cardiac arrhythmias and arrest, and resuscitation has been difficult if not impossible (Levinson et al 1987).

Pregnancy may sensitise the mother to bupivacaine (Morishima et al 1983). Datta (Datta et al 1983) showed that the sensitivity of A and C fibres to local anesthetics is increased in pregnancy. Hormonal changes have been cited as the proposed cause (Datta et al 1983, 1986).

Lignocaine

Lignocaine (Lidocaine in the U.S.) may be used in 1%– 2% solutions. The toxic dose is 3 mg/kg without adrenaline and 6 – 7 mg/kg with the addition of adrenaline. It is also a weak base which passes rapidly from the maternal blood to the fetus and accumulates in the fetal blood due to 'ion-trapping' (Ralston 1987). Studies on the effect of lignocaine on fetal outcome have shown mixed results. A study by Scanlon in 1974 suggested neurobehavioural changes after the epidural administration of lignocaine, but subsequent controlled studies showed that these differences were subtle and not significant clinically (Abboud et al 1983).

2-chloroprocaine

This drug has a very rapid onset and a brief duration of 40 minutes. It can be used in either 2% or 3% solution. There have been several case reports of neurologic damage after chloroprocaine meant for epidural injection was given intrathecally. This was thought to be due to the action of sodium metabisulfite (a preservative) in combination with a low pH of 3.0 (Gissen et al 1984). The drug has now been reformulated without the preservative.

Paracervical block

This block is usually done by the obstetrician. A paracervical block will block the visceral afferent nerve fibres that pass through the paracervical ganglion of Frankenhauser (Chestnut 1994), which lies immediately lateral and posterior to the cervico-uterine junction. It gives good analgesia without motor blockade and does not block the progress of labour. However it does not provide any perineal analgesia. There is also a high incidence of fetal bradycardia with this block (King et al 1981), attributed to high levels of local anesthetic entering the uterine artery and reaching the fetus. Other disadvantages include trauma to the fetal scalp or maternal vagina.

Pudendal nerve block

This popular block is usually performed by the obstetrician. It provides good analgesia for somatic perineal pain in the second stage of labour, vaginal delivery, episiotomies and low forceps deliveries. Disadvantages include trauma to mother or fetus and local anesthetic toxicity. Local anesthetic infiltration of the perineum may be necessary, as one study (Arulkumaran et al 1987) showed that bilateral pudendal block was not totally effective in nearly 50 per cent of cases.

Local infiltration

This is the most commonly used local anesthetic technique for vaginal delivery. It has a fast onset and can be used to cover the failure of peripheral nerve blocks. However it provides enough anesthesia only for episiotomy and repair of the perineum. Other hazards include trauma and injection of local anesthetic into the fetal scalp.

Central nervous blockade

Lumbar epidural blockade

This is currently the gold standard for pain relief in obstetrics. Many women request epidural analgesia for labour as part of the birth plan. Indications for epidural analgesia include pregnancy-induced hypertension, cardiac and respiratory disease, premature labour, multiple pregnancy and 'incoordinate' inadequate action of the uterus. Absolute contraindications include patient refusal, bleeding diatheses, sepsis, shock, lack of experienced personnel and inadequate resuscitation facilities.

Relative contraindications include lesser degrees of hemorrhage and hypovolemia, central nervous system disease, spinal disease and previous spinal surgery.

Epidural analgesia provides the most effective form of pain relief devised so far for labour and delivery (Crawford 1972). The mother is conscious and can participate in the birth process. Levels of maternal catecholamines (Schnider et al 1983) are lowered, which may result in improved uteroplacental perfusion and better uterine contractility. The hyperventilation due to pain is reduced, limiting the leftward shift of the oxygen dissociation curve caused by hypocarbia. If labour does not progress satisfactorily and a caesarean section becomes necessary, epidural analgesia can be converted to an anesthetic by deepening the sensorimotor block. Post-operative pain can also be addressed by leaving the catheter in situ and giving epidural opiates, alone or with a local anesthetic infusion of low concentration (for example, 0.25% bupivacaine or lower).

Fetal benefits include lack of the respiratory depressant effect of parenteral opioids, and less fetal hypoxia and acidosis.

Limitations of epidural analgesia in labour include the consequences of autonomic blockade and hypotension, a possible dural tap leading to post-dural puncture headache, missed segments, and high and total spinal blockade. These will be discussed below.

Motor blockade is another significant problem. Relaxation of the pelvic diaphragm can cause malrotation of the fetal head during descent and may result in an increased need for forceps deliveries (Husemeyer 1990). If the abdominal wall muscles are paralysed, voluntary expulsive efforts in the second stage might be reduced. Finally obtundation of Fergusson's reflex might result in decreased uterine activity and an increased need for oxytocic drugs (Goodfellow et al 1979).

The establishment of an epidural service requires committed individuals and the presence of an anesthetist on the labour ward, as well as equipment and staff education.

Test dose   A test dose is a dose of local anesthetic or other drug designed to allow recognition of inadvertent intrathecal or intravenous placement of an epidural catheter.

The epidural venous plexus of Batson deserves special mention. This plexus is most dense anterolaterally, and thus vessels are more easily punctured when using the paramedian approach. Raised intra-abdominal pressures cause a corresponding rise in inferior vena caval pressure, which is transmitted to the epidural plexus of veins. Hence in pregnancy, and especially when labour begins, the plexus becomes very engorged and diminishes the volume of the epidural space. Smaller volumes of drugs cause higher levels of blockade and veins are more easily punctured and cannulated with epidural catheters.

The dose of local anesthetic should be large enough to produce a clinical subarachnoid block but not so large that it causes an excessively high spinal. 3 to 4.5 ml of 1.5% lignocaine (Abraham et al 1984; Moore et al 1981) have been recommended. It is necessary to wait at least five minutes for any intrathecal block to develop. This dose of local anesthetic may not however be enough to produce the symptoms of local anesthetic toxicity that allow recognition of intravenous placement.

The addition of 15 to 20 µg of adrenaline to the doses of local anesthetic given above, if given intravenously, will cause a rise in the heart rate of over 25 beats per minute. Test dose studies were done by Moore and Batra in 1981 in surgical patients. Extrapolating the use of an adrenaline test dose to an obstetric population gives rise to some concern. The maternal ECG must be monitored as the rise in heart rate is fleeting. Tachycardia resulting from an intravenous injection of adrenaline may be confused with tachycardia from other obstetric causes. Adrenaline may cause uterine hypoperfusion (Hood et al 1986). This does not last long though, and is only as severe as the hypoperfusion caused by a normal uterine contraction.

An alternative to the addition of adrenaline might be a larger second dose of local anesthetic (not bupivacaine) such as 100–150 mg lignocaine (Albright et al 1986) which will produce systemic symptoms of local anesthetic toxicity (for example, tinnitus, circumoral numbness, giddiness).

Most authors agree that the addition of adrenaline is useful and that the benefits outweigh the hazards.

Maintenance of anesthesia   New concepts in epidural analgesia are aimed at reducing motor blockade and reducing the risk of high or total spinals. The use of lower concentrations of local anesthetics has helped to reduce the problems while maintaining satisfactory analgesia. The addition of opioids has been helpful in allowing better analgesia at very low concentrations of local anesthetics (Niv et al 1986).

Additional doses of local anesthetics usually have to be given to maintain analgesia. These can be given as boluses or as a continuous infusion.

Boluses may be given by a physician or by a midwife. Boluses administered by a physician require him to be constantly present on the labour ward. Midwife top-ups are feasible but require that the midwifery staff are educated in the physiology of epidural analgesia and resuscitation. Boluses are usually given when the previous dose of local anesthetic has worn off, and top-up by bolus on demand may result in uneven analgesia, with periods of pain alternating with periods of analgesia. Top-ups on a regular schedule have been tried, but were found to result in greater doses of local anesthetic being administered (Purdie et al 1992).

Continuous infusions of dilute local anesthetics with and without opioids are increasingly used for maintenance. Concentrations of bupivacaine from 0.05% to 0.25% have been used, and provide stable levels of analgesia. The total amount of local anesthetic is reduced by the infusion technique (D'Athis et al 1988), and motor block is also decreased, allowing the mother to push more effectively.

As labour progresses and the end of the first stage is reached, the patient should be placed in a more vertical position to allow the local anesthetic solution to reach the sacral nerve roots to provide analgesia for the distending perineum.

Monitoring   The blood pressure is recorded before starting the epidural. It is then taken every five minutes for 20 minutes, along with the fetal and maternal heart rates. Subsequently blood pressure should be taken every half an hour until delivery.

The sensory level of the block should be tested 15 minutes after the administration of the first dose. The upper and lower sensory limits of the block should be determined and rechecked periodically. Motor block and ease of respiration should be verified from time to time.

Complications   The commonest problem is autonomic blockade which causes vasodilation and hypotension (defined as a 20–30% drop in blood pressure (Glosten 1994)). The patient must be kept in the lateral position. The head should be lowered and the feet elevated, and oxygen given by mask. 500 ml to 1 litre of lactated Ringer's solution should be run rapidly. Ephedrine has been shown to be the vasopressor which least affects the uterine blood flow (Tong et al 1992). The level of the block should be assessed and if found to be high (above T6), the infusion of local anesthetic should be temporarily stopped until the block recedes. If the sympathetic outflow to the heart has been blocked (T1 to T4) it may be necessary to give atropine to treat bradycardia. α-agonists like phenyl-ephrine, metaraminol and methoxamine are best avoided as they cause a severe decrease in the uterine blood flow (Ralston et al 1974).

Fetal bradycardia may be caused by local anesthetic toxicity or maternal hypotension. Fluid should be run rapidly, and the mother turned to the full lateral position. Oxygen must be given by mask and the obstetrician should be informed. The blood pressure should be checked, and if it is below baseline, 5 to 10 mg ephedrine should be given. A vaginal examination might be useful to assess the progress of labour and to find out whether the second stage has been reached. If delivery needs to be expedited, it may be advisable to do a forceps delivery.

A dural tap can occur either at the time of needle insertion or during insertion of the epidural catheter. If the dural tap occurs with the Tuohy needle, the alternatives are either to resite the catheter at another interspace, or to insert a catheter intrathecally and use it to give small boluses of local anesthetic to produce anesthesia. Intrathecal catheters do not increase the risk of post-dural puncture headaches (Norris et al 1990).

Post-dural puncture headache (PDPH) is caused by continued loss of CSF through the breach in the dura, with lowering of intracranial pressure and traction on intracranial vessels. The bigger the rent, the higher the incidence of PDPH: there is a 70% incidence with a 16 gauge needle, and an incidence of 2% with a 25 gauge hole. Post-dural tap headaches are worse when the patient is sitting up and are ameliorated when the patient lies down. The headache is usually fronto-occipital. Tinnitus, photophobia and diplopia may occur. The headache occurs typically 1–2 days after dural puncture, and most headaches last up to a week.

Once a dural tap has been recognised the patient must be informed and options discussed. The resited catheter can be left in the epidural space and 1 to 1.5 litres of saline can be infused into it over 24 hours (Crawford 1972). Some researchers have injected a bolus of 10 to 30 ml of normal saline after delivery and then removed the catheter. Prophylactic blood patches have not been been proven totally effective (Loeser et al 1978). Subsequently, the patient must be seen frequently and explanations and moral support freely given. Bed rest does not decrease the incidence of PDPH, but may aid patient comfort. The patient should be kept well hydrated, and analgesics should be given. Theophylline and caffeine have been known to improve the symptoms (Feuerstein et al 1986; Sechzer et al

1978). Other methods of treatment which have been tried include abdominal binders and the prone position.

An autologous blood patch can be done after 48 to 72 hours and is effective in most patients. The patient should be afebrile and should not be septic. 15 to 20 ml of blood are drawn aseptically from the patient and injected slowly into the epidural space. Some of the blood drawn from the patient at that time can be placed in blood culture bottles for culture in case of post blood patch fever. The most frequent complication of this technique is back pain. Neck and lower radicular pains and a transient temperature rise are other complications.

Missed segments with incomplete analgesia occasionally occur. These could be due to anatomical barriers like connective tissue bands, the presence of air or blood in the epidural space, or malposition or migration of the epidural catheter. Therapeutic options are resiting or withdrawing the epidural catheter slightly, using more concentrated local anesthetic solutions, larger volumes of a weak solution (Glosten 1994), opiates, or the addition of adrenaline.

Total spinal or extremely high spinal block, can occur if a large volume of local anesthetic solution is given unintentionally intrathecally or subdurally. It can also occur if the catheter migrates intrathecally. The patient presents with a very high sensory level, blockade, upper limb weakness, and difficulty in breathing. 100% oxygen should be given with intermittent positive pressure ventilation through a bag and mask. The patient should be intubated with a rapid-sequence induction if there is difficulty in breathing. Fluids should be run rapidly and the patient placed in the Trendelenburg position with a lateral pelvic tilt. Ephedrine and other vasoconstrictors may be necessary.

New techniques   New techniques using low concentrations of bupivacaine (for example, 0.1% or 0.125%) with the addition of opioids may allow the patients to walk during epidural analgesia (Morgan et al 1994). There is an ongoing debate about the mother's ability to ambulate safely during an epidural (Buggy et al 1994).

Patient-controlled epidural analgesia shows promise, both with local anesthetics by themselves or in combination with opioids. This works on the ability of the patient to identify periods of pain and to administer the analgesic herself. A study done in 1992 by Purdie showed high maternal satisfaction with the technique, although the lock-out time resulted in longer painful episodes.

Caudal extradural block

This block is useful in the late first stage and second stage of labour. It provides good relaxation of the perineal muscles. Most caudals are performed as a single injection, but catheter techniques are also possible. Problems include a relatively high forceps rate, attributed to abnormalitites of the rotation of the fetal head due to relaxation of the pelvic floor. Other complications are increased technical difficulty, high local anesthetic dosage if given in the first stage of labour, trauma to the fetal scalp and maternal infection. Doses suitable for caudal extradural analgesia include 12 to 15 ml of 0.25% bupivacaine, 1.0% or 1.5% lignocaine or 2% 2-chloro-procaine (Glosten 1994).

Intrathecal block

Single-shot spinals have limited utility in early labour, as they have to be repeated. This block is more useful in the second stage for low and mid-cavity forceps deliveries, for the performance and repair of episiotomies, for internal or external version and for removal of retained placentas. A block reaching S1 is needed for vaginal delivery or low forceps. Blocks should reach T10 for intrauterine manipulation and removal of retained placentas. It is an easier block than the epidural blockade, has a definite end-point and allows use of lower local anesthetic doses and less local anesthetic toxicity in mother and baby. It also provides good relaxation for the pelvic musculature. Disadvantages cited include post-dural puncture headaches. However the incidence of post-dural puncture headaches is low with the use of pencil-point needles and Quincke needles smaller than 25 gauge (Ross et al 1992).

Intrathecal block can be done in the lateral or sitting position, and should be performed at the L2-3 interspace or below, as the spinal cord terminates at L1-2. Small doses of local anesthetics such as 0.5–2.5 millilitres of 0.25% isobaric bupivacaine or 1 ml of 1% lignocaine may be used (Huckaby et al 1991; McHale et al 1992). Fluids should be given rapidly as the onset of hypotension can be fast. Ephedrine should be given as needed, in boluses of 5–10 mg, and it may be useful to add 50 mg of ephedrine to 500 ml of electrolyte solution (Jouppila et al 1984).

Combined techniques   Double-catheter techniques have been described, with one epidural catheter in the lumbar regions and another inserted through the sacral hiatus (Schnider et al 1987). The lumbar catheter allows segmental block from T10 to L1 for the first stage of labour and the caudal catheter allows perineal analgesia for the second stage. However, the use of this technique has the added hazard of two needle and catheter insertions.

Combined spinal and extradural analgesia via a single puncture is a technique which is becoming more popular. The spinal block provides a rapid onset and dense analgesia, and the epidural catheter provides the means to top up or extend the block if surgical intervention becomes necessary (Carrie 1990, Stacey et al 1993). Analgesia was reported to be better with a combined technique than with extradural anesthesia alone (Rawal et al 1988). The incidence of post-dural puncture headaches was reported to be very low (Brownridge 1987).

Many methods have become available for pain relief in labour. Several factors affect the choice of technique: the mother's awareness and preferences, cultural biases, equipment, staff education and the available medical expertise. In employing any method of analgesia however the dictum 'First of all, do no harm' should always be remembered.

References

Abboud TK, Khoo SS, Miller F et al 1982. Maternal, fetal and neonatal responses after epidural anesthesia with bupivacaine, 2-chloroprocaine or lidocaine. *Anesth Analg* 61:638-44.

Abboud TK, Sarkis F, Blikian A et al 1983. Lack of adverse neonatal neurobehavioural effects of lidocaine. *Anesth Analg* 62:473-5.
Abraham RA et al, April 13 1984. Rationale and effectiveness of 1.5% lignocaine with dextrose

and epinephrine as a routine epidural test dose. (Abs) Annual meeting for the Society of Obstetric Anesthesia and Perinatology, San Antionio, Texas.

Akamatsu TJ, Bonica JJ, Rehmet R 1974. Experiences with the use of ketamine in parturition. *Anesth Analg* 53:284-7.

Albright GA et al 1986. Anesthesia in obstetrics: maternal, fetal and neonatal aspects, 2nd edition, Boston: Butterworths, p 297.

Arulkumaran S, Ingemarsson I, Hamlett JD, et al, Pudendal block 1987. An obstetric procedure that needs critical evaluation. *Asia Oceania J Obstet Gynecol* 13:37-42.

Atkinson RS, Rushman GB, Lee JA 1987. A Synopsis of Anaesthesia, 10th Edition, John Wright & Sons Ltd, p 523.

Atkinson RS, Rushman GB, Lee JA 1987. A Synopsis of Anaesthesia, 10th Edition, John Wright & Sons Ltd, p 680.

Baraka A, Maktabi M, Noueihid R 1982. Epidural meperidine-bupivacaine for obstetric analgesia. *Anesth Analg* 61:652-6.

Bonica JJ 1975. The nature of pain in parturition. *Clin Obstet Gynecol* 2:499.

Brownridge P 1987. Epidural and subarachnoid analgesia for elective caesarean section. *Anesthesia* 36:70.

Brownridge P, Plummer J, Mitchell J, Marshall P 1992. An evaluation of epidural bupivacaine with and without meperidine in labor. *Reg anesth* 17:15-21,

Buggy D, Hughes N, Gardiner J 1994. Posterior column sensory impairment during ambulatory extradural analgesia in labour. *Br J Anaesth* 73:540-2.

Caldwell J, Wakile LA, Notarianni LJ 1978. Maternal and neonatal disposition of pethidine in childbirth. *Life Sci* 22:589-96.

Carrie LES 1990. Extradural, spinal or combined block for obstetric surgical anaesthesia. *Br J Anaesth* 65:225-33.

Chestnut D, Vandewalker G, Owen C et al 1987. The influence of continuous epidural bupivacaine analgesia on the second stage of labour and method of delivery in nulliparous women. *Anesthesiology* 66:774-80.

Chestnut DH 1994. In: Chestnut DH, ed. Obstetric Anesthesia, principles and practice. Mosby, p 420.

Chia YT, Arulkumaran S, Chua S et al 1990. Effectiveness of transcutaneous electric nerve stimulator (TENS) for pain relief in labour. *Asia Oceania J Obstet Gynecol*; 16(2):145-51.

Crawford JS 1972. The prevention of headache consequent upon dural puncture. *Br J Anaesth* 44:598-9.

Crawford JS 1972. Lumbar epidural block in labour: a clinical analysis. *Br J Anaesth* 44:66-74.

D'Athis F, Macheboeuf M, Thomas H et al 1988. Epidural analgesia with a bupivacaine-fentanyl mixture in obstetrics: comparison of repeated injections and continuous infusion. *Can J Anaesth* 35(2):116-22.

Datta S, Hurley RJ, Naulty JS, et al 1986. Plasma and cerebrospinal fluid progesterone concentrations in pregnant and non-pregnant women. *Anesth Analg* 65:950-4.

Datta S, Lambert DH, Gregus J et al 1983. Differentiated sensitivities of mammalian nerve fibres during pregnancy. *Anesth Analg* 62:1070-2.

Dick-Read C 1933. Natural Childbirth, London: Heineman.

Dick-Read C 1944. Childbirth without fear. New York: Harper & Bros.

Feuerstein TJ, Zeides A 1986. Theophylline relieves headache following lumbar puncture. *Klin Woechenschr* 64:216-8.

Gauss CJ 1905. Zentbl Gynak, 274.

Ginsburg J 1971. *Am Rev Pharmacol*, 11:387.

Gissen AJ, Datta S, Lambert D 1984. The chloroprocaine controversy. *Reg Anesth* 9:135-45.

Glosten B 1994. In: Chestnut DH, ed. Obstetric Anesthesia. Mosby, p 354.

Golub MS, Eisele JH, Donald JM 1986. Obstetric analgesia and infant outcome in monkeys. Infant development after intrapartum exposure to meperidine or alfentanil. *Am J Obstet Gynecol* 159:1280-6.

Goodfellow CF, Studd C 1979. The reduction of forceps in primigravidae with epidural analgesia - a controlled trial. *Br J Clin Pract* 33:187-8.

Hodgkinson R, Huff RW, Hayashi RH et al 1979. Double-blind comparison of maternal analgesia and neonatal neurobehaviour following intravenous butorphanol and meperidine. *J Int Med Res* 7:224-30.

Hood DD, Dewan DM, James FM 1986. Maternal and fetal effects of epinephrine in gravid ewes. *Anesthesiology* 64:610-3.

Huckaby T, Gerard K, Scheidlinger J et al 1989. Continuous epidural infusion of alfentanil-bupivacaine vs bupivacaine for labor and delivery. *Anesthesiology* 71:A847.

Huckaby T, Skerman JH, Hurley RJ 1991. Sensory analgesia for vaginal deliveries: a preliminary report of continuous spinal anaesthesia with a 32-gauge catheter. *Reg Anaesth* 16:150-3.

Husemeyer RP 1990. In: Morgan B, ed. Controversies in obstetric anesthesia. London: Edward Arnold, p 30.

Jouppila P, Jouppila R, Barinoff T et al 1984. Placental blood flow during caesarean section performed under spinal blockade. *Br J Anesth* 56:1379-83.

King JC, Sherline DM 1981. Paracervical and pudendal block. *Clin Obstet Gynecol* 24:587-95.

Kotelko DM, Schnider SM, Dailey PA, et al 1984. Bupivacaine induced arrythmias in sheep. *Anesthesiology* 60:10.

Lamaze F 1958 Painless childbirth (Celestin LR, trans). London: Burke.

Leboyer F 1975. Birth without violence. New York: Alfred A Knopf.

Levinson G, Schnider SM 1987. In: Schnider SM, Levinson G, eds. Anesthesia for Obstetrics, 2nd edn. Williams & Wilkins, p 69.

Loeser EA, Hill GE, Bennett GM et al 1978. Time vs success rate for epidural blood patch. *Anesthesiology* 49:147-8.

Maduska AL, Hajghassemali M 1978. A double-blind comparison of butorphanol and meperidine in labour: maternal pain relief and effects on the newborn. *Can J Anaesth* 25:398-404.

McAllister CB 1980. Placental transfer and neonatal effects of diazepam when administered to women just before delivery. *Br J Anaesth* 52:423-7.

McHale S, Mitchell V, Howsam S et al 1992. Continuous subarachnoid infusion of 0.125% bupivacaine for analgesia during labor. *Br J Anaesth* 69:634-6.

Melzack R 1984. The myth of painless childbirth. *Pain.* 19:321-37.

Minnich M 1994. In: Chestnut DH, ed. Obstetric Anaesthesia, principles and practice. Mosby, p 331.

Moore DC, Batra MS 1981. The components of an effective test dose prior to epidural block. *Anesthesiology* 55:693-6.

Morgan B, Kadim MY 1994. Mobile regional anaesthesia in labour. *Br J Obstet Gynecol* 101:839-41.

Morishima HO, Pedersen H, Finster M et al 1983. Is bupivacaine more toxic than lidocaine? *Anesthesiology* 59:A409.

Munson ES, Embro WJ 1977. Enflurane, isoflurane and halothane and isolated human uterine muscle. *Anesthesiology* 46:11-4.

Niv D, Rudick V, Golan A et al 1986. Augmentation of bupivacaine analgesia in labour by epidural morphine. *Obstet Gynecol* 67:206-9.

Norris MC, Leighton BL 1990. Continuous spinal analgesia after unintentional dural puncture in parturients. *Reg Anaesth* 15:285-7.

Phillips G 1987. Epidural sufentanil/bupivacaine combinations for analgesia during labor: effect of varying sufentanil doses. *Anesthesiology* 67:835-8.

Purdie J, Reid J, Thorburn J et al 1992. Continuous extradural analgesia: comparison of midwife top-ups, continuous infusions and patient-controlled administration. *Br J Anaesth* 68:580-4.

Ralston DH, Shnider SM, de Lorimer AA 1974. Effects of equipotent ephedrine, metaraminol, mephentermine and methoxamine on uterine blood flow in the pregnant ewe. *Anesthesiology.* 40:354-70.

Ralston DH 1987. In: Schnider SM, Levinson G, eds. Anesthesia for Obstetrics. Williams & Wilkins, p 53.

Rawal N, Schollin J, Wesstrom G 1988 Epidural versus combined spinal epidural block for caesarean section. *Acta Anaesth Scand* 32:61-6.

Refstad SO, Lindbaek E.1980. Ventilatory depression of the newborn of women receiving pethidine or pentazocine. *Br J Anaesth* 52:265-71.

Ross BK, Chadwick HS, Mancuso JJ et al 1992. Sprotte needle for obstetric anaesthesia: decreased incidence of post-dural puncture headache. *Reg Anaesth* 17:29-33.

Scanlon JW, Brown WJ Jr, Weiss JB et al 1974. Neurobehavioural responses of newborn infants after maternal epidural anesthesia. *Anesthesiology* 40:121-8.

Schnider SM, Wright RG, Levinson G et al 1979. Uterine blood flow and plasma norepinephrine changes during maternal stress in the pregnant ewe. *Anesthesiolog y* 50:524-7.

Schnider SM, Abboud TK, Artal R et al 1983. Maternal catecholamines decrease during labor after lumbar epidural anesthesia. *Am J Obstet Gynecol* 147:13-5.

Schnider SM, Levinson G, Ralston DH 1987. In: Schnider SM, Levinson G, eds. Anesthesia for Obstetrics, 2nd edition. Williams & Wilkins, p 109.

Sechzer PH, Abel L 1978. Post-spinal anesthesia headache treated with caffeine. *Curr Ther Res* 24:307-12.

Stacey RGW, Watt S, Kadim MY et al 1993. Single-space combined spinal extradural technique for analgesia in labour. *Br J Anaesth* 71:499-502.

Swart F, Abboud TK, Zhu J 1991. Desflurane analgesia in obstetrics. *Anesthesiology* 75:A844.

Swayze C, Skerman J, Walker E et al 1991. Efficacy of subarachnoid meperidine for labor analgesia. *Reg Anesth* 16:309-13.

Tong C, Eisenach JC 1992. The vascular mechanism of ephedrine's beneficial effect on uterine perfusion during pregnancy. *Anesthesiology* 76:792-8.

Van Hoosen B 1928. *Anesth Analg Curr Res* 7:151.

Vella L, Francis D, Noulton P et al 1985. Comparison of the antiemetics metoclopramide and promethazine in labour. *Br Med J* 290:1173-5.

Vincenti E, Cervellin A, Mega M et al 1982. Comparative study between patients treated with transcutaneous electric stimulation and controls during labour. *Clin Exp Obstet Gynecol* 9:95-7.

Wakefield ML 1994. In: Chestnut DH, ed. Obstetric Anaesthesia, principles and practice. Mosby, p 341.

Walker JJ, Johnston J, Fairlie FM 1988. The transfer of ketorolac tromethamine from maternal to fetal blood. *Eur J Clin Pharmacol* 34:509-11.

Way WL, Costley EC, Way EL 1965. Respiratory sensitivity of the newborn infant to meperidine and morphine. *Clin Pharm Ther* 6:454-61.

Wilson CM, McClean E, Moore et al 1986. A double-blind comparison of intramuscular pethidine and nalbuphine in labour. *Anaesthesia* 41:1207-13.

4

Intrapartum Fetal Monitoring

A Biswas
C Anandakumar

'Monitoring' or surveillance during labour has three main components : monitoring the mother, monitoring the fetus and monitoring the progress of labour. The aim of monitoring the fetus during labour is to identify fetal problems which, if uncorrected, could lead to death or short or long-term morbidity in the neonate. During labour, a fetus could become unwell due to hypoxia, infection or trauma, of which hypoxia is the most common.

Pathophysiological basis

The oxygen supply to the fetus depends principally on the adequacy of uterine perfusion, placental gas transfer and fetal circulation. The oxygen tension in the umbilical venous blood returning from the placenta however remains lower than that in the uterine venous blood. Despite this relatively low oxygen tension, fetal tissue oxygenation is usually more than adequate for two main reasons. Firstly, the hemoglobin concentration in the fetus is higher than in adults and fetal hemoglobin has a higher affinity for oxygen. Secondly, at the tissue level, fetal hemoglobin delivers more oxygen than is usually required. These physiological advantages make the fetus relatively resistant to mild–moderate hypoxia. However when the decrease in umbilical venous oxygen tension becomes severe, fetal tissue requirements for aerobic metabolism exceed the oxygen supply and fetal tissue hypoxia occurs. The fetus switches to anerobic metabolism, leading to an accumulation of lactic acid and a consequent fall in tissue and blood pH.

During labour, fetal hypoxia may develop in a number of ways affecting intervillous space perfusion, placental oxygen transfer or umbilical blood flow. Chronic reduction in uteroplacental perfusion, as is seen in intrauterine growth retardation, could be worsened by reduced intervillous perfusion during repeated uterine contractions or maternal hypotension. Acute fetal hypoxia could result from the cessation of intervillous flow due to uterine hyperstimulation, from the disruption of placental oxygen transfer due to placental abruption or uterine scar rupture, or acute interference with umbilical blood flow as in cord prolapse.

The fetal response to hypoxia depends on the acuteness of onset and its severity and duration. The initial fetal response to gradually developing hypoxia is an attempt to increase and redistribute cardiac output to vital organs like the brain and the heart. The increase in cardiac output is brought about by an increase in the fetal heart rate. This may be followed by a decrease or loss of variability and an absence of accelerations due to hypoxia of the brainstem centres. With worsening oxygen supply, hypoxic depression of the myocardium occurs. The placenta of the fetus acts like the lung and interruption of the circulation on the maternal side presents with late decelerations while on the fetal side, by way of cord compression, it presents with variable decelerations. The fetal response in an individual case is modified by the compensatory mechanisms which depend upon the reserve capacity of the fetoplacental unit. However when the hypoxia is acute, the initial reflex response is a decrease in fetal heart rate (FHR), manifesting as prolonged brady-cardia or recurrent decelerations, caused initially by chemoreceptor mediated vagal stimulation, and subsequently by hypoxic myocardial depression. These changes in FHR form the basis of fetal heart monitoring as the most common method of monitoring the intrapartum welfare of the fetus.

With poor placental transfer of gases, carbon dioxide accumulates in the fetus, resulting in respiratory acidosis. The base deficit remains normal or only slightly increased. This form of acidosis is easily reversed if the carbon dioxide is eliminated (Ingemarsson and Arulkumaran 1986). However further prolongation of fetal hy-poxia leads to anerobic glycolysis and consequently, metabolic acidosis. This results in a further fall in pH and a rise in base deficit. Metabolic acidosis cannot be reversed until oxygen delivery to the fetal tissues is reestablished. Hence, when FHR monitoring suggests fetal hypoxia, biochemical monitoring of the fetal acid-base status improves the diagnostic accuracy of fetal heart monitoring.

METHODOLOGY

1. **Fetal heart monitoring**
Since the introduction of fetal heart auscultation in the early 19th century by Evory Kennedy of Rotunda Hospital, Dublin, the estimation of the FHR has evolved considerably and become the mainstay of intrapartum fetal monitoring. Prior to the introduction of electronic FHR monitors, intermittent auscultation was the usual method of fetal monitoring in labour. It is still in common use in many developing countries. Although there is no published standard technique of auscultation, the majority view is that the FHR should be counted over 15 sec (preferably for 1 min) every 15–30 min, immediately following a contraction. Continuous electronic fetal heart rate monitoring (EFM) was introduced in the late 1960s and since then has attained wide acceptance in clinical obstetrics. Although a number of different tech-niques can be used to obtain a continuous record of FHR and uterine contractions, in practice, only two methods are utilised for each. Electronic fetal monitors measure the FHR and uterine contractions either by means of external transducers using the Doppler ultrasound and a strain gauge, or by means of internal sensors using a fetal electrode and an intrauterine catheter respectively. Internal monitoring of FHR re-quires direct contact of the electrode with the fetus, and hence can only be performed after the membranes are ruptured.

Although electronic fetal monitors produce reliable recordings of FHR, the problem of FHR monitoring is in the interpretation of the tracings. During the interpretation of FHR recording, a systematic approach should be used to assess the following four aspects of FHR :

a. *Baseline rate*   This is derived from a line passing through the saw-toothed fluctuations of the trace. The normal baseline rate at term is between 110 and 150 beats/minute (FIGO guidelines, 1987).

b. *Baseline variability*   This is assessed from the band-width or amplitude of the fluctuations of the FHR, measured by the difference between two lines drawn through the highest and lowest point of the trace in any one-minute segment. Normal variability is between 10 and 25 beats/min. When the variability is < 5 beats/min, 5–10 beats/min or > 25 beats/min, it is described as absent, reduced or increased respectively.

c. *Presence of accelerations*   Accelerations are sporadic rise in FHR of > 15 beats/min from the baseline, lasting for 15 sec or more. A normal 'reactive' trace should have at least two accelerations within a 20 min observation window.

d. *Presence of decelerations and their type and severity*   Decelerations are drops in FHR by > 15 beats/min from the baseline lasting for > 15 sec. They can be further classified as :

    i.   early decelerations : These coincide with contraction, with a gradual decline and recovery, mirroring the contraction. The drop is usually < 40 beats/min and it is believed to be secondary to head compression and not a result of hypoxia. Therefore early decelerations in the early first stage of labour, when the head is not deeply in the pelvis may denote other possibilities like variants of variable decelerations.

    ii   variable decelerations : These decelerations vary in occurrence in relation to contractions, and also vary in shape and size. They show a precipitous fall and rise. They are described as severe when the drop is > 60 beats/min and lasts > 60 sec. Variable decelerations are usually secondary to cord compression.

    iii.   late decelerations : These have a delay of > 15 sec between the nadir of the deceleration and to the peak of contraction. Both the decline and recovery of the FHR have a gradual slope. It usually represents transient fetal hypoxia during contraction due to reduction of retroplacental perfusion.

A normal FHR trace is one with a baseline rate between 110 and 150 beats/min showing good variability (between 10 and 25 beats/min) with accelerations and no decelerations (Table 1). In the presence of a normal FHR trace there is only a 2% chance for the fetus to be acidotic (pH < 7.20) and a 1% chance for it to have a 5 min Apgar score of < 7 (Beard et al 1971; Steer et al 1989). A definitely 'ominous' or 'pathological' FHR trace is one with a baseline tachycardia (>150 beats/min) with absent variability and repetitive late or variable decelerations. Other sinister patterns are prolonged severe bradycardia (< 80 beats/min) for >10 min or a sinusoidal pattern without accelerations. While a definitely pathological pattern is seen very rarely, in only 40–60% of labours does the FHR remain unequivocally normal throughout labour (Ingemarsson et al 1980; Steer et al 1989). The presence of an abnormality in any one of the four aspects of FHR is usually labelled as a 'suspicious' pattern in the absence of accelerations. The significance of these suspicious patterns are more difficult to judge without further evaluation. If more than two features are abnormal the trace is termed 'abnormal'. In general, the more the four basic aspects of FHR are abnormal, the more the likelihood of the fetus to be acidotic (Table 1).

Table 1:   Classification of intrapartum CTG

1.   *Normal/Reassuring*

Baseline heart rate 110–150 bpm
Baseline variability 5–25 bpm
Presence of accelerations of at least > 15 bpm lasting > 15 sec
Absence of decelerations

2.   *Suspicious/Equivocal*

Absence of accelerations for > 40 min
Baseline heart rate 150–170 bpm or 100–110 bpm
Absent baseline variability (< 5) for > 40 min, with normal baseline
    and no decelerations
Variable decelerations < 60 bpm for < 60 sec
Transient prolonged bradycardia < 80 bpm for > 2 min or
    < 100 bpm for > 3 min

3.   *Pathological/Ominous*

Baseline FHR > 150 bpm with absent variability and/or repetitive
    late or variable decelerations
Absent baseline variability (< 5) for > 90 min
Complicated variable decelerations (> 60 bpm lasting > 60 sec)
Repetitive late decelerations
Prolonged bradycardia (< 80 bpm for > 10 min)
Sinusoidal pattern with no accelerations

As subacute hypoxia develops during labour, the following FHR changes gradually develop: 1) absence of accelerations 2) gradual increase in baseline heart rate and 3) reduction in baseline variability. The presence of decelerations in the trace indicates the causative mechanism of hypoxia. While variable decelerations suggest cord compression, late decelerations indicate inadequate placental gas exchange. Many an error in the interpretation of the FHR is caused by an undue reliance on the presence or absence of decelerations and consequent disregard for the other three aspects of the FHR pattern. However during the interpretation of a suspicious FHR trace, due consideration should be given to the normal physiological 'sleep-activity cycle' of the fetus. A healthy fetus has alternating phases of quiet sleep with reduced baseline variability and absent accelerations, and phases of activity with high variability. During labour these phases could be as long as 20–40 minutes (Spencer and Johnson 1986) and a FHR trace seen during the quiet phase may be mistaken to be abnormal. In the absence of other complicating features like decelerations or thick meconium, such FHR traces should be observed for up to 60 minutes for a spontaneous reversal to the active phase. In doubtful cases, the fetus could be stimulated or aroused using an acoustic stimulation to elicit a normal response of acceleration and good baseline variability (Ingemarsson and Arulkumaran 1989). Even in the presence of a suspicious or abnormal trace, FHR accelerations evoked by external stimulation are indicative of a non-acidotic fetus (Arulkumaran et al 1987; Ingemarsson and Arulkumaran 1989).

Predictive value of abnormal CTG in labour

Using a low 5 minute Apgar score as end point (Apgar < 7), abnormal intrapartum FHR has a high negative predictive value of over 90%, but a low positive predictive value of about 30% (Grant 1989). This means that a normal trace indicates a fetus that is not hypoxic, while an abnormal trace is associated with a large number of false positives. There are a number of reasons for this low positive predictive value: a) Variable definitions of abnormal traces have been used and the diagnosis of an abnormal FHR trace is usually a 'mixed bag' including both suspicious traces and ominous traces. As mentioned earlier, the association with fetal hypoxia depends on the degree of FHR abnormality. b) The positive predictive value of any test is dependent on the prevalence of the abnormal condition. The positive predictive value is greater in 'high risk' cases (Beard et al 1971), but considerably lower when applied to all cases (Curzen et al 1984). The positive predictive value has been shown to have fallen with the decrease in prevalence due to a lower overall risk in the population of labours monitored. c) A fetus 'stressed' by hypoxia does not necessarily become 'distressed' at birth (Fig 4.1). The condition of the baby at birth depends on its reserves to tolerate hypoxia, as well as on the degree and duration of hypoxia (Fysh et al 1982). Whatever the reason for the low positive predictive value, it is obvious that a clear differentiation between significant and non-significant CTG changes in labour continues to pose great difficulties (Murphy et al 1990). If management is guided by abnormal FHR traces alone, it leads to unduly high instrumental and operative delivery rates for non-compromised infants. To reduce the number of false positives and consequently unnecessary caesarean sections, fetal scalp blood pH estimation is recommended for cases with suspicious FHR traces in labour (FIGO guidelines, 1987).

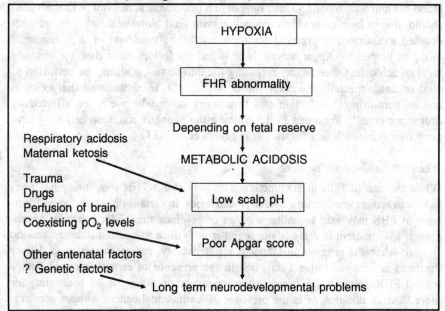

Fig 4.1 The relationship between hypoxia, intrapartum fetal monitoring and neonatal outcome.

2. **Fetal scalp blood pH estimation**

Fetal scalp blood sampling (FBS) for the estimation of pH was introduced by Saling in the 1960s before the introduction of EFM in clinical practice. When the FHR trace is normal the chance of fetal acidosis is extremely rare (Ingemarsson 1981), while abnormal FHR changes are not always associated with acidosis. Hence, in all cases of suspicious FHR trace in labour, FBS to detect acidosis (pH < 7.20) is recommended. Even in the presence of an ominous FHR pattern of tachycardia, reduced baseline variability and decelerations, only 50–60% of the fetuses are acidotic (Beard et al 1971). The reason for this discrepancy is because different fetuses have different capacities to withstand hypoxia and depends on the duration of the hypoxic insult. Hence, a single record of normal scalp blood pH does not guarantee fetal health. In the presence of a continuing abnormal FHR trace, the FBS should be repeated in 30 minutes. A downward trend suggests deteriorating fetal oxygenation and requires further evaluation, while an abnormal value indicates delivery.

Considering a low (< 7) 5 min Apgar score as an end point, the FBS has a high negative predictive value, but only a modest positive predictive value. Sykes et al (1982) in a study from Oxford, UK, showed that only 1 in 5 babies with 5 min Apgar < 7 had severe acidosis (pH < 7.1). Similarly, only 1 in 7 babies with a severe acidosis had 5 min Apgar < 7, confirming that hypoxemia and acidosis are only one of the several causes of low Apgar scores at birth (Fig 4.1). These false positive low pH (< 7.20) arise from situations where for example, a fetal respiratory acidosis develops secondary to uterine hypertonus or maternal hypotension, or when a metabolic acidosis in fetus occurs secondary to maternal ketosis (Roversi et al 1975). This has led some researchers to suggest that maternal venous blood pH and fetal blood CO_2 and base deficit (metabolic acidosis if > 13 mMol/lit) should always be measured in conjunction with fetal blood pH. Not only are such detailed evaluations impractical for routine use, the condition of the neonate at birth, as judged by Apgar scores, is modified by factors other than the absolute level of acidosis. Other factors including the duration of acidosis, the perfusion of vital organs, especially the brain, the coexisting pO_2 level, trauma (such as intracranial hemorrhage), infection and respiratory drive which may be affected by drugs, are equally important in determining the neonatal condition and long term prognosis (Chiswick and James 1979; Myers et al 1981).

When FBS should not be done

While the use of FBS in conjunction with continuous FHR monitoring has been shown to reduce unnecessary operative deliveries, in certain situations the performance of FBS may lead to undue wastage of precious time. When there is an abnormal FHR pattern in early labour together with thick meconium stained amniotic fluid or when the progress of labour is unsatisfactory, caesarean section to deliver the fetus is required rather than FBS. In the presence of certain forms of pathological FHR patterns, for example, prolonged bradycardia (< 80 beats/min) for more than 10 minutes, or in the presence of a sinusoidal pattern without accelerations, FBS will lead to unnecessary delay in delivery. Similarly, in the presence of ominous FHR patterns in the second stage of labour, where instrumental vaginal delivery can be easily accomplished, fetal scalp blood pH estimation by FBS is not indicated. FBS can increase the sensitivity of continuous FHR monitoring, if it is performed for a trace which on its own would not be considered to warrant immediate delivery.

The technique of FBS has changed little since it was first described, and remains somewhat cumbersome and time-consuming. Important as FBS undoubtedly is, it requires the immediate availability of laboratory support, and may need frequent repetition of an uncomfortable procedure. The expertise and facilities required are not available in many centres, even in the developed countries. This has led to the development of simpler fetal stimulation tests to evaluate suspicious FHR traces.

3. Intrapartum fetal stimulation tests

a. *Fetal scalp stimulation test*

Clark et al (1982) were the first to observe that FHR acceleration sometimes coincided with FBS and that the scalp blood pH tended to be normal if an acceleration occurred. This led to the development of the scalp stimulation test, in which the fetal scalp is stimulated by pinching with a tissue forceps, while the CTG is observed for an acceleration (Clark et al 1984; Arulkumaran et al 1987). If an acceleration is observed, it is highly unlikely for the scalp blood pH to be < 7.20. Of the fetuses which fail to respond, about 45% would have a pH estimation below 7.20 and only 5% would have a scalp pH > 7.25. Absence of acceleration in non-acidaemic fetuses may be related to the use of analgesia (Spencer 1991).

b. *Fetal acoustic stimulation test (FAST)*

Similar to the scalp stimulation test, sound stimulation with an artificial electronic larynx placed near the region of the fetal head results in an acceleration of FHR of most non-acidotic fetuses (Smith et al 1986). About 50% of fetuses which fail to respond with an acceleration would have a scalp pH of < 7.20. Thus the FAST has a predictive value similar to the scalp stimulation test, while it is far less invasive and carries no chance of introducing any infection (Ingemarsson and Arulkumaran 1989).

From the studies available it appears that both the scalp stimulation test and FAST can be used as useful adjuncts to continuous FHR monitoring in identifying the non-acidotic fetus, thus reducing the need for FBS. Further evaluation of non-responders by FBS would still be necessary. However these stimulation tests would be especially useful in centres with limited or no facility for FBS and help in the reduction of unnecessary operative deliveries.

Choice of cases for monitoring

Every fetus has a potential risk of intrapartum hypoxia or birth injury and an optimal outcome can be concluded only at the end of labour or occasionally, much later. Therefore every fetus deserves intrapartum monitoring. However intrapartum monitoring does not necessarily mean electronic fetal monitoring. Most patients with uncomplicated low risk pregnancies do not need EFM, and may be effectively monitored by the traditional method of intermittent auscultation of the fetal heart. From a purely 'theoretical' standpoint, a graphical record of FHR obtained during intrapartum EFM has a number of advantages over intermittent auscultation. Undoubtedly continuous EFM provides more information regarding the FHR than intermittent auscultation with a fetal stethoscope. Listening to the fetal heart for a minute every 15 minutes samples the FHR for only about 7% of the total time in labour. In addition, it provides very little information about the relationship between FHR changes and uterine contractions, or about FHR variability. However more information is not necessarily more instructive. The question is whether this increased information generated from continuous EFM during labour leads to any improvement in outcome.

The value of continuous fetal heart rate monitoring in labour in low risk gravidas remains unproven. When the results of nine prospective randomised controlled trials of the use of continuous FHR monitoring in labour were pooled for systematic meta-analysis, the results showed that continuous EFM caused higher rates of medical intervention: both caesarean section and instrumental vaginal delivery, without any accompanying decrease in perinatal mortality (Shy et al 1990). When compared with intermittent auscultation alone continuous FHR monitoring doubled rates of caesarean section for 'fetal distress' even when it was complemented by selective fetal blood sampling (FBS) and pH estimation; the rate was quadrupled when EFM was used alone (Neilson 1993). Although in the largest randomised trial involving nearly 13,000 women, carried out in Dublin, a 55% decline in the incidence of neonatal convulsions was noted in the group who had EFM, further stratified analysis showed that the reduction in neonatal convulsion occurred very largely in those women whose labours had lasted more than 5 hours (MacDonald et al 1985). This suggests that regular intermittent auscultation is sufficient and is an acceptable form of monitoring in low risk mothers who progress to delivery within five hours. Continuous FHR monitoring is more appropriate in more complicated labours, such as those that are prolonged, augmented or induced, multiple pregnancies, those with thick meconium stained amniotic fluid, and those with a known or suspected growth-retarded or preterm fetus (Table 2).

For the proper allocation of available resources, CTG machines and manpower, it is important to identify the mother who is genuinely 'low risk' for the development of intrapartum hypoxia. However risk assessment or scoring systems based on the antenatal history and clinical examination of the mother are not very satisfactory in this respect. Intrapartum fetal hypoxia usually reflects fetal compromise antedating the onset of labour. Hence some form of risk assessment at the beginning of labour or an 'admission test' should, in principle, allow one to choose the type of intrapartum fetal monitoring in a given case.

The admission test (AT)

For patients who are considered as low risk, a short 15–20 minutes external EFM on admission in labour has been suggested as a screening 'admission test' (Ingemarsson et al 1986). If no FHR changes are observed with early labour contractions and the trace is normal and reactive, the chances of fetal hypoxia due to causes other than acute events are unlikely in the next few hours of labour. In a study of over 1,000 low risk women conducted in Singapore, 40% of women with an ominous AT developed fetal distress, compared to 1.4% in those with a

Table 2: Indications for electronic fetal monitoring

A. *Risk arising from maternal medical problems*

1. Hypertension
2. Diabetes
3. Renal diseases
4. Collagen diseases
5. Severe anaemia and hemoglobinopathies
6. Cyanotic heart disease
7. Hyperthyroidism

B. *Risk arising from problems of the fetus*

1. Intrauterine growth retardation
2. Post-term
3. Preterm
4. Oligohydramnios
5. Multiple pregnancy
6. Breech presentation
7. Rhesus isoimmunisation

C. *Risk arising from problems of labour*

1. Induced labour
2. Augmented labour
3. Prolonged labour
4. Prolonged rupture of membranes
5. Previous caesarean section
6. Regional analgesia
7. Antepartum or intrapartum vaginal bleeding
8. Intrauterine infection

D. *Suspected fetal distress in labour*

1. Meconium stained amniotic fluid
2. Abnormal/suspicious 'Admission test'
3. Suspicious FHR on auscultation

reactive AT (Ingemarsson et al 1986). Thus AT helps to identify a subgroup of fetuses who would benefit from more intensive monitoring, while others can be monitored with intermittent auscultation.

In a small subgroup of patients, AT – so called suspicious test – cannot be regarded as unequivocally pathological. The fetal acoustic stimulation (FAST) to provoke accelerations can be used to evaluate these equivocal ATs. The minority with an abnormal AT with FAST are at high risk of developing fetal distress (Ingemarsson et al 1988). The FAST appears to have a better discriminatory power than AT, since when it had been abnormal even in presence of a reactive AT the incidence of fetal distress was 14.2%, compared with a 6.1% incidence of fetal distress when FAST was normal with an equivocal or abnormal AT (Ingemarsson et al 1988).

Significance of meconium staining of amniotic fluid

The presence of fresh meconium in the amniotic fluid has been 'traditionally' regarded as a sign of fetal hypoxia. The passage of meconium is associated with an increased risk of intrapartum stillbirth, neonatal morbidity of various degrees and neonatal death. Thick meconium recognised at the onset of labour with decreased amniotic fluid volume carries the worst prognosis and is associated with a five- to seven-fold increased risk of perinatal death. The first objective study associating meconium passage during labour and fetal hypoxia was that done by Walker (1954), where he found that meconium passage, especially thick meconium, was associated with a low umbilical venous pO_2. In the presence of an abnormal FHR pattern, the presence of meconium is associated with a higher chance of the baby being acidotic and asphyxiated at birth*(Miller et al 1975; Steer et al 1989). However it has been shown in a number of studies that when the FHR pattern was normal, there was no difference in scalp and cord blood pH or neonatal outcome between fetuses who had or had not passed meconium (Miller et al 1975; Shaw and Clark 1988; Baker et al 1992).

Meconium is present in the amniotic fluid in 10–15% of all deliveries (Katz and Bowes 1992). In 5% of these cases meconium is aspirated i.e., present below the vocal cords, and may lead to meconium aspiration syndrome (MAS) which is the principal cause of neonatal morbidity and mortality from the presence of meconium. Although there is no objective proof that meconium passage occurs secondary to hypoxia, it appears that meconium aspiration is principally an intra-uterine event caused by fetal hypoxia and gasping (Katz and Bowes 1992). Meconium inhaled by the fetus with normal acid base status and meconium inhaled at delivery are relatively benign in the absence of hypoxia (Danielian 1994). Fetuses with light or moderate meconium staining have a better prognosis than those with thick meconium stained amniotic fluid (Arulkumaran et al 1985).

Thus, although the cause and effect relationship between hypoxia and meconium passage seems tenuous, there is no doubt that the presence of meconium in liquor, especially thick meconium, is associated with increased perinatal risk. The risk is further compounded when FHR abnormalities are present during labour. Hence, the assessment of the amniotic fluid during labour continues to be an important clinical component of intrapartum fetal monitoring.

Newer approaches to intrapartum monitoring

As the deficiencies of FHR monitoring and of FBS and pH measurement have become apparent, other techniques of monitoring the fetus have emerged. Fetal electrocardiography, scalp blood lactate estimation and continuous biochemical monitoring are some of the methods which are currently under investigation.

Until recently, the problems of background electrical noise and signal distortion made the study of the components of fetal ECG waveform difficult. With recent technical improvements, it is now possible to obtain a representative fetal ECG signal using the fetal scalp electrode. There is renewed interest in fetal ECG waveform analysis in the hope that it will improve the specificity of detecting intrapartum fetal hypoxia when there is an abnormal fetal heart rate pattern. Two portions of the fetal ECG are potentially useful: the ST waveform (T/QRS ratio) and the PR interval correlated with the RR interval. Animal experiments suggest that changes in the ST waveform, and an increase in the T wave amplitude in particular, reflect myocardial anerobic metabolism. Clinical studies have shown poor correlation between the T wave changes and fetal heart rate changes. There is also concern that the sensitivity of the ST waveform changes for fetal acidemia may be poor. More information is required before its use is incorporated into routine clinical practice (Loh and Arulkumaran 1993). A recent randomised trial from Plymouth concluded that the addition of ECG waveform analysis to continuous FHR monitoring could halve the rate of operative deliveries for fetal distress (Westgate et al 1992).

The measurement of scalp blood lactate has a number of advantages over FBS and pH estimation. Firstly, the measurement of lactate is not affected by CO_2 levels and therefore by respiratory acidosis. Secondly, there is strong evidence that it is the level of lactic acid, rather than the pH per se which, in conjunction with cerebral perfusion levels, governs the risk of long term neurological damage (Myers et al 1981). In spite of these advantages, very few studies were done with fetal scalp blood lactate levels primarily because the available techniques for lactate estimation were time consuming and required rather large amounts of blood. A dry reagent strip method which requires only 20 µl of blood and needs about 1 min to perform is being currently evaluated in clinical studies (Nordstrom et al 1992; Nordstrom and Arulkumaran 1994).

Methods for continuous measurement of pH, pO_2 and pCO_2 have been under development for more than ten years. None of them is yet sufficiently reliable or practical for use in routine practice. Techniques for the measurement of the absorption spectra of both visible range (using pulse oximetry) and near infra-red range (using near infra-red spectroscopy, NIRS) light reflected from the fetal scalp, are currently being investigated as a means of detecting changes in the degree of oxygen saturation (SaO_2) of hemoglobin and of cytochrome oxidase aa3 in scalp tissue (Doyle 1994; Johnson et al, 1994). Recent developments in reflectance pulse oximetry techniques which utilise a specially designed probe sited on the fetal cheek and held in place by the uterine wall seems promising. However the clinical usefulness of these newer techniques remains to be determined in large randomised studies.

The use of continuous FHR monitoring has been associated temporally with a great reduction in the incidence of unexpected intrapartum stillbirths. In a recent study from Singapore, comparing perinatal mortality between 1982 and a seven-year period between 1986–1992, it was shown that a marked reduction in overall perinatal mortality was accompanied by a significant decline of deaths due to intrapartum hypoxia. While in 1982, intrapartum hypoxia was responsible for 14.5% of perinatal deaths, during 1986–1992 it was the cause in only 7.9% (Biswas et al 1995). Similar falls in perinatal mortality after the introduction of EFM have been reported by others (Edington et al 1975; Parer 1979). However the extent to which the improvement could be attributed to the monitoring itself is difficult to define.

The consensus view among obstetricians is that EFM is the method of choice in high risk pregnancies, but routine EFM in low risk cases remains controversial. Regular intermittent auscultation may be sufficient in low risk mothers who have a normal 'admission test' and who progress to delivery within five hours. Evidence from the randomised comparisons of different methods of fetal heart rate monitoring suggests that in short, low risk labours perinatal death and morbidity are equally effectively prevented by either intermittent auscultation or continuous EFM, provided that importance is attached to the prompt recognition of intrapartum FHR abnormalities, whatever the monitoring policy adopted. Improvements in the results of monitoring will be effected not only by better identification and interpretation of abnormalities in FHR patterns but also through better responses by attendants to unusual patterns. Clearly, the available techniques of intrapartum monitoring have limitations, and hence the search for better techniques of fetal assessment during labour continues.

References

Arulkumaran S, Yeoh SC, Gibb DFM, Ratnam SS 1985. Obstetric outcome of meconium stained liquor in labour. *Sing Med J.* 14:47-51.

Arulkumaran S, Ingemarsson I, Ratnam SS 1987. Fetal heart response to scalp stimulation as a test for fetal wellbeing in labour. *Asia Oceania J Obstet Gynecol* 13:131-135.

Baker N, Kilby MD, Murray H 1992. An assessment of the use of meconium alone as an indication for fetal blood sampling. *Obstet Gynecol* 80:792-796.

Beard RW, Filshie GM, Knight CA, Roberts GM 1971. The significance of changes in continuous fetal heart rate in the first stage of labour. *J Obstet Gynecol Br Cwlth.* 78:865-881.

Biswas A, Chew S, Joseph R, Arulkumaran S, Anandakumar C, Ratnam SS 1995. Towards improved perinatal care — Perinatal audit. *Ann Acad Med Singapore.* 24:211-217.

Chiswick ML, James DK 1979. Kielland's forceps — association with neonatal morbidity and mortality. *Br Med J.* i:7-9.

Clark SL, Gimovsky ML, Miller FC 1982. Fetal heart rate response to scalp blood sampling. *Am J Obstet Gynecol* 144:706-708.

Clark SL, Gimovsky ML, Miller FC 1984. The scalp stimulation test: A clinical alternative to fetal blood sampling. *Am J Obstet Gynecol* 148:274-277.

Curzen P, Bekir JS, McLintock DG, Patel M 1984. Reliability of cardiotocography in predicting baby's condition at birth. *Br Med J* 289:1345-1347.

Danielian PJ 1994. The significance of meconium in the amniotic fluid. *Contemp Rev Obstet Gynecol* 6:129-132.

Doyle M 1994. Near infra red spectroscopy used for intrapartum fetal surveillance [editorial]. *J R Soc Med.* 87:315-316.

Edington PT, Sibanda J, Beard RW 1975. Influence on clinical practice of routine intrapartum fetal monitoring. *Br Med J.* iii:341-343.

FIGO 1987. Guidelines for the use of fetal monitoring. *Int J Gynecol Obstet* 25:159-167.

Fysh WJ, Turner GM, Dunn PM 1982. Neurological abnormality after extreme birth asphyxia. *Br J Obstet Gynecol* 89:24-26.

Grant A 1989. Monitoring the fetus during labour. In: Chalmers I, Enkine M, Keirse MJNC, eds: Effective care in pregnancy and childbirth. Oxford: Oxford University Press, pp 846-882.

Ingemarsson E, Ingemarsson I, Solum T, Westgren M 1980. Influence of occipito posterior position on fetal heart rate pattern. *Obstet Gynecol* 155:301-305.

Ingemarsson E 1981. Routine electronic fetal monitoring during labor. *Acta Obstet Gynecol Scand (Suppl).* 99:1-29.

Ingemarsson I, Arulkumaran S 1986. Fetal acid base balance in low risk patients in labor. *Am J Obstet Gynecol* 155:66-69.

Ingemarsson I, Arulkumaran S, Ingemarsson E, Tambyraja RL, Ratnam SS 1986. Admission test : A screening test for fetal distress in labor. *Obstet Gynecol* 68:800-806.

Ingemarsson I, Arulkumaran S, Paul RH, Ingemarsson E, Tambyraja RL, Ratnam SS 1988. Fetal acoustic stimulation in early labour in patients screened with the admission test. *Am J Obstet Gynecol* 158:70-74.

Ingemarsson I, Arulkumaran S 1989. Reactive FHR response to sound stimulation in fetuses with low scalp blood pH. *Br J Obstet Gynecol* 96:562-565.

Johnson N, Johnson VA, McNamara H, Montague IA, Jongsma HW, Aumeerally Z, et al 1994. Fetal pulse oximetry: a new method of monitoring the fetus. *Aust NZ J Obstet Gynecol* 34:428-32.

Katz VL, Bowes WA 1992. Meconium aspiration syndrome : reflections on a murky subject. *Am J Obstet Gynecol* 166:171-183.

Loh FH, Arulkumaran S 1993. ECG waveform analysis in intrapartum fetal monitoring. *Aust NZ J Obstet Gynecol* 33:39-44.

MacDonald D, Grant A, Sheridan-Pereira M, Boylan P, Chalmers I 1985. The Dublin randomised trial of intrapartum fetal monitoring. *Am J Obstet Gynecol* 152:524-539.

Miller FC, Sacks DA, Yeh S, Paul RH, Schifrin BS, Martin CB, et al 1975. Significance of meconium during labor. *Am J Obstet Gynecol* 122:573-580.

Murphy KW, Johnson P, Moorcraft J, Pattinson R, Russel V, Turnbull A 1990. Birth asphyxia and the intrapartum cardiotocograph. *Br J Obstet Gynecol* 97:470-479.

Myers RE, Wagner KR, de Courten G 1981. Lactic acid accumulation in tissue as cause of brain injury and death in cardiogenic shock from asphyxia. In: Laursen NH, Hochberg HM, eds. Clinical perinatal biochemical monitoring. Baltimore: Williams & Wilkins, pp 11-34.

Neilson JP 1993. Cardiotocography in labour— An unsatisfactory technique but nothing better yet (editorial). *Br Med J* 306:347-348.

Nordstrom L, Persson B, Shimojo N, Westgren, M 1992. Fetal scalp and umbilical artery blood lactate measured with a new test strip method. *Br J Obstet Gynecol* 99:307-309.

Nordstrom L, Arulkumaran S 1994. Lactate in fetal surveillance. *Sing J Obstet Gynecol* 24: 87-98.

Parer JT 1979. Fetal heart-rate monitoring. *Lancet.* ii: 632-633.

Roversi GD, Canussio V, Spennacchio M 1975. Recognition and significance of maternogenic fetal acidosis during intensive monitoring of labour. *J Perinat Med* 3:53-67.

Shaw K, Clark SL 1988. Reliability of intrapartum fetal heart rate monitoring of the post-term fetus with meconium passage. *Obstet Gynecol* 72:886-889.

Shy KK, Luthy DA, Bennett FC, Whitfield M, Larson EB, van Belle G, et al 1990. Effect of electronic fetal heart rate monitoring, as compared with periodic auscultation, on the neurologic development of premature infants. *New Engl J Med* 322:588-593.

Smith CV, Nguyen HN, Phelan JP, Paul RH 1986. Intrapartum assessment of fetal wellbeing: A comparison of fetal acoustic stimulation with acid-base determinations. *Am J Obstet Gynecol* 155:726-728.

Spencer JAD, Johnson P 1986. Fetal heart rate variability changes and fetal behavioural cycles during labour. *Br J Obstet Gynecol* 93:314-321.

Spencer JAD 1991. Predictive value of a fetal heart rate acceleration at the time of fetal blood sampling in labour. *J Perinat Med* 19:207-215.

Steer PJ, Eigbe FE, Lissauer TJ, Beard RW 1989. Interrelationships among abnormal cardiotocograms in labor, meconium staining of the amniotic fluid, arterial cord blood pH, and Apgar scores. *Obstet Gynecol* 74:715-721.

Steer PJ, Danielian PJ 1993. Fetal distress in labor. In: James DK, Steer PJ, Weiner CP, Gonik B, eds. High risk pregnancy - Management options. London: WB Saunders, pp 1077-1100.

Sykes GS, Molloy PM, Johnson P, Gu W, Ashworth F, Stirrat GM, et al 1982. Do Apgar scores indicate asphyxia? *Lancet.* i:494-496.

Westgate J, Harris M, Curnow JSH, Greene KR 1992. Randomised trial of cardiotocography alone or with ST waveform analysis for intrapartum monitoring. *Lancet.* 340:194-198.

Walker J 1954. Foetal anoxia. *J Obstet Gynaecol Br Emp* 61:162-180.

5

Uterine Contractions in Labour

R Haththotuwa
S Arulkumaran

Uterine contractions are a prerequisite for the initiation and progress of labour leading to vaginal delivery. Effective uterine contractions are necessary for the normal progress of labour and to overcome minor cephalopelvic disproportion. Our knowledge of what brings about the uterine contractions that initiate labour is incomplete. They involve a number of intercellular alterations in the fetal membranes, decidua and myometrium (Barry et al 1975; Grieves and Liggins 1976) which are thought to be brought about by complex interactions between various endogenous factors or agents such as progesterone, oestrogen, oxytocin, prostaglandins, relaxin, calcium ions and cyclic AMP (Roy et al 1985; Drover and Casper 1983). The action of these agents and the role of gap junctions is discussed in another chapter. This chapter will deal with the measurement and quantification of uterine activity and its clinical implications.

Measurement of uterine activity

For the normal progress of labour with a favourable outcome the fetal heart rate parameters should be normal and adequate uterine contractions should be present. If there are no fetal heart rate changes suggestive of hypoxia and if the rate of cervical dilatation is satisfactory, there may be little need to monitor uterine contractions (Arulkumaran 1994). But to interpret changes in the fetal heart rate and to diagnose and treat poor progress of labour, monitoring of uterine activity is essential.

Traditional methods

Pain associated with uterine contractions is a poor indicator to measure their effectiveness. It is subjective. Feeble incoordinate uterine contractions with poor labour progress may be associated with severe pain, while there may be little pain with powerful coordinate contractions leading to optimal progress of labour (Arulkumaran and Ingemarsson 1989). An objective method is therefore necessary.

Traditionally, uterine contractions were measured by palpation by keeping the hand midway between the umbilicus and the uterine fundus. The frequency and duration of the uterine contractions can be quantified by this method. The frequency of contractions is assessed by the number of contractions in a 10 minute period. The duration of the contraction is from the time the contraction is first felt abdominally to the time when the contraction passes measured in seconds (Arulkumaran and Lennox 1988). This method gives little information about the strength or intensity of the contractions or the basal pressure between contractions (Arulkumaran and Ratnam 1987). However it is adequate for the management of labour in most circumstances. The method of quantification on a partograph using the clinical method is shown in the chapter dealing with the management of the first stage of labour.

Mechanical methods have been developed to make graphical records (that is, tocographs) of duration, frequency and strength of contractions. External and internal tocographic methods are used in clinical practice.

External tocography

In external tocography a transducer which is a plastic plunger or membrane is placed near the uterine fundus to detect changes resulting from uterine contractions in the anteroposterior diameter of the abdomen (Arulkumaran and Ratnam 1987). It is a noninvasive method, causes only mild discomfort to the patient and is relatively cheap. But it is difficult to use in obese and restless patients. External tocographic recordings provide a good measure of contraction frequency, a fair estimate of contraction duration but only an approximation of contraction intensity (Arulkumaran 1994). Hence this method may be useful in studies done to find the action of drugs on the uterus where a major effect is anticipated (Embrey 1940) and to note the uterine activity to predict preterm labour (Bell 1983). Though external tocography is sufficient in most instances, internal tocography is more accurate for quantifying of uterine activity in high risk situations and for scientific work (Arulkumaran 1994).

Internal tocography

Schatz in Germany in 1872 was the first to attempt the recording of intrauterine pressure (Allman and Steer 1993). He inserted a rubber bag into the uterus under anesthesia and connected it by tubing to a manometer. Caldeyro-Barcia et al in 1950 inserted a catheter into the uterus through the anterior abdominal wall and studied the uterine activity serially throughout gestation (Caldeyro-Barcia et al 1950). In 1952, Williams and Stallworthy introduced a polythene catheter with a number of terminal perforations through the vagina and cervix using the Drew Smythe catheter (Williams and Stallworthy 1952). This transvaginal intraamniotic method became the preferred method. Extensive studies done by others led to many improvements in the technology. Smaller and more flexible catheters were made which could be introduced through a small plastic introducer. Since the 1970s the catheter has been connected to electronic recording equipment (Allman and Steer 1993). Several disadvantages have been reported with fluid filled catheters. The catheter could get blocked by vernix, blood clots and meconium (Odendaal et al 1976), and thus give false readings. Recordings may also be misleading if the catheter is placed in between the uterine wall and the fetus in which case not only the intrauterine pressure but also the forces exerted by the uterine wall may also be recorded (Newman et al 1972). Although rare, complications of uterine perforations and fetal, umbilical cord or placental damage have also been reported (Arulkumaran and Ingemarsson 1989).

Steer and Carter first developed the transducer tipped catheter (GAELTEC*) which obviated the technical problems of the fluid filled device (Steer et al 1978). This catheter is safe, easily inserted, reliable (Allman and Steer 1993) and is ideal to use in the ambulant patient. The pressure transducer is mounted on the end of a 90 cm catheter with a sensing area which is recessed, thus minimising accidental damage and enabling lateral pressure measurements without impact of the head or end pressure (Arulkumaran and Ratnam 1987). The catheter tip lies in the amniotic cavity and the entire transmission passes electronically through the catheter via a 2 metre flexible extension cable connected to the contraction module of a fetal monitor. When not in use the catheter is stored in a plastic tube filled with activated 2% gluteraldehyde, attached to the monitor. Each catheter, if handled with care, may be used in more than 100 patients (Gibb and Arulkumaran 1987). The ease of the use of this catheter and its reliability are well documented (Steer 1975). Recently a fibre optic catheter has been introduced. This can be kept in the uterus even in the second stage of labour (Svenningsen et al 1986). Tham et al (1991) who compared the fibre optic catheter with the 'Gaeltec' catheter found that the fibre optic pressure transducer was safe, convenient and equally accurate in assessing the uterine activity (Fig 5.1). More recently catheters with transducers to measure the pressure as well as facilities to perform amnioinfusion have been combined in one device (Arulkumaran 1994). Its usefulness in cases of meconium stained or reduced amniotic fluid is well established (Arulkumaran et al 1991).

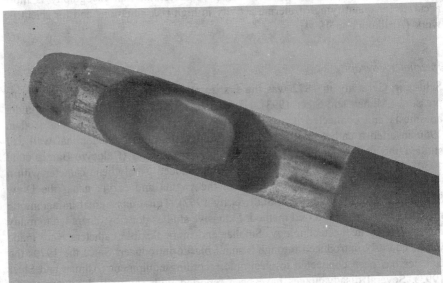

Fig 5.1   Gaeltec catheter showing the sensor tip in the recessed area to avoid end-on pressures

Reliability of intrauterine pressure measurements

Knoke et al (1976) performed a series of studies where they passed three fluid filled intrauterine catheters into the same uterus in women in labour (Knoke et al 1976). They found large differences in the readings of the three catheters on a contraction-to-contraction basis. These and other reports gave rise to doubts about the reliability of intrauterine pressure measurements. They concluded that the variations in pressure which were around 5–10 mm Hg, were due to loculation in the amniotic cavity and lack of communication between different sites in the amniotic cavity.

Steer et al (1978) compared the measurement of intrauterine pressure using a fluid filled intrauterine catheter with that using the transducer tipped catheter in four women in labour. They found only a slight difference between the two methods and it was attributed to the inherent fault of the blocking of the fluid filled catheter.

In order to assess the reliability of intrauterine pressure measurements, Chua et al (1992) did a study where they passed two catheter tipped pressure transducers tied together into the same amniotic pocket in one group and passed the two catheters into two different pockets of amniotic fluid in another group. Their results showed that in both groups there were differences in intrauterine pressures from the two catheters in the same uterus on a contraction-to-contraction basis, but in overall labour there was only a small difference. This had been the experience earlier with different catheter systems (Arulkumaran et al 1991). It is difficult to explain why there is a difference when both the catheters are tied together and are in the same pocket of amniotic fluid. For practical purposes, minor variations in the pressures on a contraction-to-contraction basis does not influence the outcome of labour. It is only the cumulative pressure over the whole duration of labour or that over a certain time segment (every ten to fifteen minutes) which is likely to have some bearing on the progress of labour (Arulkumaran 1994).

Components of uterine contractions

The main components of uterine contractions are baseline tone, active pressure, frequency and duration (Fig 5.2).

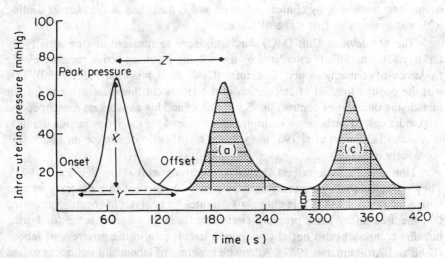

Fig 5.2 Elements and terminology of uterine contractions. X: active pressure or amplitude, Y: duration, Z: contraction interval related to frequency, (a): active contraction area, (b): basal tone, (c): total contraction area.

Active pressure or amplitude is the difference between the pressure at the peak of a contraction and the basal pressure. Baseline pressure (basal tone) is the pressure at the lowest point of the tracing existing between contractions. It may be difficult to measure if the contractions tend to merge with each other. The frequency is the number of contractions over a ten minute period and the duration is the time in seconds between the onset and offset of the contraction. Contractions are asymmetrical in shape in that they have a steeper rise than a fall. If the decreasing pressure falls to the baseline slowly it may be difficult to estimate the duration.

The reported range of the normal baseline tone varies from 0.8 to 2.6 kPa depending on the measuring technique used and the distance between the level of the transducer and the upper level of the amniotic fluid in the uterus (Allman and Steer 1993). Values over 3 kPa are likely to represent hypertonus and may compromise the maternal blood flow to the placenta and result in fetal hypoxia (Allman and Steer 1993).

The frequency of contractions in the active phase of labour is usually 4 per 10 minutes and may rise to 5 per 10 minutes in the late first stage. The duration of contractions may start with less than 20 sec, increase gradually and in the late first and second stage may last between 40 and 90 seconds.

The uterine blood flow is minimal during the ascending phase of a uterine contraction and stabilises after the peak intensity is reached (Gibb and Arulkumaran 1987). The flow then returns to the pre-contraction level or above. The blood entrapped in the intervillus space acts as a reservoir and is likely to play an important role in the oxygenation of the fetus during the periods of reduced blood flow.

Quantification of uterine activity

Over the years, several measures have been used to quantify uterine activity. The commonest method is by clinical palpation and is described in the chapter dealing with management of first stage of labour.

The Montevideo Unit (MU) was introduced to measure uterine activity by Caldeyro-Barcia. This is calculated by multiplying the mean active pressure by the frequency of contractions per 10 minutes (Caldeyro-Barcia et al 1957, 1959). This was the popular method of calculation in the 1960s but this measurement did not include the duration of contraction. So El-Sahwi and his co-workers developed the Alexandra unit by including a multiplication factor of the mean contraction duration in minutes (El-Sahwi et al 1967). As this was difficult to calculate on line it was not widely used.

Hon and Paul described the uterine activity unit (Hon and Paul 1973). They proposed that one uterine activity unit be equivalent to a contraction area with a height of 0.133 kPa lasting for 1 minute. An analysis of records suggested that the area under basal pressure contributed a large amount to the total area, but this component did not always play a useful role in the progress of labour (Gibb and Arulkumaran 1987). Adequate progress of labour did not occur unless the uterine contractions exceeded the baseline tone at least by 2 kPa (Allman and Steer 1993). Hence using the total area made the measurement less sensitive. In 1977, Steer proposed a unit based on the active contraction area derived by an electronic subtraction technique on-line (Steer 1977). Steer used the System International (SI) Units of pressure, the Pascal instead of mm of Hg (1 kPa = 7.32 mm Hg). 1 kPa of pressure existing over a duration of one second is 1 kilo Pascal second (1 kPas). The quantity was termed the Uterine Activity Integral (UAI). UAI is expressed as a 15 minute total, and thus the uterine activity is expressed as kilo Pascal seconds/15 minutes (kPas/15 min). The period of 15 minutes was decided upon as this is the time taken to establish a stable response to the short term changes in the oxytocin infusion rate.

Equipment which incorporates a uterine activity module has been developed. This module, using the information obtained from the transducer tipped or fluid filled catheter computes the active contraction area every 15 minutes and shows it in a display window on the module (Arulkumaran 1994). The same value is printed in figures and marked on the two channel chart recording paper against a vertical scale marked from 0 to 2,500 kPas/15 mins (Fig 5.3).

UTERINE ACTIVITY INTEGRAL : UAI (STEER 1977)

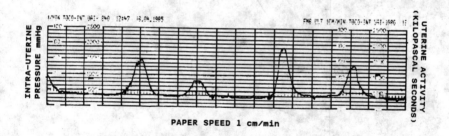

PAPER SPEED 1 cm/min

Active Contraction Area
15 minute summation of area
SI unit of pressure KILOPASCAL
   (13.3 kPa = 100 mm Hg)
1kPa for 1 sec = 1 KILOPASCAL SECOND
UAI = Active contraction area/15 minutes

Fig 5.3   Uterine activity quantified online in kPas/15 mins indicated by short dark line against a vertical axis from 0–2,500 kPas. A numerical printout of the value with paper speed, date and time is shown

Uterine activity in spontaneous labour

Uterine activity in spontaneous labour has a wide variation due to various factors: parity, age, race, fetal weight, maternal height, presentation of the fetus and multiple pregnancy. The administration of drugs, epidural anesthesia, the retention of urine, the rupture of the membranes and changes of posture could affect uterine contractions (Gibb and Arulkumaran 1987).

Uterine activity in nulliparae

Most authors have used a cervical dilatation rate of 1 cm per hour to distinguish normal from abnormal labour (Arulkumaran 1994). Cowen et al who studied labour in African women found a slow rise in uterine activity during the first stage of labour in nulliparous women with an overall median of 1,824 kPas/15 min (Cowen et al 1982). Gibb et al found in Chinese nulliparae that normal labour progress occurs when the uterine activity level is at least 650 kPas/15 min with an overall median level of 1,440 kPas/15 min (Gibb et al 1984). It was also observed that there was a slow progressive rise of pressure in the first stage of labour with a sharp rise towards the end of the first stage of labour (Fig 5.4).

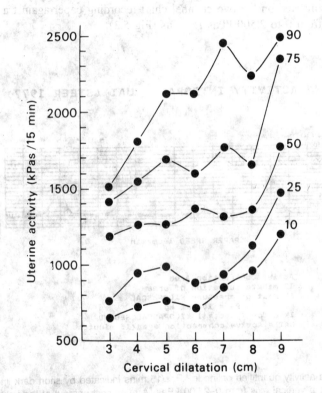

Fig 5.4   Cervical dilatation-related uterine activity kPas/15 min in spontaneous normal labour in nulliparae

A transient peak of uterine activity was noted by Gibb and others in their study, soon after the insertion of the intrauterine catheter, irrespective of whether amniotomy was performed or not (Gibb et al 1984). Release of prostaglandins during the manipulation of the lower uterine segment is a possible explanation for this observation. All the studies showed a wide range of uterine activity in nulliparae. Although this may be due to the different subject characteristics in various studies, the clinical usefulness of measurements which show a wide range becomes limited.

Uterine activity in multiparae

It has been an observation by most clinicians that multiparae who have had a vaginal delivery previously have an easier labour and delivery than their nulliparous counterparts. Whether this is due to a late admission cervical dilatation, more efficient uterine contractions, reduced cervical and pelvic tissue resistance or a combination of these factors is not known (Arulkumaran et al 1984).

Turnbull observed lower pressures and faster progress in labour in multiparae when compared with nulliparae and attributed this to the lower cervical and pelvic tissue resistance in multiparae (Turnbull 1957). Arulkumaran et al, who studied the uterine activity in multiparous Singaporean women of Chinese origin, found an overall median value of 1,130 kPas/15 min compared with 1,440 kPas/15 min observed in nulliparae (Arulkumaran et al 1984). They also observed that up to 6 cm cervical dilatation uterine activity values in the normal multiparae were significantly lower than in the nulliparous counterparts (Arulkumaran et al 1984). From 6 cm to 9 cm it rose more, with a sharp rise at 9 cm dilatation (Fig 5.5). Until the late first stage of labour most uterine activity is spent on effacing and dilating the cervix. In the late first stage and second stage, the descent of the head takes

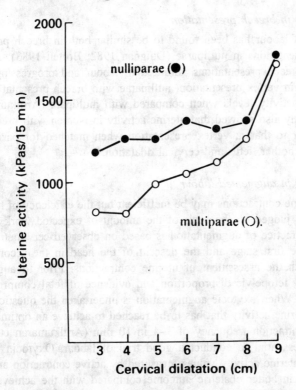

Fig. 5.5 Comparison of cervical dilatation specific median uterine activity in spontaneous normal labour in nulliparae and multiparae.

place and hence the pressure needed is greater, as reflected by the steep rise in uterine activity towards the end of the first stage of labour. The uterine activity in multiparae is significantly lower than in nulliparae till the late first stage of labour and this suggests that the parity may have a greater influence on the resistance offered by the cervix than the pelvic tissues.

Ethnic influence on uterine activity

Physiological functions in humans appear to be uninfluenced by ethnic differences when controlled for physical characteristics of the individual and environmental factors. Duignan and others showed that the progress of labour was similar in women in different ethnic groups living in the same environment (Duignan et al 1975). Arulkumaran et al compared the uterine activity in the Singaporean Malay population with that of a similar Chinese population (Arulkumaran et al 1989a). They concluded that the uterine activity profile in the Malay population was similar to that of the Chinese population in spontaneous normal labour, when controlled for parity, certain maternal characteristics and the rate of progress in labour. The presence of uterine pathology such as fibroids, short maternal stature, abnormal pelvic shape, fetal macrosomia and other pathological variables may lead to ethnic differences in uterine activity which are more apparent than real (Arulkumaran et al 1989a).

Uterine activity in breech presentation

The progress of labour has been found to be similar both in breech presentations and vertex presentations in nulliparae (Duignan 1982; Borten 1983). A study on patients with breech presentations admitted in labour and progressing normally showed that as in vertex presentation, nulliparae with breech presentation showed higher uterine activity levels when compared with multipara (Arulkumaran et al 1988). This study also showed that uterine activity in women with breech presentation is similar to that in vertex presentation when matched for parity, characteristics in the mother, fetus and cervical dilatation.

Uterine activity in augmented labour

Infrequent uterine contractions may be inefficient but the efficiency of the contractions should be judged on the basis of the amount of expected work performed. Therefore the practice of augmentation is based on observed cervimetric progress of labour in the first stage and the descent of the head in the second stage in conjunction with the assessment of uterine contractions. Prior to augmentation, malpresentation, fetopelvic disproportion and evidence of fetal compromise have to be excluded. When oxytocic augmentation is undertaken the question arises as to the target uterine activity that has to be reached to achieve an optimal obstetric outcome. A contraction frequency of 3–4 in 10 min (Arulkumaran et al 1991b) appears to be essential to conduct a good trial of labour. Oxytocin titration to achieve preset uterine activity values measured by active contraction area profiles does not result in better obstetric outcome compared with the achievement of a target frequency of 4 to 5 contractions every 10 min (each lasting > 40 sec) (Arulkumaran et al 1989b). There also appears to be no advantage in titrating oxytocin using intrauterine catheters to quantify uterine activity or the desired frequency of contractions compared with oxytocin titration based on external tocography in dysfunctional labour (Chua et al 1990).

Uterine activity in induced labour

Induction of labour is common in modern obstetric practice and can vary from as low as 3% to as high as 30% in different units even in the same country. Artificial rupture of membranes and oxytocin infusion is the commonest method employed. Generally oxytocin is titrated to achieve 4 contractions in 10 min after the rupture of the membranes. Uterine activity in induced labour is higher than that observed in spontaneous normal labour (Arulkumaran et al 1986). In order to regulate the oxytocin to achieve optimal levels of uterine activity, and to avoid any ill effects to the fetus, oxytocin infusion has been titrated to achieve the 50th centile uterine activity observed in spontaneous labour according to parity (Gibb et al 1985). The obstetric outcome with such an approach was not better compared with a group that had oxytocin titrated to achieve optimal frequency of contractions of 4–5 in

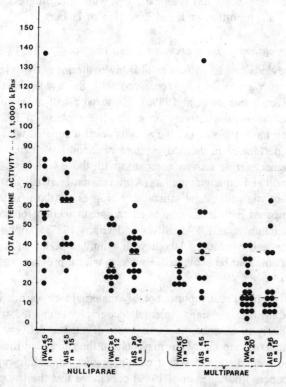

Fig 5.6   Total uterine activity according to parity, cervical score and different modes of oxytocin infusion - IVAC: manual infusion to achieve 75th centile and AIS: automatic infusion to achieve 50th centile uterine activity observed in spontaneous normal labour

10 min. In many patients who had oxytocin to achieve 50th centile uterine activity, the progress of labour was slow necessitating escalation of the oxytocin dose to achieve the optimal frequency of contractions necessary to produce acceptable progress of labour. When oxytocin was titrated to achieve 75th centile uterine activity compared with optimal frequency of contractions, each of the two methods gave an equally good outcome indicating that such quantification of uterine activity offers no advantage in induced labour (Arulkumaran et al 1987). In a recent randomised study uterine activity was quantified using an intrauterine catheter in one group and the contractions were assessed by external tocography in the second group (Chia et al 1993). The obstetric outcome was similar in the two groups, suggesting no advantage in using an intrauterine catheter in induced labour.

It is known that a uterus has to perform a given quantum of uterine activity based on the parity and cervical score in order to effect delivery in induced labour (Arulkumaran et al 1985) (Fig 5.6). The total uterine activity (TUA) is a reflection of the cervical and pelvic tissue resistance. If fetal heart rate changes are observed during induced labour associated with high uterine activity, it may be possible to reduce the uterine activity to the low levels known to be associated with the progress of labour and to achieve vaginal delivery rather than terminate the pregnancy abdominally because of fetal distress. If the expected total uterine activity for the given parity and cervical score has been exceeded with little progress, it may suggest cephalopelvic disproportion or failed induction of labour.

Uterine activity in patients with a previous caesarean scar

Women with a previous caesarean scar exhibit lower uterine activity levels if they had had a previous vaginal delivery compared with those who have not had a vaginal delivery (Arulkumaran et al 1989c). Those who had no vaginal delivery but had the caesarean done electively or in the latent phase of labour in their previous pregnancy have a higher uterine activity level compared with the women who had surgery performed in the active phase of labour. Women who are augmented exhibit higher uterine activity compared with those who have normal progress of labour and need no augmentation (Arulkumaran et al 1989d). Those who are likely to deliver vaginally show satisfactory progress in the first few hours of augmentation compared with those who need caesarean section for poor progress in labour (Arulkumaran et al 1989d; Silver and Gibbs 1987). Applying a policy of careful selection and conduct of labour with a limited period of augmentation, a satisfactory outcome can be achieved in women with a previous caesarean scar (Chua et al 1989).

The classical signs of scar rupture, notably maternal tachycardia, hypotension and vaginal bleeding are late signs. Internal tocography compared with external tocography is unlikely to enhance the success rate of vaginal delivery without additional fetal or maternal morbidity but may help in the early identification of loss of integrity of the scar in some cases. It cannot predict impending rupture of the scar. An earlier paper (Rodriquez et al 1989) concluded that the use of an intrauterine catheter was not of value in detecting early rupture of the uterus, but two recent papers (Beckley et al 1991, Arulkumaran et al 1992) have shown evidence that it may be of help. Uterine activity reflected as an increase in intrauterine pressure depends upon the increase in uterine wall tension. A breach in the scar affects wall tension and hence reduces the build up of intrauterine pressure (Gee et al 1988). This is reflected in the marked decline in the amplitude of the contractions once the scar gives way (Fig 5.7). There is no reason to expect a reduction in the frequency of contractions and it is usually not reduced with the scar rupture. In cases where uterine activity was not reduced the catheter may have been introduced posterior to the head and may have been in an isolated pool of fluid. The posterior approach is the commonest and may have been the case in the series (Rodriquez et al 1989) where no reduction in uterine activity was observed with the rupture of the uterus. This is exemplified by a case where reduction in uterine

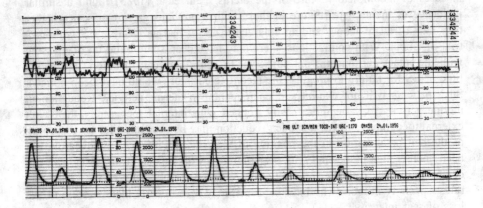

Fig 5.7   Decline in uterine activity with loss of integrity of caesarean scar. Baseline pressure and frequency were not affected

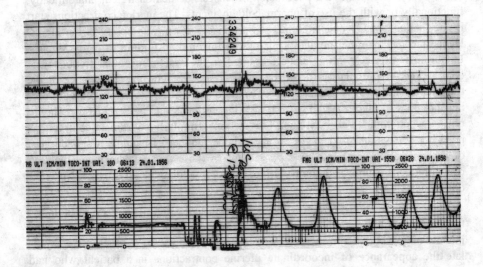

Fig 5.8   Predehiscence uterine activity recorded when the catheter was reinserted into another amniotic fluid pocket

activity was noticed (Fig 5.7). It was thought that the catheter had slipped into the cervix as the patient had no signs or symptoms of scar rupture. On reinsertion of the catheter posterior to the head, contractions with the amplitudes seen earlier were observed (Fig 5.8). Subsequently, the uterine rupture involving the bladder was seen when the patient had a caesarean for failure to progress. In those who showed a decline in pressure the catheter tip might have been situated in the anterior lower segment or in an amniotic fluid pool in the posterior portion of the uterus which communicated with the anterior pocket. The location of the catheter and the extent of loss of integrity of the scar may determine the change in the uterine activity observed.

There may be another reason for there being no reduction of uterine activity in cases of incomplete rupture of the uterus. Paul et al (1985) found a similar incidence of incomplete rupture in those with a previous caesarean scar whether they had a trial of labour and an emergency CS or had an elective CS without a trial of labour. With contractions, there may have been some build up of pressure with the intact peritoneum, not sufficient to cause cervical dilatation, and at the time of CS for failure to progress the incomplete rupture would have been noticed. Such patients will not exhibit sudden reduction in uterine activity. Reduction in uterine activity may be more easily noticed with internal tocography than with external tocography, where a sudden reduction may be accounted for by loosening of the belt or alteration in the position of the patient. Prolonged bradycardia has been another sign associated with scar rupture (Arulkumaran et al 1992). The use of an intrauterine catheter and continuous electronic monitoring of the fetal heart rate, especially in those who have oxytocin, may help in early identification of the loss of scar integrity.

Incoordinate uterine contractions

The uterus does not have a pacemaker which can be demonstrated, anatomically, functionally or with the use of pharmacologic agents. The uterine contractions start in the fundus, usually near a cornu, and propagate down to the body of the uterus. Hence incoordinate uterine activity is not an uncommon finding in many labours. Incoordinate uterine contractions are defined on the basis of irregular frequency of contractions or irregularity of the shape of contractions on the appearance of the tocographic tracings. Wide variation of incoordinate activity is associated with normal progress of labour (Gibb et al 1984). Incoordinate uterine contractions should not be synonymous with inefficient contractions. Similarly coordinate contractions need not always be efficient. In an appreciable number of patients minor degrees of incoordination are found in early labour. In those cases where incoordination of contractions is observed, the pattern of incoordination generally persists throughout labour.

Incoordinate uterine contractions are not an indication to use oxytocics unless they are found to be inefficient. The use of oxytocics may or may not correct the incoordination but should increase the efficiency. The use of oxytocin may stimulate the appearance of incoordinate uterine contractions in a patient who had coordinate uterine contractions, but if the contractions have been inefficient it may improve their efficiency. Though internal tocography is likely to delineate incoordinate uterine activity better, it is not required in cases suspected to have incoordinate uterine contractions because this phenomenon is not directly linked to the efficiency of contractions. Various degrees of incoordinate uterine activity during labour in women who had normal progress resulting in unassisted vaginal delivery is described in the chapter dealing with the management of the first stage of labour.

Tetanic contractions, hypertonic uterine activity and hyper– or polysystole

A few contractions merging together to form a sustained contraction lasting for a few minutes (3 min) is called a tetanic contraction. Such contractions are usual in the third stage after the oxytocic administration. It is not seen in spontaneous normal labour and is usually brought about by the use of oxytocics during the induction or augmentation of labour. When the contractions do not merge but the baseline pressure is elevated more than 20 mmHg for more than 3 min, it is called hypertonic (increased tone of the uterus) uterine activity. The tetanic contractions will cut off the perfusion to the retroplacental pool of blood and hypertonic uterine activity will reduce the perfusion. Such action can cause transient fetal heart rate changes unless remedial action is taken by stopping the oxytocin and/or by giving a uterine relaxant especially if it is associated with severe FHR changes (Ingemarsson et al 1985). If the contraction frequency is greater than one every 2 min it is called polysystole or hypersystole and is usually caused by higher than necessary levels of oxytocin. If remedial action is not taken and the dose of oxytocin is further increased it usually results in hypertonic uterine activity and further excess in the drug infusion results in tetanic contraction. Such uterine hyperstimulation can occur without the dose of oxytocin being increased due to the increase in sensitivity of the uterus to oxytocin with the advance of labour (Sica Blanco and Sala 1961).

Polysystole is also observed in some patients with abruptio placentae. If a woman is admitted with bleeding and abdominal pain and on cardiotocography there is evidence of polysystolic contractions of small amplitude and an abnormal fetal heart rate pattern, one should not hesitate to entertain the diagnosis of abruptio placentae. The polysystolic contractions indicate the uterine irritability caused by the seeping of blood into the myometrium.

Internal tocography and quantification of uterine activity by active contraction area measurements is of little value in spontaneous normal labour. In augmented labour, internal tocography has not been shown to be associated with reduction in duration of labour, the dose of oxytocin, the incidence of operative deliveries or better neonatal outcome compared with external tocography. Whether internal tocography offers any advantage over external tocography in difficult cases of augmentation, that is, in those who do not show satisfactory progress of labour in the first few hours of augmentation, needs further study. Obstetric outcome has not improved with the use of internal tocography and quantification of uterine activity in induced labour. The knowledge of total uterine activity (TUA) computed with internal tocography may be of value in selected cases where fetal heart rate changes are observed with high uterine activity or in those who fail to progress despite having achieved the total uterine activity according to parity and cervical score. However the cases that are likely to benefit from such an exercise may be too few in number to justify routine internal tocography in induced labour.

In those with a previous caesarean section scar, the uterine activity in augmented labour is higher than that observed in spontaneous normal labour. Those who are likely to deliver vaginally show satisfactory progress within the first few hours of augmentation. A limited period of augmentation should limit total uterine activity and may reduce the chance of scar rupture. Internal tocography may be of value in detecting excessive uterine activity which may not be obvious with external tocography. A sudden decline in uterine activity may be the earliest sign to indicate loss of integrity of a previous caesarean scar. Where difficulty arises in recording uterine contractions by external tocography, as in an obese or restless patient, internal tocography is of value. The routine use of internal tocography and quantification of uterine activity compared with external tocography does not lead to better obstetric outcome in spontaneous, augmented or induced labour. There may be a limited role for the selective use of internal tocography where recordings on external tocography are unsatisfactory, in cases of difficult augmentation or induction and in those with a previous caesarean scar and oxytocin infusion. Almost all labour can be managed by clinical palpation of uterine contractions and by quantifying the frequency and duration of contractions. Modern technology has simplified clinical evaluation and has provided an on-line recording but there is little proof that it has significantly improved the clinical outcome.

References

Allman ACJ, Steer PJ 1993. Monitoring uterine activity. *Br J Hosp Med* 49:649-653.

Arulkumaran S 1994. Uterine activity in labour. In: Chard T, Grudzinskas JG, eds. The Uterus. Cambridge: Cambridge University Press, pp 356-377.

Arulkumaran S, Gibb DMF, Lun KC, Heng SH, Ratnam SS 1984. The effect of parity on uterine activity in labour. *Br J Obstet Gynecol* 91:843-848.

Arulkumaran S, Gibb DMF, Ratnam SS, Heng SH, Lun KC 1985. Total uterine activity in induced labour – an index of cervical and pelvic tissue resistance. *Br J Obstet Gynecol* 92:693-697.

Arulkumaran S, Gibb DMF, Heng SH, Lun KC, Ratnam SS 1986. Uterine activity in oxytocin induced labour. *Asia Oceania J Obstet Gynecol* 12:533-540.

Arulkumaran S, Ratnam SS 1987. Current trends in monitoring uterine contractions in labour. *Sri Lanka J Obstet Gynecol* 13:114-127.

Arulkumaran S, Ingemarsson I, Ratnam SS 1987. Oxytocin titration to achieve preset active contraction area values does not improve the outcome of induced labour. *Br J Obstet Gynecol* 94:242-248.

Arulkumaran S, Lennox C 1988. The Partograph Section II. *A user's manual.* WHO Publication p 12.

Arulkumaran S, Ingemarsson I, Gibb DMF, Ratnam SS 1988. Uterine activity in spontaneous labour with breech presentation. *Aust NZ J Obstet Gynecol* 28: 275-278.

Arulkumaran S, Ingemarsson I 1989. Methods for measurement of uterine activity in labour. *Int J Feto-Mat Med* 2:22-28.

Arulkumaran S, Gibb DMF, Chua S, Piara Singh, Ratnam SS 1989a. Ethnic influence on uterine activity in spontaneous normal labour. *Br J Obstet Gynecol* 96:1203-1206.

Arulkumaran S, Yang M, Ingemarsson I, Piara S, Ratnam SS 1989b. Augmentation of labour: Does quantification of active contraction area to guide oxytocin titration produce better obstetric outcome? *Asia Oceania J Obstet Gynecol* 15:47-51.

Arulkumaran S, Gibb DMF, Ingemarsson I, Kitchener CH, Ratnam SS 1989c. Uterine activity during spontaneous normal labour after previous lower segment caesarean scar. *Br J Obstet Gynecol* 96:933-938.

Arulkumaran S, Ingemarsson I, Ratnam SS 1989d. Oxytocin augmentation in dysfunctional labour after previous caesarean scar. *Br J Obstet Gynecol* 96:939-941.

Arulkumaran S, Yang M, Chia YT, Ratnam SS 1991. Reliability of intrauterine pressure measurements. *Obstet Gynecol* 78:800-802.

Arulkumaran S, Chua TM, Chua S, Yang M, Piara S, Ratnam SS 1991b. Uterine activity in dysfunctional labour and target uterine activity to be aimed with oxytocin titration. *Asia Oceania J Obstet Gynecol* 17:101-106.

Arulkumaran S, Chua S, Ratnam SS 1992. Symptoms and signs with scar rupture – value of uterine activity measurement. *Austr NZ J Obstet Gynecol* 32:208-212.

Barry E, Schwarz F, Schultz M, MacDonald PC, Johnston JM 1975. Initiation of human parturition. III. Fetal membrane content of prostaglandin E₂ and F₂α precursor. *Obstet Gynecol* 46:564-568.

Beckley S, Gee H, Newton JR 1991. Scar rupture in labour after previous lower segment caesarean section; the role of uterine activity measurement. *Br J Obstet Gynecol* 98:255-269.

Bell R 1983. The prediction of preterm labour by recording spontaneous antenatal uterine activity. *Br J Obstet Gynecol* 90:884-887.

Borten M 1983. In: Friedman EA, Cohen WR, eds. Breech presentation in management of labour. Baltimore: University Park Press, p 253.

Caldeyro-Barcia R, Alvarez H, Reynolds SRM 1950. A better understanding of uterine contractility through simultaneous recording with an internal and seven channel external method. *Surg Gynecol Obstet* 91:641-650.

Caldeyro-Barcia R, Sica-Blanco Y, Poseiro JJ, Gonzalez-Panizzau, Mendez Bauer C, Feilitz C, Alvarez M, Pose SV, Hendricks CM 1957. A quantitative study of the action of synthetic oxytocin on the human uterus. *J Pharmacol Exp Ther* 121:18-31.

Caldeyro-Barcia R, Poseiro JJ 1959. Oxytocin and contractility of the human uterus. *Ann NY Acad Sci* 75:813-830.

Chia YT, Soon B, Arulkumaran S, Ratnam SS 1993. Induction of labour: Does internal tocography result in better obstetric outcome than external tocography? *Austr NZ J Obstet Gynecol* 33:159-161.

Chua S, Arulkumaran S, Piara S, Ratnam SS 1989. Obstetric outcome in patients with previous caesarean section. *Austr NZ J Obstet Gynecol* 29:12-17.

Chua S, Kurup A, Arulkumaran S, Ratnam SS 1990. Augmentation of labour: Does internal tocography result in better obstetric outcome than external tocography? *Obstet Gynecol* 76:164-167.

Chua S, Arulkumaran S, Yang M, Ratnam SS, Steer PJ 1992. The accuracy of catheter-tip pressure transducers for the measurement of intrauterine pressure in labour. *Br J Obstet Gynecol* 99:186-189.

Cowen DB, Van Middelkoop A, Philpott RH 1982. Intrauterine pressure studies in African nulliparie: Normal labour progress. *Br J Obstet Gynecol* 89:364-369.

Drover JW, Casper RF 1983. Current review: Initiation of parturition in humans. *Can Med Assoc J* 128:387-391.

Duignan NM, Studd KWW, Hughes OA 1975. Characteristics of normal labour in different racial groups. *Br J Obstet Gynecol* 82:593-601.

Duignan NM 1982. The management of breech presentation. In: Studd JWW, ed. Progress in Obstetrics and Gynecology, Vol 2. London: Churchill Livingstone, p 73.

El-Sahwi S, Gaafar A, Toppozada HL 1967. A new unit for evaluation of uterine activity. *Am J Obstet Gynecol* 98:900-903.

Embrey MP 1940. External hysterography. A graphic study of the human parturient uterus and the effect of various therapeutic agents on it. *J Obstet Gynecol Br C'wealth* 371-390.

Gee H, Taylor EW, Hancox R 1988. A model for the generation of intrauterine pressure in the human parturient uterus which demonstrates the critical role of the cervix. *J Theor Biol* 133:281-292.

Gibb DMF, Arulkumaran S, Lun KC, Ratnam SS 1984. Characteristics of uterine activity in nulliparous labour. *Br J Obstet Gynecol* 91:220-227.

Gibb DMF, Arulkumaran S, Ratnam SS 1985. A comparative study of methods of oxytocin infusion for induction of labour. *Br J Obstet Gynecol* 92:688-692.

Gibb DMF, Arulkumaran S 1987. Uterine contractions and the fetus. In: John Studd, ed. Progress in Obstetrics and Gynecology, Vol 6, pp 133-135.

Grieves SA, Liggins GC 1976. Phospholipase A activity in human and ovine uterine tissues. *Prostaglandins* 12:229-241.

Hon EH, Paul RH 1973. Quantitation of uterine activity. *Obstet Gynecol* 42:368-370.

Ingemarsson I, Arulkumaran S, Ratnam SS 1985. Bolus injection of terbutaline in term labour. 2. Effect on uterine activity. *Am J Obstet Gynecol* 153:865-869.

Knoke JD, Tsao LL, Neumen MRI, Roux JF 1976. The accuracy of intrauterine pressure during labour: a statistical analysis. *Comp Biomed Res* 9:177-186.

Newman MR, Jorden JA, Roux JF, Knoke JD 1972. Validity of intrauterine pressure measurement with transcervical intraamniotic catheters and an intraamniotic miniature pressure transducer during labour. *Gynecol Obstet Invest* 3:165-175.

Odendaal JH, Neves Dos Santos LM, Henry MJ, Crawford JW 1976. Experiments in the measurement of intrauterine pressure. *Br J Obstet Gynecol* 83:221-224.

Paul RH, Phelan JP, Yeh SH 1985. Trial of labor in the patient with a prior caesarean birth. *Am J Obstet Gynecol* 151:297-304.

Rodriquez MH, Masaki DT, Phelan JP, Diaz FG 1989. Uterine rupture: are intrauterine pressure catheters useful in diagnosis? *Am J Obstet Gynecol* 161:666-669.

Roy AC, Kottegoda SR, Ratnam SS 1985. Another look at initiation of human parturition. *Aust NZ J Obstet Gynecol* 25:94-100.

Sica Blanco Y, Sala NL 1961. Oxytocin. Proceedings of an International Symposium. London: Pergamon Press, p 127.

Silver KR, Gibbs RS 1987. Predictors of vaginal delivery in patients with a previous caesarean section who require oxytocin. *Am J Obstet Gynecol* 156:57-60.

Steer PJ 1975. Uterine activity in labour and the effects and regulation of oxytocin infusion. In: Sonicaid Operating Handbook, Sonicaid Ltd, pp 21-45.

Steer PJ 1977. The measurement and control of uterine contractions. In: Beard RW, Campbell S, eds. The Current Status of Fetal Heart Rate Monitoring and Ultrasound in Obstetrics. London: Royal College of Obstetricians and Gynecologists, pp 48-68.

Steer PJ, Carter MC, Gordon AJ, Beard RW 1978. The use of catheter tip pressure transducers for the measurement of intrauterine pressure in labour. *Br J Obstet Gynecol* 85:561-566.

Svenningsen L, Jensen O, Dodgson BS 1986. A fibreoptic pressure transducer for intrauterine monitoring. In: P Rolfe, ed. Fetal and Neonatal Physiological Measurements, London: Butterworths, pp 15-21.

Tham KF, Arulkumaran S, Chua S, Anandakumar C, Singh P, Ratnam SS 1991. A comparison between fibreoptic and catheter-tip bridge strain gauge transducers for measurement of intrauterine pressure in labour. *Asia Oceania J Obstet Gynecol* 17:83-87.

Turnbull AC 1957. Uterine contractions in normal and abnormal labour. *J Obstet Gynecol Br Emp* 64:321-332.

Williams EA, Stallworthy JA 1952. A simple method of internal tocography. *Lancet* 1:330-332.

6

The Management of
Intrapartum Fetal Distress

Y C Wong
S Arulkumaran

It is logical to deliver a distressed fetus as quickly as possible in the most appropriate way either abdominally or vaginally. Unfortunately the diagnosis of fetal distress is not always precise compared with the diagnosis of placenta previa or anemia in pregnancy (Steer 1982; Gibb and Arulkumaran 1992). By common usage and for want of a better term the situation where the clinician feels that the baby might be hypoxic and acidotic is termed fetal distress. The fetus may also get distressed by infection or injury associated with labour. Many babies are delivered operatively for fetal distress in excellent condition (Sykes et al 1983). It could be argued that action was taken long before the fetus was actually distressed and that hence the baby was born in good condition.

In practice the fetal condition is monitored by continuous cardiotocography, intermittent auscultation and by the colour and quantity of amniotic fluid. In centres where facilities exist and when it is technically feasible fetal scalp blood sampling (FBS) is performed to determine the acid base balance, when there is a suspicion of fetal acidosis based on the fetal heart rate findings and/or the findings of the amniotic fluid. Before performing FBS, consideration should be given to the clinical picture and the stage and rate of progress of labour. In some cases, with intrauterine resuscitation, no further action may be needed because the FHR returns to normal. In others with the resuscitative measures FBS may have to be undertaken to verify the fetal condition. Prompt delivery may have to be undertaken in a few without unnecessary delay associated with FBS (Arulkumaran and Ingemarsson 1990). Even in this latter group resuscitative measures would permit the fetus to be born in a better condition.

The electronic equipment used does not indicate fetal distress but exhibits a fetal heart rate (FHR) pattern which may indicate the possibility of stress to the fetus with or without hypoxia. Anemia is not treated rationally without due consideration being given to its etiology. Once the etiology is known the management varies. A similar approach should be taken when fetal distress is suspected based on the clinical picture and the abnormal FHR pattern. The appropriate management may vary from the simple step of altering the position of the mother to a complicated one of immediate delivery, if needed by an abdominal route. In between these two extremes, there are certain steps which can be tried according to the situation; like hydration, the cessation of oxytocic drugs, amnioinfusion, a bolus dose of a tocolytic drug and administration of 100% oxygen to the mother. If corrective measures do not bring about an acceptable FHR pattern, FBS may become necessary. In order to achieve a precise diagnosis of fetal hypoxia and acidosis, newer methods like ECG waveform analysis, PR - RR interval analysis, continuous fetal pO_2, Doppler blood velocity waveform in the umbilical artery and continuous fetal pH measurements are being pursued (Arulkumaran et al 1990, Fleming et al 1986, Johnson et al 1991, Malcus et al 1991) . However these methods do not appear to achieve the same degree of reliability in different centres and some of them are still in the experimental stage and are not in clinical use (MacLachlan et al 1992, Loh and Arulkumaran 1993, Westgate et al 1992). Since electronic FHR monitoring is the main method of intrapartum fetal surveillance in many centres, the main discussion will centre around abnormal FHR patterns and their management.

The concept of fetal distress and the difficulty in establishing a definitive diagnosis

To understand the concept of fetal distress in relation to the observed FHR pattern, some salient points have to be understood. The FHR trace has four recognisable features. The baseline FHR is calculated by drawing a line through the wiggliness of the trace where there are no accelerations or decelerations. The normal baseline FHR at term is 110 to 150 bpm. Accelerations are a rise in the baseline rate for > 15 beats lasting for > 15 secs from the onset to the offset. Decelerations are a drop in the baseline rate for > 15 beats for > 15 sec. Decelerations < 30 sec that immediately follow an acceleration are accepted as normal. Baseline variability is the bandwidth of the wiggliness of the trace and is best identified when the fetus is active, that is, during a period when the baby has accelerations (Fig 6.1). Normal baseline variability is 10–25 bpm, reduced baseline variability is 5–10 bpm, and the silent pattern is < 5 bpm. A normal trace will have a normal baseline rate of 110–150 bpm, two accelerations in 20 min (reactive), no decelerations and normal

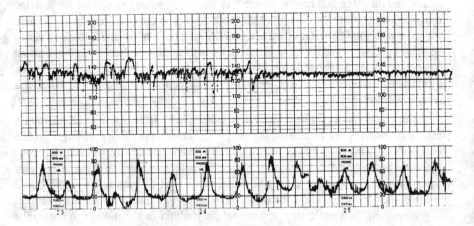

Fig 6.1   A FHR trace showing features of normal baseline rate, normal baseline variability and accelerations. An active period with accelerations and good baseline variability alternates with a quiet period with reduced baseline variability and no accelerations in a healthy fetus.

baseline variability of 10–25 bpm. Accelerations and normal baseline variability are hallmarks of fetal health. In labour, the fetus can get gradually hypoxic and acidotic if the maternal or fetal circulation to the placenta is compromised.

When there is uterine contraction there is cessation of blood flow into the uterus but the fetus continues to get its oxygen from the retroplacental pool of blood. If the oxygen in the retroplacental area is not adequate the FHR decelerates, mediated by a chemoreceptor mechanism and this classically occurs after a contraction presenting as late decelerations. Once the perfusion to the retroplacental bed is reestablished and the fetus gets an adequate oxygen transfer from the retroplacental pool of blood the FHR returns to the baseline rate (Fig 6.2).

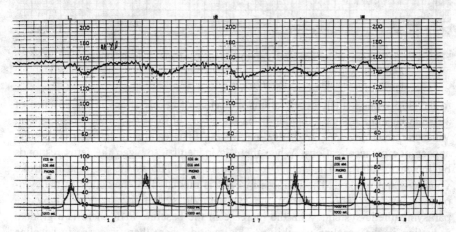

Fig 6.2   A FHR trace with repeated late decelerations. Baseline FHR is 150 bpm, there are no accelerations and the baseline variability is < 5 bpm. An abnormal trace in labour. This case needs FBS if labour is to be allowed to continue.

When the umbilical cord gets compressed, the vein being thin-walled gets occluded first whilst blood from the fetus still leaves via the arteries which are not occluded. The resultant hypotension causes slight acceleration of the FHR. Soon the umbilical arteries get constricted which causes relative hypertension. This results in a sudden fall in the FHR mediated by the baro-receptor mechanism. Once the pressure is released the artery due to its thicker wall opens first and the fetus pumps the blood away from the body, causing a relative hypotension which makes the FHR rise even slightly above the baseline FHR. This results in the characteristic pre- and post-deceleration humps of the variable decelerations. With uterine relaxation the pressure on the cord becomes less, the vein opens, the perfusion to and fro from the fetus becomes reestablished and the FHR returns to normal (Fig 6.3). Early decelerations which mirror the contractions are due to head compression and occur in the late first and second stages of labour. These are vagally mediated and do not suggest hypoxemia.

In labour, gradually developing hypoxia can either be due to occlusion of the umbilical cord (shown by variable decelerations) or decreased perfusion to the placental bed or an inadequate retroplacental pool of blood for oxygen exchange during contractions (shown by late decelerations). In labour, hypoxia is unlikely

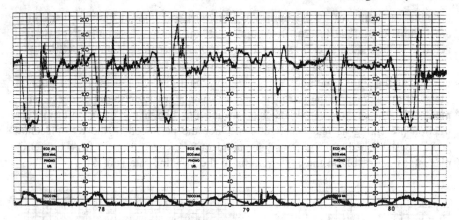

Fig 6.3   FHR trace with repeated variable decelerations. The baseline FHR is
           140 bpm with normal baseline variability (10–25 bpm), a suspicious trace in
           labour. Amnioinfusion is indicated.

to develop without FHR decelerations. Presence of decelerations in the absence of
a rise in baseline rate or reduction in baseline variability is called the stress pattern.
When hypoxia develops gradually, one of the first features to be seen is the disappearance of accelerations. When there is inadequate oxygen the fetus responds
by increasing the cardiac output by a rise in the FHR as the increase in stroke
volume is not marked. The increase in FHR is mediated by the action of the sympathetic system. The action of the sympathetic system is antagonised by the
parasympathetic system. With the increase in the baseline FHR there is a gradual
reduction in the baseline variability. This period where there is a rise in baseline
rate and a reduction in baseline variability is termed stress to distress interval.
When the fetus has reached the maximum achievable baseline FHR the baseline
variability becomes < 5 bpm (Silent pattern or flat baseline variability). This stage
indicates that the fetus may be hypoxemic or acidemic or that it is going to be
acidemic soon. If no intervention is made within a reasonable time the fetus will
be born with severe hypoxia and acidosis. This period is called the distress period
and cannot be predicted by observing the FHR pattern. FBS is useful at this stage.
In extreme instances when the situation is ignored a stillbirth may result. The
staircase-like drop in the FHR pattern to the point when the fetus dies is termed
'distress to death interval', and is usually short (for example, 20–60 min). Figs
6.4–6.9 show a series of FHR tracings of a fetus in labour at intervals from the
time of admission to labour till fetal demise. The trace, with accelerations and no
decelerations developed variable decelerations and an absence of accelerations.
With the progress of time the baseline rate increases and the baseline variability
decreases prior to fetal bradycardia and demise.

The rise in baseline FHR, reduction in baseline variability finally becoming
a flat baseline (baseline variability < 5 bpm) is the usual presentation in a case of
gradually developing hypoxia in a fetus which has exhibited accelerations and good
baseline variability.

A fetus with chronic hypoxia prior to the onset of labour shows a flat baseline
(baseline variability < 5 bpm) and may exhibit shallow decelerations of < 15 beats

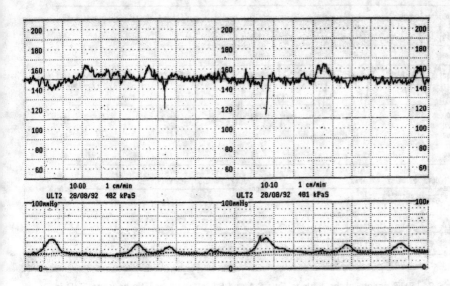

Fig 6.4 FHR pattern at 10.00 hr. The baseline rate is 150 bpm, accelerations are present, the baseline variability 5–10 bpm, with repetitive decelerations — signs of a healthy fetus. The patient was hydrated when the baseline FHR came to 140 bpm.

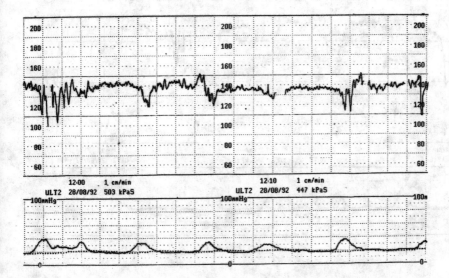

Fig 6.5 FHR pattern of the fetus as in Fig 6.4 at 12.00 hr. Appearance of repetitive variable decelerations but the baseline FHR remains at 140 bpm. If positioning the patient brings no relief this is a good point of time to try amnioinfusion. Amnioinfusion was not attempted.

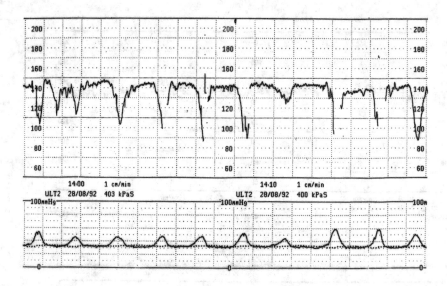

Fig 6.6   FHR pattern of the fetus in Figs 6.4 and 6.5 at 14.00 hr. The baseline FHR is still 140 bpm but variable decelerations are more obvious.

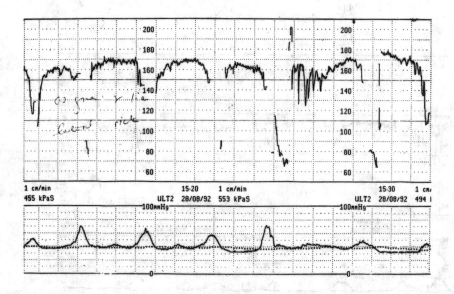

Fig 6.7   FHR pattern of the fetus as in Figs 6.4, 6.5 and 6.6 at 15.20 hr. The baseline rate has increased to 170 bpm with reduced variability and more ominous variable decelerations (depth > 60 beats, duration > 60 sec). This is a good point of time to perform FBS or to plan delivery if the delivery is not in sight within one hour. This step was not taken.

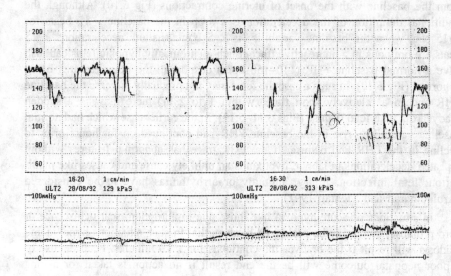

Fig 6.8   FHR pattern of the fetus as in Figs 6.4 to 6.7 at 16.20 hr. The baseline is
dropping gradually from 170 bpm to 80 bpm with attempts to recover. There
is no response to lateral position or oxygen inhalation. A trace too late to try
resuscitative measures or to wait without taking action.

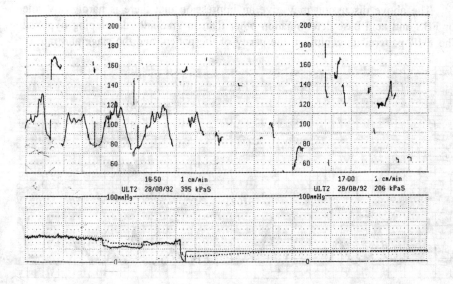

Fig 6.9   FHR pattern of the fetus as in Figs 6.4 to 6.8 at 17.00 hr. The baseline rate
has dropped to 60 bpm without recovery and fetal death was confirmed by
ultrasound scan.

from the baseline with the onset of uterine contractions (Fig 6.10). Although the traditional definition of the deceleration is a drop in the baseline > 15 beats for > 15 sec, when the baseline variability is < 5 bpm, shallow decelerations < 15 beats are ominous in a nonreactive trace. Such a chronically hypoxic fetus can also have a normal baseline FHR (110–150 bpm) despite all the other features being abnormal (Fig 6.10). In such a case the fetus may not gradually increase the baseline FHR and in a relatively short time (within 1 to 2 hr) there may be a sudden bradycardia with fetal demise (Figs 6.11–6.13). In the earlier case which had normal baseline variability, rise in the baseline FHR had continued on for hours prior to decline in the FHR and demise. If the FHR trace has abnormal features without repeated decelerations in labour, hypoxia is an unlikely cause and causes like medication, fetal infection, injury, anomaly or arrhythmias have to be considered (Arulkumaran and Montan 1991).

In situations of acute hypoxia like those due to abruption, scar dehiscence or cord prolapse, there may be prolonged bradycardia. In such situations hypoxia and acidosis will result if the bradycardia continues for > 10 minutes. Fetal demise or a poor neonatal outcome will be the end result if no action is taken for a long period (Figs 6.14 and 6.15).

At times there is subacute hypoxia where acidosis develops within 1–2 hours. It is shown by prolonged decelerations where the FHR stays a very short time at its normal baseline rate and is below it most of the time, with each deceleration lasting > 60 sec. There is no shift in the baseline rate till the terminal bradycardia (Fig 6.16).

The above discussion may give an impression that there is hardly any role for FBS and acid base determination other than in gradually developing hypoxia. The FHR pattern, its evolution, the parity of the patient and the stage and rate of

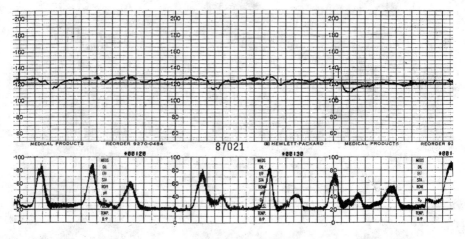

Fig 6.10 A FHR trace with no accelerations showing normal baseline rate but silent pattern (baseline variability < 5 bpm) and shallow (< 15 beats) late decelerations. Baseline rate of 128 bpm, although the baseline rate is in the normal range (110–150 bpm). An ominous pattern suggestive of chronic hypoxia.

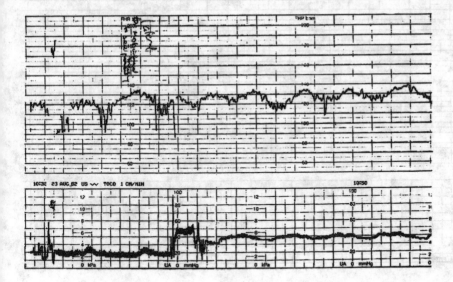

Fig 6.11 FHR trace at 10.36 hr on admission. Baseline rate of 135 bpm and silent pattern (baseline variability < 5 bpm). Increased baseline variability at troughs of decelerations.

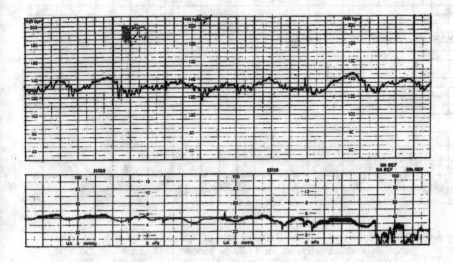

Fig 6.12 FHR trace of the fetus as in Fig 6.11 at 11.00 hr. Baseline rate of 140 bpm. The baseline variability is progressively decreasing without increase in the baseline rate. The decelerations are shallow and the baseline variability in the trough of decelerations is also decreasing.

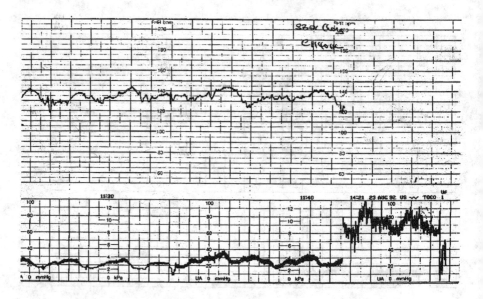

Fig 6.13 FHR trace of the fetus as in Figs 6.11 and 6.12 at 11.30 hr. The baseline
rate is still around 140 bpm with hardly any baseline variability. After 11.42
hr the FHR could not be traced. Ultrasound confirmed fetal death.

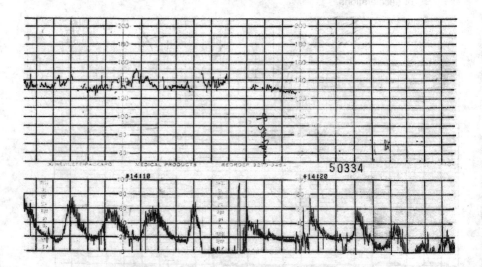

Fig 6.14 FHR pattern at 14.10 hr. Baseline rate of 130 bpm with good baseline
variability and accelerations. At 14.20 hr sudden bradycardia and the fetal
monitor is finding difficulty in picking the FHR signal.

progress of labour should determine the necessity for FBS. The trace has to be
taken in the context of the clinical picture. Special attention has to be paid to those
who are likely to get acidotic faster, for example, fetuses which are IUGR, preterm,
post-term, infected and those with thick meconium and scanty amniotic fluid

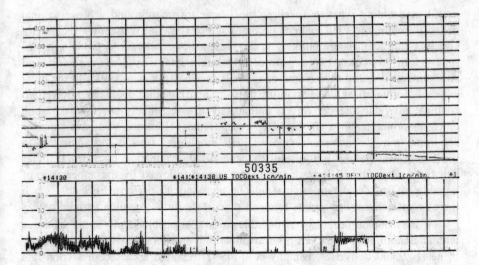

Fig 6.15 FHR pattern of the fetus as in Fig 6.14 from 14.30 to 14.50 hr. The bradycardia did not disappear. CS after 15.00 hr showed scar rupture and the fetus was born in poor condition. The neonate died after three days having had convulsions.

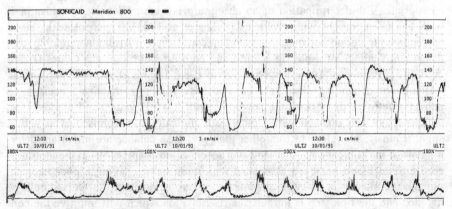

Fig 6.16 FHR trace showing prolonged decelerations (> 60 sec) with the trace recovering to baseline rate for a brief period (< 15–30 sec). No shift in baseline rate - hypoxia and acidosis tends to occur within 40 to 60 min ('subacute hypoxia').

(Arulkumaran and Montan 1991). Other factors in labour which have a significant influence on the rate of decline of pH are the use of oxytocin, epidural anesthesia, difficult instrumental delivery and acute events like cord prolapse, scar rupture or abruptio placentae. In these clinical high risk situations the FHR pattern can become ominous in a short time, and when abnormalities of baseline rate and variability start to appear acid base determinations by FBS will be of value except when associated with acute events (cord prolapse, abruptio and scar dehiscence), bradycardia or patterns with subacute hypoxia where delivery should be expedited. When the rate of progress of labour is good in the presence of an abnormal FHR pattern with reduced baseline variability (5–10 bpm), the determination of pH will be useful in deciding whether to allow the labour to progress and achieve vaginal delivery before the FHR pattern becomes worse (baseline variability < 5 bpm). Hypoxia and acidosis are unlikely in the presence of accelerations (whether spontaneous or provoked) and normal baseline variability (Ingemarsson and Arulkumaran 1989; Arulkumaran et al 1987; Ingemarsson et al 1993). In the presence of normal baseline variability (10–25 bpm) labour could be allowed to continue provided the delivery is anticipated in a reasonably short time despite other abnormal features in the FHR trace. If the FHR trace was suspicious or abnormal from the commencement of FHR monitoring (that is, on admission to the labour ward) then it is useful to have pH determination by FBS. In other situations when the FHR trace has been reactive followed by the appearance of variable or late decelerations, it would be necessary to perform FBS only when there is an increase in baseline rate and a decrease in the baseline variability.

It may not be necessary or possible to do a scalp blood pH in all the cases with an abnormal FHR pattern prior to embarking on operative delivery. In a study of nearly 9,400 deliveries, Dunphy et al (1991) reported a caesarean section rate of 1.1% for fetal distress of whom only 31% had fetal scalp blood sampling. Nevertheless there were more babies with low Apgar scores and those who needed admission to the neonatal intensive care unit for asphyxia in this group. This suggests that the decision made based on the FHR tracing and the clinical picture was appropriate. The determination of an absolute pH value to decide on acidemia at birth has been fraught with problems (Sykes et al 1983). Transient scalp blood acidemia with a good outcome in labour (Ingemarsson and Arulkumaran 1986) and discordant findings of asphyxia at birth and cord arterial blood gas values (Beard et al 1971; Page et al 1986; Ruth and Ravio 1988; Dennis et al 1989) explain the difficulty of depending absolutely on acid base values in making a decision to deliver a fetus in distress. Some newborns with low pH values and marked base deficits adopt and do well whilst others are clinically compromised even with a slight acidosis. Therefore factors other than acid base balance are important determinants of the clinical outcome. However severe acidosis (pH< 7.0) in the umbilical cord arterial blood has been associated with more babies having a poor neonatal outcome (Goldaber et al 1991). In practice severe acidosis in the fetus should be avoided and the first step is intrauterine resuscitation which will improve the condition of the fetus and prevent unnecessary intervention. Even if intervention becomes necessary, such resuscitative measures would contribute to a better outcome in the neonate.

Management of fetal distress

Alteration of maternal position   The fetus receives its oxygen and excretes the carbon dioxide via the placenta. Blood from the maternal side perfusing the placenta and the blood which is brought into the placenta from the fetus via the umbilical arteries are quite important for the maintenance of fetal oxygenation. Problems to the fetus surface when the maternal or fetal perfusion to the placenta is altered. Only a minority of labouring women exhibit hypotension when they are in the supine position (Howard et al 1953). But in the majority of women there is decreased venous return due to the pressure of the pregnant uterus on the inferior vena cava and the increased intraabdominal pressure. The decreased venous return leads to a reduced cardiac output which leads to diminished uterine blood flow. Therefore the position of the patient in labour is an important consideration especially when there is an abnormality of the FHR pattern like late decelerations indicating reduced perfusion in the retroplacental area. Correction to the left or right lateral position of the mother may alleviate the problem. This fact is of greater importance when patients have epidural anesthesia. The anesthesia may cause peripheral vasodilatation and further reduce the venous return and hence the cardiac output and uterine blood flow (Clark 1976). In these situations, in addition to adequate hydration, importance should be given to the positioning of the patient.

Altering the position of the patient may be adequate management in some cases of late decelerations provided they do not reappear. Variable decelerations due to cord compression are usually due to reduced amniotic fluid and appear with uterine contractions when the cord gets compressed against its own body, limbs or uterine wall. It may be feasible to alter the position of the mother and to avoid the cord compression and thus the variable decelerations in a few cases. Amnio-infusion is becoming a popular mode of therapy for variable decelerations and will be discussed later.

Hydration   It is clear that in a vast majority of cases fetal hypoxia and acidosis are due to inadequate utero-placental or umbilico-placental perfusion. In conditions where hypotension is expected (for example, epidural anesthesia, maternal bleeding) it is important to hydrate the patients well in order to prevent FHR changes. It is known that although there may not be overt maternal hypotension the uterine perfusion can be affected due to epidural. FHR changes are commoner with epidural analgesia than with other forms of pain relief (Schifrin 1972, Cohen and Schifrin 1978). In labour it is not unusual to find a shift in the baseline rate without any decelerations. This could be due to under hydration, ketosis, pain or anxiety in the mother. Adequate hydration will alleviate these FHR changes if they are due to inadequate hydration. Other abnormalities of the FHR like late decelerations may improve with improved placental perfusion. Hydration should constitute an integral part of intrauterine resuscitation unless there is a contraindication for infusing reasonable amounts of fluid (for example, 180–200 ml/hr). The consequence of infusing such volumes of fluid are discussed elsewhere.

Use of oxygen   Administering 100% oxygen by mask to the mother has been shown to be beneficial when fetal distress is encountered (Althabe et al 1967; Morishima et al 1975; Khazin et al 1971). Although it may increase the fetal oxygen concentration considerably in certain circumstances (Jackson and Piasecki 1983), the oxygen transfer at the placental interphase is more dependent on the perfusion on the fetal and maternal side of the placenta rather than on the lack of oxygen in maternal blood in most instances. Inhalation of oxygen by the mother will not increase the maternal oxygen level significantly. Even if it does there will not be any significant improvement in fetal oxygenation if the placental perfusion is affected. Therefore it is of primary importance to increase the perfusion on both sides of the placenta in order to increase the amount of oxygen to the fetus.

More information is available regarding oxygen therapy in the antenatal period than in labour. There is some worry about oxygen supplementation at least in growth retarded fetuses (Harding et al 1992). In the animal model, oxygen supplementation restores fetal pO_2 level in moderately but not severely growth retarded fetuses. It has also been observed that fetal oxygenation was worse than it had been before, immediately after discontinuation of oxygen therapy. This may be the reason for FHR decelerations after the discontinuation of hyperoxia in growth retarded fetuses (Bekedam et al 1991). Increase of cerebrovascular resistance as opposed to a decrease in the periphery during maternal oxygenation has been observed by Doppler velocimetry in human fetuses which are hypoglycemic (Arudini et al 1988). This might divert the greatly needed oxygen from the brain to other areas. Based on the available data it appears that at least in severely growth retarded fetuses additional oxygen may cause more harm than good. In fetuses which are not growth retarded the response might be different. Based on the available information it appears that oxygen therapy may result in a little improvement in selected patients and no improvement in severe IUGR fetuses. Oxygen should be used with other measures like hydration, positioning of the mother and tocolysis. It is best avoided in severely growth retarded fetuses. It is also important to recognise that the fetus does not benefit in any way if the decelerations are still persistent despite oxygen therapy. In such situations alternate action like hydration, amnioinfusion, FBS, or delivery should be considered.

Intravenous hypertonic dextrose   In the past, bolus doses of hypertonic dextrose were part of the management when fetal distress was diagnosed as it was thought to improve the fetal condition. But the use of dextrose and many other substrates has been shown to be of little value (Mann et al 1970). On the other hand, a rapid infusion of large amounts of dextrose has been reported to be associated with an impaired acid-base balance in the human fetus. Hyperglycemia and hyperlacticemia in both maternal venous and fetal scalp blood have been demonstrated if a glucose infusion is given for 30 min to maintain the maternal glucose levels at 10–13 mmol/l (Gardmark et al 1974). A 5% dextrose infusion prior to caesarean section has been shown to produce maternal and fetal hyperglycemia, hyperinsulinism and a fall in cord pH (Kenepp et al 1982; Morton et al 1985; Philipson et al 1987). These observations suggest that moderate hyperglycemia in a healthy normoxic fetus induces a reactive hyperinsulinemia leading to an increased glucose uptake, increased cellular oxidation, increased oxygen consumption and thus a relative hypoxemia and a lower pH. Studies on several animal models also bear witness to the association between hyperglycemia and hypoxemia (Robillard et al 1978; Carson et al 1980; Philips et al 1982; Philips et al 1984). In the fetal lamb, profound hyperglycemia (> 16 mmol/l) leads to hyperinsulinemia and severe lactic acidosis (Philips et al 1984). Alternatively, infusion of insulin leads to increased glucose uptake and decrease in fetal arterial oxygen concentration (Carson et al 1980). There appears to be little doubt about the association between profound hyperglycemia, lacticemia and hypoxia. It is estimated that an adverse metabolic effect is unlikely if the blood glucose concentration does not exceed 8.3 mmol/l (Robillard 1978).

In most labour wards, 5% dextrose or 5% dextrose saline infusion is used for hydration or as a vehicle for oxytocin infusion. To find out whether this would have any influence on the acid base balance, 5% dextrose was administered at a rate of 180 ml/hr (9g/h). The metabolic effects were compared with those seen when 0.9% normal saline was given at the same rate (Nordstrom and Arulkumaran 1993). Hyperglycemia was observed in the mother and fetus but hyperinsulinemia only in the mother. The dextrose infusion lowered the level of β-hydroxybutyrate in maternal and cord blood, but no differences were seen in lactate levels or the acid base balance in the cord arterial blood. The effect on β-hydroxybutyrate may have been due to the antiketogenic effect of hyperglycemia and hyperinsulinemia (Williamson 1992). It can be concluded that there is no risk of neonatal lactacidosis or hypoglycemia in the normoxemic normally grown fetus when 5% dextrose is given at a rate of 180 ml/hr (Nordstrom and Arulkumaran 1993). But in severe intrauterine growth retardation the lack of insulin response to hyperglycemia may block the cellular glucose uptake and promote an anerobic metabolism with sub-sequent acidosis (Nicolini et al 1990). Based on these studies, hydration or correction of hypovolemia by increasing the 5% dextrose infusion rate up to 180 ml/hr when fetal distress is encountered is unlikely to affect the acid base balance, but the administration of bolus doses of hypertonic dextrose may aggravate acidosis.

Amnioinfusion   In the presence of oligohydramnios the umbilical cord can get compressed with uterine contractions and the FHR trace may show variable decel-erations. If the trace shows good baseline variability the fetus is likely to be in good health. However if the decelerations continue the fetus may get hypoxic and acidotic and this condition will usually be reflected by a rising baseline rate and a reduction in the baseline variability (Figs 6.4–6.8). In order to abolish the variable decelerations the position of the mother could be altered. If the decelerations persist despite such a manoeuvre and if oligohydramnios was the cause as determined by a scan, amnioinfusion with warm normal saline may alleviate the cord compression and the variable decelerations will not appear. By such a manoeuvre it may be possible to deliver the fetus vaginally without compromising it.

Studies on prophylactic and therapeutic amnioinfusion in labour are encour-aging. A recent report claims amelioration of variable decelerations in 51% in the amnioinfusion group compared with only 4.2% in the control group (Miyazaki and Navarez 1985). In a randomised study where amnioinfusion was performed (n=43) for post-term pregnancy, variable decelerations, preterm labour and oligohydram-nios associated with intrauterine growth retardation, a lower incidence of caesarean section for fetal distress was recorded compared with the control group (n=57) (Owen et al 1990). In a similar study consisting of 60 patients where the recruitment for the trial was an amniotic fluid index of < 5 cm, the amnioinfusion group had significantly lower rates of meconium passage, severe variable decelerations, end stage bradycardias, and operative intervention for fetal distress (Strong et al, 1990). Amnioinfusion has also been used in the presence of meconium and it has been reported that it effectively decreases the frequency of thick meconium, neonatal acidemia, meconium below the vocal cords and the need for positive pressure ven-tilation (Sadovsky et al 1989; Wenstrom and Parsons 1989). Based on these studies it appears that amnioinfusion should be considered when there are simple variable decelerations or thick meconium stained amniotic fluid.

Reduction or abolition of uterine activity   Transient inhibition of uterine ac-tivity can be brought about by a bolus dose of a tocolytic drug. Inhibition of uterine activity is useful when there is abnormal uterine activity, fetal distress (Arias 1978) or prolonged fetal bradycardia (Ingemarsson et al 1985). It has also been used during complicated caesarean sections, external cephalic version at term (Arulkumaran et al 1986) and during the transport of a labouring woman (Ingemarsson 1982). It may be beneficially used when a theatre or anesthetist is not available for an emergency caesarean section. The bolus dose of a Beta mimetic drug used is small and is not associated with the adverse side effects which are reported with a prolonged infusion of such drugs used for inhibition of preterm labour (Ingemarsson and Arulkumaran 1985). The use of terbutaline, a selective β-2 receptor agonist has found favour in some centres but ritodrine, salbutamol and magnesium sulphate have been used in a similar manner (Lipshitz 1977; Reece et al 1984; Cohn et al 1982; Parer 1983).

An immediate (within 1–2 min) and pronounced inhibition of uterine activity in term labour can be achieved by an intravenous dose of 250 ug terbutaline diluted in 5 ml of saline and given over 5 min (Ingemarsson et al 1985). The mean duration for which the contractions are abolished vary, being 17.0 min in spontaneous labour and 14.6 min in augmented labour. A 83.7% reduction in uterine activity was observed in the first 15 min after the bolus dose of terbutaline in spontaneous labour. In augmented labour when the oxytocin was stopped and followed immediately by the bolus dose of terbutaline, a 75.3% reduction of uterine activity was observed in the first 15 min (Fig 6.17). The recovery of the uterine activity was gradual and was 50% of the preinjection value in spontaneous labour and 44% in augmented labour after 90 min. In augmented labour the cessation of the oxytocin infusion without the use of a tocolytic drug did not abolish uterine contractions, reduced the uterine activity gradually to 50% and sustained it at that level after 75 min (Fig 6.17).

In the presence of grossly abnormal FHR patterns the fetal scalp blood pH can drop drastically within 20–30 min in the presence of contractions (Fig 6.18). In these situations and in cases where fetal distress is related to uterine hyperactivity, inhibition of uterine activity may be of value as a temporary expedient.

The side effects of such therapy to the mother were mild and well tolerated. There was a slight drop in the systolic and diastolic blood pressure; the mean pulse rate increased from 84 to 109 per min in the first 15 min followed by a decline after that period. A pulse rate of 120–130 per min was observed in 25% of women for a short period (< 5 min) but none had a pulse rate > 130/min. None had signs of pulmonary edema but less than 10% experienced palpitations, tremors or shortness of breath. There was a slight rise in the FHR for a few min in < 20% of cases (Ingemarsson et al, 1985). It appears that the advantage gained by the abolition and reduction in uterine activity in situations of fetal distress far outweighs the minor side effects experienced. Since fetal cardiac output is largely dependent on the heart rate, prolonged bradycardia and repeated decelerations would compromise it. The use of a bolus dose of a tocolytic drug produces maternal tachycardia (mostly from peripheral vasodilatation) and increased cardiac output and thus increases uteroplacental perfusion. In addition, inhibition of uterine contractions reduces the interruption of blood flow to the placental bed.

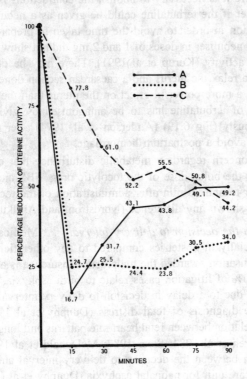

Fig 6.17 Percentage reduction of uterine activity in groups A, B and C. A: spontaneous
labour, terbutaline given. B: augmented labour, oxytocin infusion stopped,
terbutaline given. C: augmented labour, oxytocin infusion stopped, terbutaline
not given.

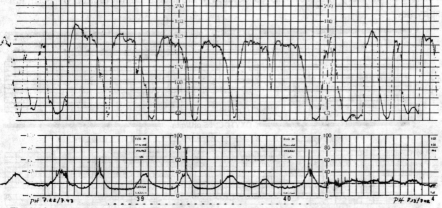

Fig 6.18 An abnormal FHR pattern with baseline rate of 150–160 bpm, no
accelerations, flat baseline (baseline variability < 5 bpm) and ominous
decelerations. Note the rapid decline of pH from 7.22 to 7.13 within 30 min.
Fetus with such a trace would benefit by a bolus dose of terbutaline which
would abolish the uterine contractions and prevent interruption of
uteroplacental perfusion as well as prevent cord compression.

A situation where it is necessary to abolish the contractions is an emergency and it would be easier if the terbutaline could be given as a nebuliser instead of an intravenous injection in order to avoid the time taken to prepare the injection. Terbutaline used as a nebuliser in doses of 1 and 2 mg did not show any significant inhibition of uterine activity (Kurup et al 1991). There may be occasions where terbutaline is given to relax the uterus and a caesarean section done within a short time. Terbutaline has a more powerful effect on the uterus than the oxytocic drug. Therefore the effect of terbutaline has to be antagonised by giving 1 to 2 mg propranalol intravenously (Fig 6.19) (Anderson et al, 1974) after the delivery of the baby in order to avoid a postpartum hemorrhage.

There is also concern regarding metabolic disturbance that can be brought about in the fetus by the bolus dose of the tocolytic drug. FBS and measurement of lactate levels prior to and 30 min after administration of the tocolytic drug for fetal distress has not shown any difference (Nordstrom and Arulkumaran 1993).

Reduction of delay in the decision to delivery interval   Medical litigation is on the increase especially in obstetrics compared to any other field of medicine. Parallel to the compensation awarded the malpractice insurance is also on the rise. It is estimated that 80% of litigation cases relate to birth asphyxia. Of these, two-third of the cases are due to a delay in decision to delivery interval rather than to the problem with the diagnosis of fetal distress (Dunphy et al 1991). Although there is a lack of correlation between fetal heart rate patterns and long term outcome for the neonate (Curzen et al 1984; Steer 1987; McDonald et al 1985), there is a significant association between the decision to delivery interval and admission to a neonatal intensive care unit for neonatal asphyxia. Dunphy et al (1991) reported the relative risk to be doubled between a 10 and 35 min interval although no correlation was found between the decision interval and 1 or 5 min Apgar scores or cord arterial and venous acid-base results. Similar observations have been made in the past (Choate and Lund 1968) and a more than 15 minutes delay between decision to delivery interval was associated with increased incidence of perinatal asphyxia.

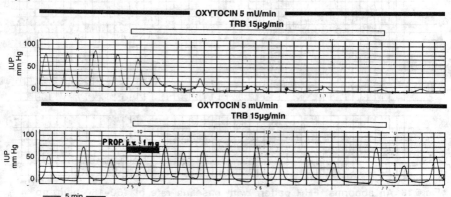

Fig 6.19   Record of intrauterine pressure (IUP). Infusion of terbutaline (TRB) 15 ug/min, effectively inhibits oxytocin stimulated (5 mu/min) uterine contractions (upper panel). Terbutaline infusion has no effect after pre-treatment with propranolol (PROP) 1 mg i.v. (lower panel).

The concept of immediate caesarean section   It is best that caesarean delivery be achieved within 10–15 min in cases of fetal distress in order to reduce the incidence of perinatal hypoxia. But this is not practical in most institutions due to the difficulty in getting a theatre or an anesthetist or because of the delay caused by the difficulty in intubating the patient. An effort should be made to deliver the fetus within 30 min of decision making. In certain circumstances like abruption, scar dehiscence, prolonged bradycardaia (FHR < 80 bpm for > 10 min) and cord prolapse it is best to deliver the fetus within 15 min. The request for immediate caesarean section as opposed to emergency caesarean section, meaning that the fetus needs to be delivered within 15 min, will make everyone concerned aware of the urgency. This may help to reduce severely hypoxic babies being born by shortening the decision to delivery interval.

Fetal distress is not a precise diagnosis in most instances, especially when it is based on an abnormal fetal heart rate pattern without the supportive evidence of acidosis by FBS. Even in situations where intervention is a must and where fetal distress like that due to cord prolapse is likely, some resuscitative measures must be undertaken. The aim should be to keep the cord warm and moist by reducing it into the vagina (to prevent the vessels going into spasm) and alleviate the pressure on the cord by the presenting part by adopting a knee chest position and filling the bladder with 500 cc saline using a Foley's catheter. Care must be taken to drain the bladder just prior to surgery. If the patient is fully dilated and instrumental delivery is possible it should be undertaken. If a caesarean delivery is indicated, a bolus dose of terbutaline will relax the uterus and prevent the contractions causing pressure on the cord.

Hypoxia and acidosis increase with progress of time with an abnormal FHR pattern. The rate of deterioration increases with an increasing number of abnormal features on the trace. Based on the FHR pattern and the suspected degree of hypoxia and acidosis, many resuscitative measures can be undertaken. Subsequent management would vary depending on the improvement of the FHR pattern, the clinical picture (for example, IUGR, thick meconium with scanty fluid, suspicion of abruption), parity, stage of labour and the rate of progress of labour. Interim measures would vary from simple manoeuvres like alteration of the maternal position or hydration to more complex procedures like amnio infusion or abolition of contractions by a bolus dose of a tocolytic drug. In the most severe cases of fetal distress, immediate operative delivery may be the only answer but resuscitative measures would improve the neonatal condition at birth. For optimal outcome to the fetus there must be team work between midwives, obstetricians, the theatre staff, the anesthetist and the neonatal pediatrician.

Acknowledgements
Authors would like to acknowledge Prof I. Ingemarsson (Department of Obstetrics and Gynecology, University of Lund, Sweden) for providing the Figs 6.1, 6.2, 6.17 and 6.18. Authors would like to thank Professor W Dunlop, Editor of *Fetal and Maternal Medicine Review* and the publishers Cambridge University Press for granting permission to reproduce the author's article with a few modifications.

References

Althabe O Jr, Schwarez RL, Pose SV et al 1967. Effects on fetal heart rate and fetal pO_2 of oxygen administration to the mother. *Am J Obstet Gynecol* 98:858-870.

Anderson KE, Ingemarsson I, Persson CGA 1974. Effects of terbutaline on human uterine motility at term. *Acta Obstet Gynecol Scand Suppl* 1-8.

Arias F 1978. Intrauterine resuscitation with terbutaline: a method for the management of acute intrapartum fetal distress. *Am J Obstet Gynecol* 131:39-.

Arudini D, Rizzo G, Mancuso S, Romanini C 1988. Short term effects of maternal oxygen administration on blood flow velocity waveforms in healthy and growth retarded fetuses. *Am J Obstet Gynecol* 159:1077-1080.

Arulkumaran S, Chua S, Ingemarsson I 1986. External cephalic version in current obstetric practice. *Sing J Obstet Gynecol* 17:78-81.

Arulkumaran S, Ingemarsson I, Ratnam SS 1987. Fetal heart rate response to scalp stimulation as a test of fetal wellbeing in labour. *Asia Oceania J Obstet Gynecol* 13: 131-135.

Arulkumaran S, Ingemarsson I 1990. Appropriate technology in intrapartum fetal surveillance. In: John Studd, ed. Progress in Obstetrics and Gynecology. Vol 8. London: Churchill Livingstone, pp 127-140.

Arulkumaran S, Lilja H, Lindecrantz K, Ratnam SS, Thavarasah AS, Rosen KG 1990. Fetal ECG waveform analysis should improve fetal surveillance during labor. *J Perinat Med* 18:13-21.

Arulkumaran S, Montan S 1991. The fetus at risk in labour - identification and management. In: Ratnam SS, Ng SC, Sen DK, Arulkumaran S, eds. Contributions to Obstetrics and Gynecology, Vol 1. Singapore: Churchill Livingstone, pp 179-190.

Arulkumaran S, Montan S, Ingemarsson I, Gibb DMF, Paul RH, Schiffrin B, Spencer JAD, Steer PJ 1993. Traces of you - Clinician's guide to fetal trace interpretation. Hewlett Packard GmbH, Germany. Publication No. 50 gn - 7 n 35 EE.

Beard RW, Filshie GM, Knight CA, Roberts GM 1971. The significance of the changes in the continuous fetal heart rate in the first stage of labour. *J Obstet Gynaecol Br C'wlth* 78:865-881.

Bekedam DJ, Muller EJH, Snijders RJM, Visser GHA 1991. The effects of maternal hyperoxia on fetal breathing movements, body movements and heart rate variation in growth retarded fetuses. *Early Hum Dev* 27:223-232.

Carson BS, Philipps AF, Simmons MA, Battaglia FC, Meschia G 1980. Effects of a sustained insulin infusion upon glucose uptake and oxygenation of the ovine fetus. *Pediatr Res* 14:147-152.

Choate JW, Lund CJ 1968. Emergency caesarean section. An analysis of maternal and fetal results in 177 operations. *Am J Obstet Gynecol* 100:703-714.

Clark RB 1976. Prevention of spinal hypotension associated with caesarean section. *Anesthesiology* 45:67-674.

Cohen WR, Schifrin BS 1978. Clinical management of fetal hypoxemia. In: Friedman E, ed. Management of Labor. pp 163-188.

Cohn HE, Piasechi GJ, Jackson BT 1982. The effect of β adrenergic stimulation on fetal cardiovascular function during hypoxemia. *Am J Obstet Gynecol* 144:810.

Curzen P, Bekir JS, McLintock DG, Patel M 1984. Reliability of cardiotocography in predicting a baby's condition at birth. *Br Med J* 289:1345-1347.

Dennis J, Johnson A, Mutch L, Yudkin P, Johnson P 1989. Acid base status at birth and neurodevelopmental outcome at four and one-half years. *Am J Obstet Gynecol* 161:213-220.

Dunphy BC, Robinson JN, Sheil OM, Nicholls JSD, Gillmer MDG 1991. Caesarean section for fetal distress, the interval from decision to delivery, and the relative risk of poor neonatal condition. *J Obstet Gynecol* 11:241-244.

Fleming JEE, Raymond SPW, Smith GCS, Whitfield CR 1986. The measurement of fetal systolic time intervals; lessons from ultrasound. *Eur J Obstet Gynecol Reprod Biol* 23:289-294.

Gardmark S, Gennser G, Jacobson L, Rooth G, Thorell J 1974. Influence on fetal carbohydrate and fat metabolism and on acid base balance by glucose administration to the mother during labour. Thesis, Malmo, Sweden 1974, Sweden: Studentlitteratur Lund.

Gibb DMF, Arulkumaran S 1992. Fetal Monitoring in Practice. Oxford: Butterworth Heineman, p 21.

Goldaber GK, Gilstrap LC, Leveno KJ, Dax JS, McIntire DD 1991. Pathologic fetal acidemia. *Obstet Gynecol* 78:1103-1106.

Harding JE, Owens JA, Robinson JS 1992. Should we try to supplement growth retarded fetuses? A cautionary tale. *Br J Obstet Gynecol* 99:707-710.

Howard BK, Goodson JH, Mengert WF 1953. Supine hypotensive syndrome in late pregnancy. *Obstet Gynecol* 1:371-377.

Ingemarsson I, Ingemarsson E, Spencer JAD 1993. Practical guide to fetal heart rate monitoring. Oxford: Oxford University Press.

Ingemarsson I, Arulkumaran S 1989. Reactive fetal heart rate response to vibroacoustic stimulation in fetuses with low scalp blood pH. *Br J Obstet Gynecol* 96:562-565.

Ingemarsson I, Arulkumaran S 1986. Fetal acid base balance in low risk patients in labor. *Am J Obstet Gynecol* 155:66-69.

Ingemarsson I, Arulkumaran S, Ratnam SS 1985. Single injection of terbutaline in term labor. I. Effect on fetal pH in cases with prolonged bradycardia. *Am J Obstet Gynecol* 153:859-865.

Ingemarsson I, Arulkumaran S 1985. Beta receptor agonists in current obstetric practice. In: Chiswick M, ed. Recent Advances in Perinatal Medicine Vol 2. London: Churchill Livingstone, pp 39-58.

Ingemarsson I 1982. Beta receptor agonists in obstetrics. *Acta Obstet Gynecol Scand: (Suppl)* 108: 29.

Ingemarsson I, Arulkumaran S, Ratnam SS 1985. Single injection of terbutaline in term labor. II.

Effect on uterine activity. *Am J Obstet Gynecol* 153:865-869.

Jackson BT, Piasecki GJ 1983. Fetal Oxygenation. In: Cohen WR and Friedman EA., eds. Management of Labor. Baltimore, USA: University Park Press, pp 117-142.

Johnson N, Johnson VA, Fisher J, Jobbings B, Bannister J, Lilford RJ 1991. Fetal monitoring with pulse oximetry. *Br J Obstet Gynecol* 98:36-41.

Kenepp NB, Shelley WC, Gabbe SG, Kumar S, Stanley CA, Gutsche BB 1982. Fetal and neonatal hazards of maternal hydration with 5% dextrose before caesarean section. *Lancet* 1:1150-1152.

Khazin AF, Hon EH, Hehre FW 1971. Effects of maternal hyperoxia on the fetus. *Am J Obstet Gynecol* 109:628-637.

Kurup A, Arulkumaran S, Tay D, Ingemarsson I, Ratnam SS 1991. Can terbutaline be used as a nebuliser instead of intravenous injection for inhibition of uterine activity? *Gynecol Obstet Invest* 32:84-87.

Lipshitz J 1977. Use of a B sympathomimetic drug as a temporizing measure in the treatment of acute fetal distress. *Am J Obstet Gynecol* 129:31.

Loh FH, Arulkumaran S 1993. ECG waveform analysis in intrapartum fetal monitoring. *Austr NZ J Obstet Gynecol* 33:39-44.

MacLachlan NA, Spencer JAD, Harding K, Arulkumaran S 1992. Fetal acidemia, the cardiotocograph and the T/QRS ratio of the fetal ECG in labour. *Br J Obstet Gynecol* 99:26-31.

Malcus P, Gudmundsson S, Marsal K, Ho HK, Vengadasalam D, Ratnam SS 1991. Umbilical artery doppler velocimetry as a labour admission test. *Obstet Gynecol* 77:10-16.

Mann LI, Prichard JW, Symmes D 1970. The effect of glucose loading on the fetal response to hypoxia. *Am J Obstet Gynecol* 107:610-618.

McDonald D, Grant A, Sheridan Pereira M, Boylan P, Chalmers I 1985. The Dublin randomised controlled trial of intrapartum fetal heart rate monitoring. *Am J Obstet Gynecol* 152:524-539.

Miyazaki FS, Navarez F 1985. Saline amnioinfusion for relief of repetitive variable decelerations; a prospective randomised study. *Am J Obstet Gynecol* 153:301-306.

Morishima H, Daniel S, Richards R, James LS 1975. The effect of increased maternal pO$_2$ upon the fetus during labor. *Am J Obstet Gynecol* 123:257-264.

Morton KE, Jackson MC, Gillmer MDG 1985. A comparison of the effects of four intravenous solutions for the treatment of ketonuria during labour, *Br J Obstet Gynecol* 92:473-479.

Nicolini U, Hubinont C, Santolaya J, Fisk NM, Rodeck CH 1990. Effects of fetal glucose challenge in normal and growth retarded fetuses. *Hormon Meta Res* 22:426-430.

Nordstrom L, Arulkumaran S 1993. Lactate in fetal surveillance. *Sing J Obstet Gynecol* 24:87-97.

Owen J, Henson BV, Hauth JC 1990. A prospective randomised study of saline solution amnioinfusion. *Am J Obstet Gynecol* 162:1146-1149.

Page FO, Martin JN, Palmer SM et al 1986. Correlation of neonatal acid base status with Apgar scores and fetal heart rate tracings. *Am J Obstet Gynecol* 154:1306-1311.

Parer JT 1983. The influence of β adrenergic activity on fetal heart rate and the umbilical circulation during hypoxia in fetal sheep. *Am J Obstet Gynecol* 147:592-.

Philips AF, Dubin JW, Matty PJ, Raye JR 1982. Arterial hypoxemia and hyperinsulinemia in the chronically hyperglycemic fetal lamb. *Pediatr Res* 16:653-658.

Philips AF, Porte PJ, Stabinsky S, Rosenkrantz TS, Raye JR 1984. Effects on chronic hyperglycemia upon oxygen consumption in the ovine uterus and conceptus. *J Clin Invest* 74:279-286.

Philipson EH, Satish C, Kalhan MB, Margo M, Riha RN, Pimentel R 1987. Effects of maternal glucose infusion on fetal acid base status in human pregnancy. *Am J Obstet Gynecol* 157:866-873.

Reece EA, Chervenak FA, Romero R, Hobbins JC 1984. Magnesium sulfate in the management of acute intrapartum fetal distress. *Am J Obstet Gynecol* 148:104.

Robillard JE, Sessions C, Kennedy RL, Smith FG 1978. Metabolic effects of constant hypertonic glucose infusion in well-oxygenated fetuses. *Am J Obstet Gynecol* 130:199-203.

Ruth VJ, Ravio KO 1988. Perinatal brain damage: predictive value of metabolic acidosis and the Apgar score. *Br Med J* 297:24-27.

Sadovsky Y, Amon E, Bade ME, Petrie RH 1989. Prophylactic amnioinfusion during labor complicated by meconium: A preliminary report. *Am J Obstet Gynecol* 161: 613-617.

Schifrin BS 1972. Fetal heart rate patterns following epidural anesthesia and oxytocin infusion during labour. *J Obstet Gynecol Br C'wlth* 79:332-339.

Steer PJ 1982. Has the expression 'fetal distress' outlived its usefulness? *Br J Obstet Gynecol* 89:690-693.

Steer PJ 1987. Fetal monitoring - present and future. *Eur J Obstet Gynecol Rep Biol* 24:112-117.

Strong TH, Hetzler G, Sarno AP, Paul RH 1990. Prophylactic intrapartum amnioinfusion; a randomised clinical trial. *Am J Obstet Gynecol* 162:1370-1374.

Sykes GS, Molloy PM, Johnson P, Stirrat GM, Turnbull AC 1983. Fetal distress and the condition of the newborn infants. *Br Med J* 287:943-945.

Wenstrom KD, Parsons MT 1989. The prevention of meconium aspiration in labor using amnioinfusion. *Obstet Gynecol* 73:647-651.

Westgate J, Harris M, Gurnshow JSH, Green KR, 1992. Randomised trial of cardiotocography alone or with ST waveform analysis for intrapartum monitoring. *Lancet* 34:194-198.

Williamson DH 1992. Ketone body production and metabolism in the fetus and newborn. In: Polin RA and Fox WW, eds. Fetal and neonatal physiology. London: WB Saunders Co.

7

Fluid Management in Labour

V Annapoorna
S Arulkumaran

Mothers in labour may require intravenous fluid therapy for various reasons. The choice of fluid and the amount administered should be appropriate to the clinical situation. Colloids, crystalloids and many drugs used in therapy cross the placenta readily and equilibrate with the fetal vascular compartment. Volume, energy, hematological and electrolyte imbalance may occur with fluid administration because of the pre-existing blood volume and hematological changes brought about by the pregnancy. Any such imbalance could affect the mother and the fetus during labour and in the immediate post-delivery period. The fluid selected should be of maximum benefit with minimum side effects. Consideration should be given to additive drugs in the fluid and to medical or obstetric disorders in the mother. This chapter evaluates the use of various intravenous solutions used in labour in reference to the points stated above.

Blood volume

It is important to understand the various maternal hematological changes that occur in normal and abnormal pregnancy in order to provide supportive and coordinated care during pregnancy and the intrapartum period. Plasma volume, red cell mass and cardiac output are all increased in pregnancy. Plasma volume increases by 40% compared to the red cell mass which increases by 20–30%. This hypervolemia per se helps in combating the hazards of acute blood loss which cause dramatic changes in the blood volume immediately after delivery.

Ketonuria and dehydration

Maternal ketonuria is a common indication for fluid administration during labour. Increased energy consumption coupled with partial starvation gives rise to ketonuria. Maternal ketonuria was thought to cause impaired myometrial function and dysfunctional labour (Dumouline and Foulkes 1984), although correction of ketonuria does not improve the progress of labour (Dahlenburgh et al 1980; Singhi et al 1982). Treating ketonuria during labour with infusions of 10% dextrose in water, or excessive volumes of 5% dextrose has been shown to be dangerous, causing hyponatremia in the mother (Evans et al 1986) and causing rebound hypoglycemia (Kenepp et al 1982) and hyponatremia (Tarnow-Mordi et al 1981) in the neonate. Hyponatremia in infants impairs erythrocyte membrane function. This alters the intracellular electrolyte content and pH, predisposing to hemolysis (Zeilder and Kim 1979), and thus increasing bilirubin levels. An increased osmotic fragility (Arieff and Guisado 1976), impaired erythrocyte, leucocyte and neuronal functions were also noted (Kenepp et al 1980).

Morton et al (1985) compared the effects of one litre of normal saline, Hartmann's solution, 5% dextrose and 10% dextrose in women in whom ketonuria was detected during the first stage of labour. They concluded that the rapid infusion of dextrose or Hartmann's solution produced significant elevation in blood lactate and pyruvate concentrations, and therefore recommended that normal saline be used. However in 1989 Piquard et al showed that these adverse events did not occur if the glucose infusion rate was restricted to 30 g per hour. If more than 500 ml of a 5% dextrose solution are required, it would be wiser to use fluids containing sodium (Spencer et al 1981).

Regional analgesia

The chemical sympathectomy that follows epidural blockade can cause hypotension, especially if the mother is hypovolemic. Kenepp et al (1982) in a randomised study concluded that the infusion of dextrose in normal saline gave no advantage over a 5% dextrose infusion, and neither of them decreased the incidence of hypotension. They inferred that rapid infusions of dextrose are not advisable if delivery is imminent and in diabetic patients because they increase fetal insulin levels. It is common practice to preload with 500–1000 ml normal saline to limit the fall in blood pressure when the vascular compartment expands in response to sympathetic blockade.

Induction and augmentation of labour

Induction and augmentation of labour is by far the most common indication for the use of intravenous fluids. The pharmacologic agents for induction include oxytocin and prostaglandin. The widespread use of these drugs and the understanding of the associated complications are essential for the care of the women undergoing induction or augmentation. Hyperstimulation of the uterus may occur either as a result of high dosage or increased sensitivity of the uterus to these drugs with progress of labour. Another important property of oxytocin to be considered is its antidiuretic effect.

When oxytocin infusions are prolonged and the infusion rate approaches 40 mμ/min, there is a dramatic drop in the urinary output and potential exists for water intoxication (Musacchio 1990). Rapid intravenous infusion of oxytocin has been noted to cause severe maternal hypotension, increased heart rate, venous return and cardiac output and electrocardiographic changes that are indicative of cardiac ischaemia (American Society of Hospital Pharmacists 1993). However these effects should not occur when oxytocin is properly diluted and administered by an infusion pump.

Allergic reactions including anaphylaxis can occur and may be fatal. The injudicious use of oxytocin has resulted in maternal deaths due to a hypertensive episode and subarachnoid hemorrhage (American Society of Hospital Pharmacists 1993). Derangements of neonatal biochemistry leading to neonatal seizures can occur in severely disturbed cases.

Prior to initiating infusion, baseline vital signs (that is, temperature, pulse, respiration, and blood pressure) and fetal and uterine status should be assessed. The use of continuous cardiotocographic monitoring permits the evaluation of the fetal heart rate and strength of uterine activity. With current technology, fetal scalp electrode is rarely necessary whilst use of the intrauterine pressure catheter gives more accurate information about uterine activity but may not be necessary in routine clinical practice (Arulkumaran 1994).

It has been a tradition in most obstetric units to use glucose solution of a 5% strength for oxytocin infusion. Intravenous electrolyte free solution significantly decreases maternal serum sodium levels, and the concurrent use of oxytocin further reduces them (Spencer et al 1981). Cord sodium levels are reduced with the use of oxytocin and electrolyte free solutions. When oxytocin is used for the induction of labour, more than 500 ml of fluid vehicle may be required, hence the use of fluids containing sodium is advisable (Spencer et al 1981). Higher strength oxytocin solutions would limit the volume of infusion to the mother, but precise control of the infusion by a syringe or a peristaltic infusion pump becomes mandatory to avoid hyperstimulation of the uterus, fetal distress and the remote possibility of uterine rupture. Oxytocin-induced hyperstimulation has become a major subject of litigation in the USA (Fuchs 1985). To avoid such problems the ideal dose of oxytocin which would effect vaginal delivery in optimal time without compromising the fetus should be infused. The medication sticker on the oxytocin solution should reflect the concentration of oxytocin used.

The infusion should be initiated with a low dose since the effective dose varies greatly among women. Oxytocin infusion rates normally start at 2–6 mU/min and variably (arithmetically or logarithimically) increase at 15–30 min intervals, often to a maximum of around 32 mU/min or until satisfactory labour has been established. Oxytocin infusion is titrated by determining the frequency and duration of uterine contractions. The intensity may be considered when an intrauterine catheter is used. Three factors are continually assessed in order to determine a patient's therapeutic oxytocin dose: uterine activity, fetal response, and cervical effacement and dilatation. The optimal uterine activity to be achieved consists of uterine contractions with a frequency of one every 2 to 3 minutes with each contraction lasting for 40 to 90 sec (Arulkumaran et al 1991). If facilities permit use of an intrauterine catheter, an intensity of 40 to 90 mm Hg may be aimed for (Petrie and Williams 1986) and a resting tone of less than 20 mm Hg. Should hyperstimulation occur, the infusion is decreased or discontinued. The definitive measurement of the response to adequate oxytocin dosage is cervical dilatation which should progress by at least 1 cm/hour.

Water intoxication, a complication of prolonged high dose oxytocin administration, is prevented by using balanced salt intravenous solutions, limiting the total dose of oxytocin, monitoring fluid intake and output, and observing patients at risk for signs and symptoms of weakness, restlessness, nausea, vomiting, diarrhoea, polyuria or oliguria and seizures.

In summary, the ongoing assessment of the patient undergoing induction or augmentation of labour consists of maternal vital signs, uterine activity, fetal response, cervical dilatation, and observation for conscientious fluid management.

Work on induction of labour spanning the last three decades has found that 11 to 12 mU/min of oxytocin satisfies the above requirement in most cases (Caldeyro-Barcia et al 1957, Steer et al 1985, Arulkumaran et al 1985). Based on these studies, an oxytocin regime is suggested to avoid possible hyperstimulation due to a higher strength, and fluid overload due to a dilute solution (Thavarasah and Arulkumaran 1988) (Table 1).

Table 1: Oxytocin regime for induction or augmentation of labour

---

Oxytocin 2.5 U in 500 cc of normal saline

Perform cardiotocography for 20 min to check fetal condition and frequency of contractions

Start with 10 drops/min (2 or 2.5 mu/min)

- Escalation of dose every 30 min is advised as follows using a peristaltic infusion pump until 4–5 painful contractions are achieved every 10 min

Giving set 1 cc = 20 drops   1 cc = 15 drops

2.5 units oxytocin in 500 cc of N Saline

10 drops/min = 2.5 mu/min	10 drops/min = 3.3 mu/min	
20 drops/min = 5.0 mu/min	20 drops/min = 6.6 mu/min	
30 drops/min = 7.5 mu/min	30 drops/min = 9.9 mu/min	
40 drops/min = 10.0 mu/min	40 drops/min = 13.2 mu/min	
50 drops/min = 12.5 mu/min	50 drops/min = 16.5 mu/min	

5 units oxytocin in 500 cc of N Saline

30 drops/min = 15 mu/min	30 drops/min = 19.8 mu/min
40 drops/min = 20 mu/min	40 drops/min = 26.4 mu/min
50 drops/min = 25 mu/min	50 drops/min = 33.0 mu/min

10 units oxytocin in 500 cc of N Saline

30 drops/min = 30 mu/min	30 drops/min = 39.9 mu/min
40 drops/min = 40 mu/min	40 drops/min = 26.3 mu/min
50 drops/min = 50 mu/min	50 drops/min = 33.0 mu/min

Escalation of dose undertaken despite 4–5 contractions in 10 min if the progress in cervical dilatation is unsatisfactory at 3 hourly review. The dose is limited, halved (even to 5 drops/min) or discontinued if signs of hyperstimulation or evidence of fetal distress occur.

Normal saline had less risk of hyponatremia and fetal acidosis. Check input/output every 4 to 6 hours and urine albumen and ketones with every specimen of urine passed.

If intrauterine catheter is used, oxytocin can be titrated till activity values increase to 1,500 kPas/15 minutes in multiparae and 1,750 kPas/15 minutes in nulliparae unless limited by hyperstimulation or fetal heart rate changes.

Fetal distress

Romney and Gabel (1966) suggested that the infusion of hypertonic dextrose is therapeutic in the treatment of fetal distress. Plasma lactate concentration in the fetal lamb rises and the pH falls with increasing glucose concentrations, especially when there is fetal hypoxia, due to its influence on the carboxylic cycle (Shelley et al 1975). Similar observations were made by Kenepp et al (1982). Myers (1978) demonstrated that a hypoxic insult to the fetal rhesus monkey is less damaging to the fetal brain when this follows a period of maternal starvation compared with its effect after glucose infusion. Oxygen therapy to the mother improves the fetal heart rate changes (Pearson 1982) but its value as a definitive therapeutic modality is questioned (Arulkumaran 1994b). Current opinion forbids the use of hypertonic glucose or fructose infusions in situations of fetal distress.

Tocolytic therapy for preterm labour

Betamimetics are potent drugs and require vigilant maternal and fetal assessment during intravenous use. Pulmonary edema is a serious and potentially fatal complication and the reported incidence has been studied by Ingemarsson and Arulkumaran (1985). Although the cause is not completely understood, most reported cases had normal saline as the fluid vehicle for tocolytic therapy, fluid overload and polypharmacy. The use of betamimetics causes an increase in circulating volume due to its effect in causing increased activity of the renin aldosterone system (Lamminstanta and Erkolla 1979) and increased production of antidiuretic hormone with resultant retention of water and sodium (Schrier et al 1972). The occurrence of side effects may be more frequent during increases in the infusion rate than during the maintenance of infusion (Caritis et al 1980).

To prevent side effects, an assiduous follow up of mother and fetus is necessary. Vital signs are monitored at least half hourly during infusion, saline should be avoided and the quantity of fluid infused closely monitored. Monitoring of the fetal heart rate and uterine activity should continue throughout the infusion. The patient must have nothing orally during the tocolytic infusion. Output records should be maintained and auscultation of lung fields should be done. The tocolytic infusion should be discontinued or decreased if there is maternal tachycardia (a pulse rate of more than 130/min), chest pain, discomfort or breathlessness. Diuretics should be administered when there are symptoms of overload.

Fetal tachycardia, arrhythmias, neonatal hypoglycemia, hypokalemia, and hyperinsulinemia following the maternal use of beta receptor agonists have been reported (Brazy and Pupkin 1979; Epstein et al 1979). Fetal heart rate monitoring during infusion and a close neonatal check up over the first 24 hours following delivery is advisable.

Diabetes

Adequate control of maternal blood sugar levels immediately before and during labour is essential to prevent diabetic ketoacidosis in the mother and excessive fetal insulin secretion, causing hypoglycemia in the neonate (Light et al 1972).

Generally, a 5% dextrose saline solution to provide 5–10 g of glucose and 75–150 ml of fluid per hour is administered throughout labour (Nelson 1984) and the patient has nothing orally. Glucose utilisation during labour is about 2.5 mg/kg/

min (Jovanovic et al 1981). Careful monitoring of blood glucose during labour is important in order to determine the need for insulin therapy. Often well controlled diabetics do not require insulin during labour. The blood sugar values are generally kept at 80–120 mg/dl (or 4.4–6.6 mmol/l) in order to prevent ketosis. If the blood glucose level exceeds 140 mg/dl (7.8 mmol/l) and continues to rise, an intravenous infusion of insulin should be considered. The dose of insulin varies and is based on blood glucose determinations 4 to 6 hourly and if necessary on an hourly basis. Only soluble (regular) insulin is administered intravenously because of its rapid half life. To prevent the development of hypoglycemia after delivery, the glucose infusion should be continued and the administration of insulin discontinued. Further insulin requirements would depend on the blood sugar levels of the mother.

The use of oxytocin for induction or augmentation should follow appropriate protocols. When used concomitantly with insulin, oxytocin should be mixed in a separate intravenous bottle and not with insulin. Two separate infusion control devices will be necessary; one for the insulin containing fluid and one for the oxytocin containing fluid.

Diabetic ketoacidosis represents a state of acutely decompensated diabetes and is classified as mild, moderate, or severe (Table 2). Immediate goals include the replacement of insulin, fluids, and electrolytes. After the patient is rapidly assessed and blood glucose and urine ketones are evaluated, large amounts of intravenous fluids without glucose are rapidly administered to reduce dehydration and to replace electrolytes. Normal saline is the usual fluid of choice, and 1 to 2 litres are administered over .30 to 60 minutes. Intravenous fluids are then administered at 200 to 250 ml/hour while assessment continues for intravascular volume. Invasive hemodynamic monitoring is preferable to monitor fluid replacement and to prevent shock from decreased intravascular volume or pulmonary edema from excessive replacement. Glucose containing fluids (for example, 5% to 10% dextrose in water) is administered when blood glucose falls to 200 mg/dl, to prevent hypoglycemia.

Table 2:   Diabetic ketoacidosis classification

	Total CO_2	*pH*
Mild	21–22 mEq/litre and/or	> 7.30
Moderate	11–20 mEq/litre and/or	7.10–7.30
Severe	< 10 mEq/litre and/or	< 7.10

Intravenous insulin is administered concomitantly with a starting dose of 12 U/hour but must be titrated according to blood glucose levels. Once blood glucose falls to 200 mg/dl, intravenous insulin is continued at a lower infusion rate. Bicarbonate and potassium replacements are often necessary and are started if the pH is less than 7.10 and/or the potassium level is < 3.0 mEq/l respectively.

Preeclampsia and hypertensive disorders
Maternal blood volume increases progressively with an increasing gestational period (Hytten and Paintin 1963; Pirani et al 1973) and is generally in proportion to

the size of the conceptus in normal pregnancy. In preeclampsia the blood pressure is elevated, there is little if any increase in blood volume and albumin is low in plasma (Studd et al 1970, Horne et al 1970). Renal leak of albumin is known, but extravascular leak has not been substantiated (Chesley 1978). This leads to low oncotic pressure (Benedetti and Carlson 1979), resulting in fluid loss from the vascular compartment.

Although the incidence of renal damage may be rare, this should be taken into consideration before initiating fluid administration in cases of preeclampsia. Oliguria may result from three underlying mechanisms (Clark et al 1986). The first subset includes patients whose oliguria is secondary to intravascular fluid volume depletion. Hemodynamic monitoring in this subset characteristically demonstrates a low wedge pressure, moderately increased systemic vascular resistance, a low-to-normal cardiac output, and hyperdynamic left ventricular function. Volume infusion raises the wedge pressure and cardiac output, decreases systemic vascular resistance and may increase the urine output. The second subset includes patients with isolated renal arterial spasm. These patients demonstrate a persistent oliguria when the measured intravascular volume would normally be sufficient to perfuse the kidneys. Those in whom systemic vascular resistance measurements remain in the normal range can be managed with pharmacologic pre- and/or afterload reduction. The third subset includes patients with increased systemic vascular resistance, elevated wedge pressure and a low cardiac output. Oliguria develops from vasospasm in preeclampsia with depressed left ventricular function and low cardiac output. Volume restriction and afterload reduction will be helpful in correcting oliguria in this group. Preload refers to the initial myocardial muscle fibre length and is determined by intraventricular volume and pressure. As preload increases in a normal heart, the cardiac output increases. A higher preload than normal is required to maintain adequate cardiac output in a failing heart. *Afterload* refers to ventricular wall tension during systole and is dependent primarily on pulmonary and systemic vascular resistance. In a normal heart, there is an inverse relationship between afterload and cardiac output.

Sodium retention with increase of total body sodium occurs in preeclampsia (Chesley 1966), but sodium restriction and administration of sodium free solutions are ineffective in mobilising edema, because of the good compensatory capacity of the intrarenal regulation mechanism and humoral control by the renin aldosterone system (Chesley 1978). Hyponatremia is usually a consequence of salt restriction or the use of diuretics. Arias (1984) advocates a 50% correction of the sodium deficit by using a 3% sodium chloride solution. Full correction may not be advisable, as sodium excretion is delayed to twice the normal time in preeclamptic patients compared with normal pregnant women when hypertonic saline solution is infused (Chesley et al 1958).

Crystalloid solutions are the mainstay of fluid therapy in the preeclamptic patient even if the central oncotic pressure is low. Administration of colloid solutions can transiently elevate oncotic pressure but may compound the problem by allowing the intravascular fluid into interstitial space through the damaged capillaries.

Oxytocin has been used to advantage without complications despite its anti-diuretic properties. Close monitoring of fluid intake and output must be undertaken in order to prevent an imbalance of hydrostatic and oncotic forces that can potentiate the occurrence of pulmonary edema.

Hypovolemia

Bleeding in obstetric patients requires prompt and adequate treatment to prevent disseminated intravascular coagulopathy which could otherwise result in maternal mortality and morbidity. Even though the rational treatment is blood transfusion, the risks of blood administration include transfusion reaction, transmission of infectious disease, and circulatory overload.

At times, the situation may be so acute that transient restoration of blood volume by other fluids becomes necessary to prevent shock due to hypovolemia. The choice of intravenous fluids lies between crystalloids such as normal saline, Hartman's or Ringer lactate, or colloidal solutions like dextran, hydroxyethyl starch or gelatin. If crystalloids are used, they must be three to four times the volume of estimated blood loss, because they stay in the vascular compartment for a shorter time than colloids. Plasma substitutes such as dextran, gelatin and starch solutions may cause severe reactions including anaphylactic shock and cardio-respiratory arrest (Doenicke et al 1977) even though this is rare. Dextran is known to affect platelet function and to interfere with blood grouping and cross matching. Moss (1972) and Carey et al (1970) suggested that hypovolemic shock should be managed initially by transfusing a crystalloid solution like normal saline followed by blood or fresh frozen plasma. More recent work by Hauser et al (1980) has shown that solutions containing albumin are superior to crystalloids in patients postoperatively shocked by hypovolemia.

Letsky (1985) advocates polygeline (Hemacel solution) as the first method of fluid resuscitation, because it is iso-oncotic, does not interfere with platelet function or affect subsequent blood grouping and cross matching and improves renal function. Although polygeline is considered to be non-immunogenic and does not trigger the production of antibodies in humans (Letsky 1985), reactions due to histamine release have been reported with the use of this compound (Lorenz et al 1976), hence caution should be exercised if it is to be used. Freeman (1979) reported a fatality following its use. It is easily available and has a long shelf life with minimal storage requirements. Regardless of the substitute used, a central venous pressure line is useful for optimal replacement of the lost blood volume.

Platelet transfusion is generally not recommended except as a prophylaxis in the clinically stable patient with a count of less than 10 to 20,000/L or in the postoperative patient with a count of under 50,000/L (FDA Drug Bulletin 1989). Transfusion of fresh frozen plasma strictly for volume replacement is not indicated; however it is advocated for the replacement of clotting factors (FDA Drug Bulletin 1989). Cryoprecipitate provides an alternative for the replacement of clotting factors by fresh frozen plasma for the volume restricted patient, since each unit is only 15–20 ml. The disadvantage posed by cryoprecipitate is that it does not contain antithrombin III. More discussions regarding the use of crystalloids, colloids, clotting factors and blood are discussed on the chapters dealing with postpartum hemorrhage and eclampsia.

AIDS

With regard to universal practices, nursing care for patients identified with HIV infection does not differ from that for nonidentified patients. Universal precautions were recommended by the CDC for use with all patients in 1987 (MMWR supplement 1987). Patients with AIDS have increased incidence of multisystem compromise. For patients with gastrointestinal complications, accurate monitoring of intake and output are essential, and laboratory values are monitored for electrolyte imbalance. Adequate hydration and acid base balance maintenance is essential throughout labour.

In present day obstetrics, induction rates of 30% and augmentation rates reaching 50% are not uncommon (McNaughton 1980; O'Driscoll et al 1984). Induction of labour with an unfavourable cervix leading to long labour with dehydration, ketonuria and fetal distress is commonplace (Arulkumaran et al 1985). Fluids are administered for these conditions and for similar obstetric interventions, along with potent pharmacological agents. The appropriate type and quantity of fluids in these situations must be carefully controlled to avoid complications. Hence the selection must be based on the knowledge of the physiological circulatory volume changes during pregnancy and of any obstetric or other medical disorders in the mother that could affect the fluid balance of the internal milieu. Lack of such knowledge and inappropriate fluid administration may be detrimental to maternal, fetal or neonatal health.

References

American Society of Hospital Pharmacists 1993. *AHFS Drug Information*. Bethesda, MD, ASHP. 2039-2041.

Arieff AI, Guisado R 1967. Effects on CNS of hyponatremic states. *Kidney International* 10:104-109.

Arias F 1984. Hypertension during pregnancy. In: Arias F, Mosby CV, eds. High Risk Pregnancy and Delivery comp. Toronto.

Arulkumaran S, Gibb DMF, Ratnam SS, Lun KC, Heng SH 1985. Total uterine activity in induced labor - index of cervical and pelvic tissue resistance. *Br J Obstet Gynecol* 92:693-697.

Arulkumaran S, Gibb DMF, Thambyraja RL, Ratnam SS 1985. Failed induction of labor. *Austr NZ J Obstet Gynecol* 25:190-193.

Arulkumaran A, Chua S, Chua TM, Yang M, Piara S, Ratnam SS 1991. Uterine activity in labour and target uterine activity to be aimed with oxytocin titration. *Asia Oceania J Obstet Gynecol* 17:101-106.

Arulkumaran S 1994. Uterine activity in labour. In: Chard T, Grudzinskas JG, eds. The Uterus. Cambridge: Cambridge University Press, ii:356-377.

Benedetti TJ, Carlson RW 1979. Studies of colloid osmotic pressure in pregnancy induced hypertension. *Am J Obstet Gynecol* 35:308-311.

Brazy JE, Pupkin MJ 1979. Effects of maternal isoxsuprine administration on preterm infants. *J Pediatr* 94:444-448.

Caldeyro-Barcia R, Sica-Blanco Y, Poseiro JJ et al 1957. A quantitative study of the action of synthetic oxytocin on the pregnant human uterus. *J Pharmacol* 121:18-23.

Carey LC, Coumer CT, Loasery BD 1970. The use of balanced electrolyte solution for resuscitation. In: Body Fluid Replacement in Surgical Patients. New York: Grune and Stratton.

Caritis S, Lin L, Toig G, Wong LK 1980. Pharmaco-dynamics of ritodrine in pregnant women during preterm labor. *Am J Obstet Gynecol* 56:7-12.

Centres for Disease Control 1987. Recommendations for prevention of HIV transmission in healthcare settings. *MMWR Suppl* 37:3S-17S.

Chesley LV, Valenti C, Rein H 1958. The excretion of sodium loads by nonpregnant and pregnant, normal, hypertensive and preeclamptic women. *Metabolism* 7:575.

Chesley LC 1966. Sodium retention and preeclampsia. *Am J Obstet Gynecol* 95:127-132.

Chesley LC 1978. Hypertensive Disorders in Pregnancy. New York: Appleton-Century-Crofts, pp 215-221.

Clark SL, Greenspoen J, Aldahl D 1986. Severe preeclampsia with persistent oliguria: Management of hemodynamic subsets. *Am J Obstet Gynecol* 154:490-494.

Dahlenburg GW, Burnell RH, Braybrook R 1980. The relation between cord serum and sodium levels in newborn infants and maternal intravenous therapy during labor. *Br J Obstet Gynecol* 87:519-522.

Doenicke A, Grote B, Lorenz W 1977. Blood and blood substitutes. *Br J Anesth* 49:681-684.

Dumouline JG, Foulkes J 1984. Commentary: Ketonuria during labour. *Br J Obstet Gynecol* 91:97-98.

Epstein MF, Nicholls E, Stubblefield PG 1979. Neonatal hypoglycemia after beta-sympathomimetic tocolytic therapy. *J Pediatr* 94: 449-456.

Evans SE, Crawford JS, Stevens ID, Durbin GM, Daya H 1986. Fluid therapy for induced labor under epidural analgesia: Biochemical consequences for mother and infant. *Br J Obstet Gynecol* 91: 97-98.

FDA Drug Bulletin 1989. 19:14.

Freeman M 1979. Fetal reaction to Haemacel. *Anesthesia* 34:34.

Fuchs F 1985. Cautions on using oxytocin for induction. *Contemp Obstet Gynecol* 25:1315.

Goodlin R, Holdt D, Woods R 1982. Pregnancy-induced hypertension associated with hypervolemia; case report. *Am J Obstet Gynecol* 142:114-115.

Hauser CJ, Shoemaker WC, Turpin I, Goldberg SJ 1980. Oxygen transport responses to colloids and crystalloids in critically ill surgical patients. *Surgica Gynecologica Obstetrica* 159:181-186.

Henhall WR 1979. Differences in albumin distribution and dynamics between toxemia and nontoxemic pregnant women. *Br J Obstet Gynecol* 86:463-467.

Horne CHW, Howie PW, Goudie RB 1970. Serum alpha2 - macro globulin, transferrin, albumin and IgG levels in preeclampsia. *J Clin Pathol* 23:514-518.

Hytten FE, Paintin DB 1963. Increase in plasma volume during normal pregnancy. *J Obstet Gynecol Br Cwlth* 70:402-407.

Ingermarsson I, Arulkumaran S 1985. Beta receptor agonists in current obstetric practice. In: Malcolm Chiswick, ed. Recent Advances in Perinatal Medicine. London: Churchill Livingstone, pp 45-57.

Jovanovic L, Druzin M, Peterson CM 1981. Effect of euglycemia on the outcome of pregnancy in insulin-dependent diabetic women as compared with normal control subjects. *Am J Med.* 71: 921-927.

Kenepp NB, Shelley WC, Kumar S, Stanley CA, Gutsche BB 1980. Effects on newborn of hydration with glucose in patients undergoing caesarean section with regional anesthesia. *Lancet* i:645.

Kenepp NB, Shelley WC, Gabbe SG, Kumar S, Stanley CA, Gutsche BB 1982. Fetal and neonatal hazards of maternal hydration with 5% dextrose before caesarean section. *Lancet* i:1150-1152.

Lamminstanta R, Erkolla R 1979. Effect of long-term salbutamol treatment on renin aldosterone system in twin pregnancy. *Acta Obstet Gynecol Scand* 58:447-451.

Letsky EA 1985. Disseminated intravascular coagulation. In: Lind T, ed. Coagulation problems during pregnancy. London: Churchill Livingstone, pp 62-87.

Light IJ, Keenan WJ, Sutherland JM 1972. Maternal intravenous glucose administration as a cause of hypoglycemia in the infant of the diabetic mother. *Am J Obstet Gynecol* 113:345-350.

Lorenz W et al 1976. Histamine release in human subjects by modified gelatin (Hemoccel) and dextran: An explanation for anaphylactoid reactions observed under clinical conditions. *Br J Anesth* 48:151-165.

McNaughton MC 1980. Induction of labor. The case for a high rate In: Beard RW, Paintin DB, eds. Obstetric Intervention in Britain. London: RCOG publication, p.137.

Morton KE, Jackson MC, Gillmer MDG 1985. A comparison of the effects of four intravenous solutions for the treatment of ketonuria during labor. *Br J Obstet Gynecol* 92:473-479.

Moss GS 1972. An Arguement in Favor of Electrolyte Solution for Early Resuscitation. *The Surgical Clinics of North America.* 52:3-17.

Musacchio MJ 1990. Oxytocins for Augmentation and Induction of Labor. New York: March of Dimes.

Myers RE 1978. Experimental models of perinatal brain damage relevance to human pathology. In: Gluck L, ed. Intrauterine Asphyxia and the Developing Fetal Brain. Chicago: Year Book Medical, p 37.

Nelson DM 1984. Diabetes and pregnancy. In: Arias F, ed. High Risk Pregnancy and Delivery. Toronto: C.V.Mosby Company.

O'Driscoll K, Folley M, MacDonald D 1984. Active management of labor as an alternative to caesarean section for dystocia. *Obstet Gynecol* 63:485-490.

Pearson JF, 1982. Monitoring high risk pregnancy. In: Bonnar J, ed. Recent Advances in Obstetrics and Gynecology No 14, London: Churchill Livingstone, pp 3-11.

Petrie RH, Williams AM 1986. Induction of labor. In: Knuppel RA, Drukker JE, eds. High Risk Pregnancy: A Team Approach. Philadelphia: Saunders, pp 303-315.

Pirani BBK, Campbel DM, Macgillivary I 1973. Plasma volume in normal first pregnancy. *J Obstet Gynecol Br Cwlth* 80:884-887.

Pritchard JJA 1978. Summary of management of pregnancy-induced hypertension at Parkland Memorial Hospital. In: Beller, Macgillivary I, eds. Hypertensive Disorders in Pregnancy. Struttgart: Thieme.

Piquard F, Hsiunh R, Haberey P 1990. Does fetal acidosis envelop with maternal glucose infusions during normal labor? *Obstet Gynecol* 74: 909-914.

Romeny SL, Gabel PV 1966. Maternal glucose loading in the management of fetal distress. *Am J Obstet Gynecol* 96:698-709.

Schrier RW, Lieberman R, Ufferman RC 1972. Mechanism of antidiuretic effect of beta adrenergic stimulation. *J Clin Invest* 51:977-1003.

Shelley HJ, Bassett JM, Milmer RDG 1975. Control of carbohydrate metabolism in the fetus and newborn. *Br Med Bull* 31:37-43.

Singhi S, Choo-Kang E, Hall JST 1982. Hazards of maternal hydration with 5% dextrose. *Lancet* ii:335-336.

Spencer SA, Mann NP, Smith ML, Woolfson AMJ, Benson S 1981. The effects of intravenous therapy during labour on maternal and cord serum sodium levels. *Br J Obstet Gynecol* 88:480-483.

Steer PJ, Carter MC, Choong K, Hanson M, Gordon AJ, Pradhan P 1985. A multicentre prospective randomised controlled trial of induction of labor with an automatic closed loop feedback-controlled oxytocin infusion system. *Br J Obstet Gynecol* 92:1127-1133.

Studd JWW, Blainey JD, Bailey DE 1970. Serum protein changes in the preeclampsia-eclampsia syndrome. *J Obstet Gynecol Br Cwlth* 77:796-801.

Tarnow-Mordi WO, Shaw JC, Liu D, Gardner DA, Flynn FV 1981. Iatrogenic hyponatremia of the newborn due to maternal overload: A prospective study. *Br Med J* 283: 639-642.

Thavarasah AS, Arulkumaran S 1988. Administration of intravenous fluids in labor - a critical evaluation. *Int J Feto-Mat Med* 1:42-50.

Zeilder R B, Kim H D 1979. Effect of low electrolyte media on salt loss and hemolysis of mammalian red blood cells. *J. Cell Physiol* 100:551-561.

8

Management of the Second Stage of Labour

V Annapoorna
S Arulkumaran

The second stage of labour lasts from the end of the first stage, when the cervix has reached full dilatation, to the birth of the baby. The successful outcome of the second stage culminates the hopes and fears of a pregnancy. The journey, from the ischial spines to the perineum, is short but full of anxiety with the two main hazards of hypoxia and trauma. Normal labour is characteristically progressive in nature and second stage is no exception. Hasty intervention in the second stage with an instrumental delivery is unnecessary and may be more difficult than expected. Excessive delay on the other hand may lead to fetal morbidity and mortality. Therefore the aim must be to strike the correct balance between expectancy and intervention so that a healthy baby is born and the mother attains emotional satisfaction from the process of her delivery. This chapter seeks to highlight some of the uncertain events of the second stage of labour and to create guidelines for safer and more definitive management.

Fetal response to the second stage

Subjected to the stressful conditions of the second stage, it is common for the fetal heart rate (FHR) pattern to change dramatically, becoming more complex and more difficult to interpret. The obstetrician may either wrongly interpret FHR changes to do a hasty intervention or do nothing about it, either way causing damage to the fetus at birth. Therefore it is vitally important to assess the fetal condition accurately from the FHR pattern and to determine which features indicate that fetal stress has progressed to the point of hypoxic distress. Stewart and Philpott (1980) in their study of the fetal response to cephalopelvic disproportion, noted that prolonged early decelerations were due to fetal head compression and late decelerations were due to placental insufficiency. The latter type of FHR pattern was noted by Stewart (1984) in the normal second stage of labour but with lesser intensity.

Early decelerations in the second stage indicate head compression rather than fetal compromise. Late decelerations on the other hand indicate the possibility of the onset of hypoxia with impaired uteroplacental perfusion which may well proceed to established acidosis if it is allowed to persist for too long. The most critical feature is the evolution of the cardiotocographic trace with time. A change in the baseline heart rate and baseline variability are indicative of developing hypoxia and acidosis (Gibb and Arulkumaran 1992). During labour, as long as the normal variability is maintained and the recovery of the deceleration to the baseline is immediate, the pattern is considered benign. An ominous pattern is that of reduced baseline variability, tachy or bradycardia, late decelerations or end stage decelerations with baseline heart rate gradually falling to bradycardia. These features suggest hypoxic distress and demand delivery.

Uterine contractions and placental perfusion

The normal uterine contraction pattern increases through labour and reach a zenith with the urge to push, the added maternal effort causing a considerable expulsive force. Uterine contractions occur four to five times in 10 min with an amplitude of 70–85 mmHg each lasting for 50–75 seconds. Caldeyro-Barcia (1979) found that with bearing down efforts the peak pressure may even reach upto 165 mmHg. This increase in intrauterine pressure will reduce uteroplacental perfusion leading to a drop in the pO_2 of the fetal blood (Morishima et al 1975). The ability of the fetus to tolerate hypoxemia will depend on its nutritional reserves. In the second stage, even with a well functioning uteroplacental unit, a prolonged period of rhythmic uterine contractions can lead to impairment of the uteroplacental and umbilical blood flow leading to anerobic metabolism (Rooth 1973) and lactic acidosis (Modanlow et al 1974).

Pelvic and perineal phases of the second stage of labour

The second stage of labour consists of two phases : the pelvic and the perineal phase. During the pelvic phase the head rotates as it is pressed on the gutter shaped, forward-sloping levator ani muscles, but the presenting part may still be high and thus may not give rise to the sensation of bearing down. In the perineal phase, the head is on the thinning pelvic floor and perineum, which exerts pressure on the rectum and the woman feels the sensation of bearing down. At crowning, the occipital prominence escapes under the symphysis pubis and the head no longer recedes between contractions.

Clinical identification of the second stage

The contractions become more frequent and more painful. The patient will bear down with each contraction and there is an increase in bloodstained discharge. The woman will feel the pressure on the rectum accompanied by the desire to defecate. Before encouraging the woman to bear down, the condition of the cervix and the station of the presenting part must be confirmed by vaginal examination. At times a small lip of the cervix may be felt anteriorly, posteriorly or laterally in between contractions but may not be felt with the contraction and in the opening bearing down effort. Observation of the lengthening of the perineum with contractions and a gradual increase in the opening of the anal orifice exhibiting the pink/red anterior mucosal wall of the anal canal indicates that the head is low and indicates the probability of the second stage. It is not uncommon to see the head at the introitus with bearing down efforts. In a considerable proportion of women, especially in those with epidural analgesia, the second stage is identified whilst performing the routine three to four hourly vaginal examination. Advice to these women to bear down should be given only when the head has reached the perineal phase in order to avoid maternal exhaustion.

Assessment of the second stage

Progress in the second stage is monitored by the descent of the fetal head. The uterine contractions are monitored with attention to their duration and frequency within a period of 10 minutes. The head level must be assessed by abdominal as well as pelvic examination. The head level felt abdominally (Chrichton 1952; Simons and Philpott 1973; Studd 1973) describes the number of fifths palpable above the brim. Clinical accuracy can be increased by estimating the number of finger breadths palpable above the pubic symphysis (Notelovitz 1972). At the point of 'engagement' the bony part of the vertex is at the ischial spines. When it is in the 'midcavity' it will be 1/5th to 2/5th palpable. As the head is wholly in the pelvic cavity, the leading point will be 2 cm below the ischial spines and when it is 4 cm below the ischial spines it is in the 'low cavity' and outlet.

It is important to establish the time of onset of the second stage of labour on the partogram. Vaginal examination should be carried out when necessary or when there is concern about the fetal condition, to assess the descent of the fetal head while pushing. At vaginal examination the position of the fetal head, the degree of flexion, the amount of moulding and caput formation is determined.

Management of the second stage

The management of the second stage of labour is crucial for both the mother and the fetus. It is only prudent to discuss here the optimum delivery position for the mother, the maximum permitted duration, pain relief and important techniques in management.

Position for delivery

There are considerable variations in the delivery positions used by various cultures. The requirements for an optimal position should prevent fetal hypoxia, create an efficient uterine contraction pattern, improve the pelvic dimension, allow easy access for monitoring the FHR, should expose the perineum well to present a clear field for delivery and should also be comfortable for the mother.

The upright or vertical position

Included are the standing, sitting, squatting and kneeling positions in gravity assisted delivery. Russell (1969) pointed out that radiologically the squatting position increased both transverse and anteroposterior diameters by 28% compared with the supine position. A woman can increase the efficiency of the forces of labour by pulling her knees upward especially in the squatting position. The disadvantages are that it is difficult for the accoucheur to control the birth and to manage complications. Administration of sedatives and regional analgesia precludes the parturient from adopting such positions.

The horizontal or semihorizontal position

In this group are the lateral, prone, semirecumbent, knee-elbow, and dorsal positions. The advantages of the lateral position include ease, convenience, and comfort and precludes the supine hypotensive syndrome. It relaxes the pelvic muscles, and facilitates the descent of the fetal head. It is easier to control the delivery of the head. In the dorsal (supine) position, the woman lies on her back with the knees flexed. The dorsal position is advantageous for those who do not need an episiotomy. It is potentially harmful for the mother and fetus if supine hypotension develops. A pillow placed behind the back to produce lateral tilt should reduce the incidence of hypotension. In the lithotomy position, the woman lies on her back, her legs in stirrups, and her buttocks close to the lower edge of the couch. The advantages include easy monitoring of fetal heart, efficient analgesia, a good position to conduct assisted delivery and repair of an episiotomy or lacerations. Semi-reclining positions came into vogue because of the advantages of the upright and horizontal delivery posture. Women are more comfortable with their backs raised at an angle of between 30° and 45° from the horizontal position. The efficiency of the expulsive forces are increased by directing them toward the pelvis and by making use of the forces of gravity. The introduction of birthing beds has helped women to deliver in sitting and semi-reclining positions.

Duration of the second stage

The length of the second stage is important and still remains controversial with regard to what action is to be instituted and when; particularly when epidural analgesia is used. Several factors influence the duration of the second stage such as birth weight (Kadar and Romero 1983), occipitoposterior position (Philips and Freeman 1974), parity and use of regional analgesia. Philpott and Castle (1972) and Studd (1973) arrived at the conclusion that 45 min for primis and 15 min for multis represent the normal duration of the second stage. Paterson et al (1993) in their study showed that in women for whom epidural analgesia is used, the duration of the second stage was longer than reported previously, possibly reflecting a more conservative approach to operative intervention. They concluded that so long as maternal and fetal conditions are satisfactory, intervention should be based on the rate of progress rather than on the time elapsed since full cervical dilatation. Saunders et al (1992) in their findings also agreed with the above study and inferred that in the absence of factors suggesting fetal compromise, a second stage labour of up to 3 hr duration does not seem to carry undue risk to the fetus. However they concluded that the duration of the second stage of labour had a significant independent association with the risk of both postpartum hemorrhage and maternal infection after adjustment for other factors. A review of the literature by Derham et al (1991) indicates that prolonged duration of the second stage, that is, from full dilatation of the cervix until delivery, with or without epidural analgesia, has little adverse effect on the perinatal outcome.

Some guidelines have to be followed in the management of the second stage. Ideally the patient should be encouraged to bear down only in the perineal phase. If the onset of the second stage is identified in the pelvic phase (especially when the patient has an epidural analgesia) time should be given (approximately 1–2 hr) for the uterine contractions to effect the descent of the head. If the expected progress is not achieved in one hour, the uterine contractions should be checked and if necessary oxytocin infusion commenced. With one hour of good uterine contractions if the head does not descend, bearing down efforts may be encouraged. Despite such management if the head does not descend a decision should be made as to whether to allow more time, with the view of achieving an instrumental vaginal delivery. If not, a careful decision should be made to deliver the baby abdominally.

Pain relief

Pain in the second stage is the worst pain of the whole labour because of the crescendo of contractions. But a friendly atmosphere, the support of a companion, homely surroundings (Chapman et al 1986) and a good midwife (Waldenstrom 1988) are all believed to reduce the need for analgesia in labour.

Intramuscular pethidine in the second stage of labour is not commonly used because of its respiratory depressant effect on the neonate. It reduces the baseline variability of the fetal heart rate pattern which is difficult to distinguish from that caused by hypoxia. If a woman progresses rapidly to the second stage after the administration of pethidine, accelerations in the FH may not be evident and the baseline variability may become reduced as in the quiet or sleep phase. The difference in the effects of pethidine on the fetal heart rate pattern from hypoxia is that the FHR after pethidine will neither show decelerations nor an increase in the baseline heart rate as in hypoxia, despite the fact that there are no accelerations and there is decreased baseline variability. When the baby is born, it may not cry and may need stimulation or assisted ventilation because the drug affects the central nervous system and causes respiratory depression, but the fetus will have good cord arterial blood gas status and pH indicating that there was no intrauterine hypoxia.

Entonox in the second stage is considered invaluable with no adverse effect on neonatal condition (Stefani et al 1982). Entonox usage has its shortcomings if it has to be used for long hours with poor analgesic effects (Levack and Tunstall 1984). The woman might hyperventilate herself, with resultant hypocapnia leading to dizziness and even tetany.

Epidural analgesia is the most effective technique of pain relief during labour. The catheter through which injections are given at intervals or continuously is usually inserted in the left lateral position (Crawford 1972; Steel 1972) although the sitting position is also sometimes employed. Bupivacaine is the drug most commonly used in a strength of 0.25%. It blocks pain impulses passing along the thin posterior nerve routes but does not block the larger anterior motor fibres. The intention is to relieve pain in the second stage caused by the passage of the head distending the cervix, vagina and perineum.

The prolongation of the second stage is common with the use of epidural anesthesia (O'Driscoll and Meagher 1980; Paintin and Vincent 1980). This has been attributed to reduced uterine activity due to the absence of the normal surge of oxytocin secretion seen in the second stage (Vascika et al 1978), secondary to the abolition of the Ferguson reflex (stretching of the cervix and upper vagina) (Ferguson 1941). Studd et al (1980) had shown that epidural analgesia increases the incidence of instrumental delivery, particularly the use of the rotational forceps. The correct epidural dosage is judged by the woman's ability to retain leg movements, which means that it leaves the patient with effective abdominal muscle power with which to bear down.

Self hypnosis has anecdotally been found successful in individual cases while acupuncture, which is time consuming with inconsistent results, has been practised in some centres.

Second stage techniques

Bearing down

The woman with an urge to push usually starts bearing down in the second stage with the onset of pain. It is routine practice to advise the woman to 'take a deep breath, hold it and push' in the second stage of labour, but there is no scientific evidence to support this. Caldeyro-Barcia (1979) showed that with organised pushing the second stage lasted twice as long compared with spontaneous pushing and that the former practice increased fetal hypoxia. Pushing against a closed glottis increases the intrathoracic pressure with reduction in venous return, cardiac output and uteroplacental perfusion with further reduction in fetal oxygen supply. Thomson (1993) in a randomised trial of spontaneous versus directed pushing in the second stage, found no adverse effects of spontaneous pushing on the mother or baby. There was a negative correlation between the duration of the second stage and the venous cord blood pH at delivery in the directed pushing group, but no such association was found in the spontaneous pushing group, despite the fact that the women in this group had a significantly longer mean second stage. Stewart (1984) recommended that bearing down should be restricted to 5 sec efforts with four or five per contraction, without closing the glottis and with one or two breaths of entonox in between.

Spontaneous birth of the head

With each contraction the head advances and then recedes as the uterus relaxes. The pressure of the head thins out the perineum. With descent, the occiput comes to lie under the pubic symphysis. With each contraction the head descends and the largest diameter of the head passes through the vulva after crowning. By a process of extension the head is born, as the bregma, forehead, nose, mouth and chin appear over the perineum. Then the head restitutes as the neck untwists followed by external rotation to bring the shoulders to the anteroposterior diameter of the pelvis.

Assisted delivery of the head

Some women may need assistance in the delivery of the head. Gradual birth of the head reduces the incidence of injury to the fetus and perineal lacerations in the mother. Timely episiotomy should be performed when necessary. Correct management of the bearing down efforts of the parturient and also gentle manual pressure to flex the fetal head at delivery are important to guard against a sudden extension of the head which may cause vestibular and anterior vaginal wall lacerations. A Ritgen manoeuvre, which encourages extension of fetal head is performed when the suboccipitofrontal diameter is ready to be born. The obstetrician's left hand is placed on the most superior aspect of the fetal head while the right hand is placed over the perineum posteriorly and pressed against the baby's chin so that the bregma, forehead and face are born in that order.

Episiotomy

Episiotomies need to be performed if a perineal tear is imminent. In current obstetric practice, the rate of episiotomy in primigravidas has risen from 21% in 1958 to 91% in 1978 (Buchan and Nicholls 1980). There is no concensus of opinion as to whether mediolateral episiotomy is better than midline episiotomy. Clinical research in this area has been deficient but the clinical impression is that the midline episiotomy is much less painful, much easier to repair accurately and gives much better cosmetic results (Nicholas Kadar 1985). The fear of extension of the episiotomy into the rectum is the major objection to midline incision, but it is easy to repair and rarely breaks down. Mediolateral episiotomy which is widely practised has been shown to have a higher incidence of pain in the immediate postpartum period, and pain and difficulty with sexual activity later, requiring medical help especially in primigravidas (Reading et al 1982). The shorter the distance between the fourchette and the anus (short perineum), the better it is to give a more mediolateral episiotomy to avoid the episiotomy extending into the anus or rectum, damaging the sphincteric muscles or causing a third degree tear. Episiotomy is not needed as a routine. When there is urgency in delivering the fetus for fetal (for example, fetal distress) or maternal (severe cardiac disease) reasons and if an episiotomy would shorten the delivery process, it is indicated. In a preterm cephalic, in assisted breech delivery (term or preterm) and in multiple pregnancy, use of an episiotomy would assist the delivery process by reducing soft tissue resistance and allowing more space. Bleeding from within the vagina before the head is delivered indicating a vestibular or anterior vaginal wall tear and the appearance of multiple tears at the perineum is an indication for episiotomy in order to avoid anterior vaginal wall and/or multiple perineal tears. Instrumental vaginal delivery will be facilitated by an episiotomy and the apex of the episiotomy should be high enough to visualise the periphery of a vacuum cup or the shank of the forceps in order to avoid spiral tears or apical extensions due to the distension of the vaginal canal above the apex of the episiotomy.

Delivery of the shoulders and body

The head should be supported as it restitutes and rotates externally. The face should be wiped gently and mucus aspirated from the mouth and throat by a small rubber or plastic catheter with a rounded tip. If the cord is loose around the neck it can be left alone or slipped over the head easily. If not, then it must be clamped doubly, cut between the clamps and then unwound. By this time the shoulders are ready for delivery. During a contraction the parturient is asked to bear down with uterine contraction. At the same time, the baby's head is depressed toward the rectum which enables the anterior shoulder to emerge under the symphysis pubis. Then the head is raised so that the posterior shoulder appears over the perineum. Undue force should not be exerted while delivering the shoulders, as this carries with it the risk of damaging the nerve plexuses in the neck. Once the head and shoulders have been delivered, the rest of the body slips out easily, usually with a gush of amniotic fluid. The head being pushed against the perineum (turtleneck sign) with difficulties in palpating the fetal neck indicates the possibility of shoulder dystocia and is discussed in another chapter.

Complications in the second stage of labour
Inefficient uterine action

Just as in the first stage, inefficient uterine action can develop in the second stage, either primary or secondary to cephalopelvic disproportion. If cephalopelvic disproportion is excluded in a primigravid patient with a healthy fetus, oxytocin is started to augment the uterine contractions. However in a multigravida, inefficient uterine action is uncommon and greater caution is required in augmenting labour because of the risk of uterine rupture. Also care must be taken not to overstimulate the uterus and produce contractions that are frequent resulting in fetal hypoxia.

Malposition

In the presence of malposition, the second stage of labour is often prolonged and the head may be high. There may be minimal disproportion due to various degrees of extension of the head. In addition the uterine activity may be unsatisfactory. In these cases augmentation with oxytocin should be considered with great care. With good uterine contractions, malposition may correct itself by further flexion, rotation, moulding and pelvic give resulting in normal delivery. If despite augmentation, malposition persists with a high head, caesarean section may be necessary. Instrumental vaginal deliveries for poor progress or malposition in the second stage are not without danger. This is discussed further in the chapter dealing with instrumental delivery. The possibility of disproportion should be considered before attempting an instrumental vaginal delivery. Clinically or ultrasonically estimated fetal size > 4 kg, and instances where two fifths or more of the head are palpable above the pelvic brim indicate that there may be disproportion. On vaginal examination, if the bony part of the head is above the ischial spines, there is excessive caput and moulding and if the head fails to descend with contractions and bearing down effort, difficulties will be encountered with instrumental vaginal delivery. An attempt should be made to palpate the baby's ear when there is a contraction and bearing down effort. If felt easily it indicates that the head is adequately low to attempt an instrumental delivery. The ears being below the parietal eminences indicates that the maximal diameter of the head is adequately low and also describes the position of the vertex.

Supine hypotensive syndrome

The clinical picture of this syndrome is one of hypotension when the parturient lies on her back, compressing the aorta and vena cava by the gravid uterus. This leads to an increased volume of blood in the lower limbs, decreased venous return to the heart, lowered pressure in the right atrium, diminished cardiac output, and systemic hypotension. Reduced uteroplacental perfusion leads to fetal hypoxia and changes in the fetal heart rate pattern. There is rapid recovery when the parturient turns on her side or is propped up in bed. Other symptoms of supine hypotension include nausea, shortness of breath, faintness, pallor, tachycardia, and increased femoral venous pressure. Complete relief of symptoms occur when the baby is delivered.

Fetal distress — fetal monitoring

Meconium

Meconium aspiration in the baby can lead to mild or severe respiratory compromise and care should be taken to prevent its occurrence. The passage per vaginum of meconium or meconium stained amniotic fluid when the fetal presentation is cephalic may be a sign of fetal distress. It is believed to result from relaxation of the anal sphincter and/or increased peristalsis as a consequence of fetal hypoxia. However, the presence of meconium may represent nothing more than fetal maturity. In most cases no cause is found.

When thick meconium has been passed there is danger that the baby will aspirate it during the first postnatal cry which follows a deep breath. Therefore in cases where meconium is present the following steps should be taken:

a) The paediatrician should be on standby at delivery.

b) As soon as the head is born, and before the baby breathes, the mouth, hypopharynx, nostrils and nasopharynx are suctioned thoroughly in that order to prevent the neonate attempting to sneeze and inhaling the meconium.

c) After the delivery is complete and the above step has been performed the laryngoscope is employed to see whether there is meconium at or below the level of the vocal cords.

d) If there is, all the meconium should be suctioned out before any resuscitative measures, such as positive pressure ventilation, are performed. This is discussed further in the chapter dealing with neonatal resuscitation.

Fetal heart rate

Intermittent and continuous recording of fetal heart rate (FHR) are the methods available for fetal monitoring and each method has its advantages and disadvantages. O'Driscoll (1980) maintains that intermittent auscultation with a stethoscope is sufficiently accurate for the majority of mothers. A fetal stethoscope is used on the maternal abdomen to auscultate FH in between contractions to obtain the baseline heart rate. Although accelerations and decelerations can be detected during and immediately after contractions, baseline variability cannot be measured using intermittent auscultation.

Intermittent and continuous electronic recording of FHR can be obtained with a cardiotocograph (combined print out of FHR and uterine activity). The monitor measures the interval between paired beats, converts and registers it into beats per minute. Uterine activity can be assessed by an external strain gauge transducer or measured with an intrauterine catheter. A randomised study by Herbst and Ingemarsson (1994) on intermittent versus continuous electronic monitoring in women with low or moderate risk showed that the intermittent use of electronic fetal heart monitoring at regular intervals (with stethoscopic auscultation in between) appears to be as safe as continuous electronic fetal monitoring. FHR traces compatible with a normal second stage and occasions where hypoxia is likely unless there is intervention (abnormal FHR) are shown in Figs 8.1–8.5.

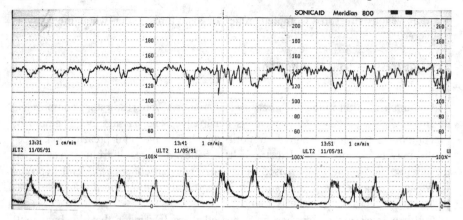

Fig 8.1   Second stage FHR pattern with early decelerations (due to head compression) but no shift in the baseline rate and baseline variability is maintained — normal for second stage.

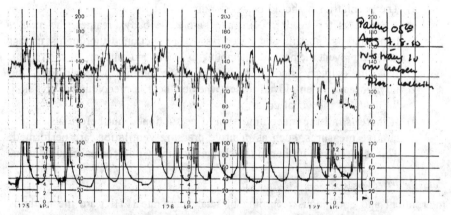

Fig 8.2   Uterine contractions show pushing spikes of the second stage. Variable decelerations but quick recovery with no shift in the baseline rate or change in variability till the head crowns and delivers — normal for second stage.

Fetal scalp blood sampling   Fetal scalp blood sampling and FHR recordings are complementary. In the event of an abnormal FHR trace, a scalp blood pH analysis at full dilatation can help plan a safe delivery. If normal, > 7.25, a vaginal delivery can be anticipated. If it is borderline, 7.20–7.25, FHR should be closely monitored and pH repeated after half an hour. If the pH is < 7.20, the fetus should be delivered either by the vaginal route or by caesarean section, whichever is appropriate.

The patient is placed in the left lateral position for fetal scalp blood sampling and the amnioscope is introduced into the vagina and fixed onto the fetal head or buttock. The fetal skin is cleaned, sprayed with ethyl chloride and smeared with silicone gel. A droplet of fetal blood is obtained by a guarded 2 mm blade during a contraction. The blood is allowed to flow into a pre-heparinised capillary tube and transferred to a blood gas analyser. The whole procedure should not take more than three minutes.

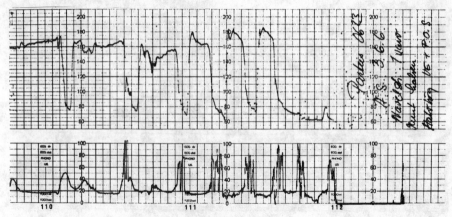

Fig 8.3   Variable decelerations but with shift in baseline rate to tachycardia (180 bpm)
and markedly reduced baseline variability (< 5 beats). Abnormal trace and
needs assistance unless spontaneous delivery is imminent.

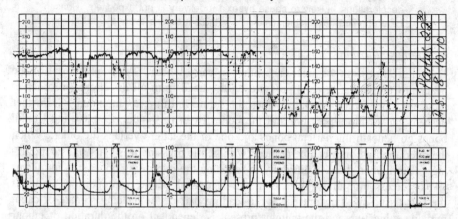

Fig 8.4   Abnormal trace with tachycardia (160 bpm) and reduced variability (< 5 beats)
and variable decelerations resulting in bradycardia/decelerations. Needs
assistance unless spontaneous delivery is imminent.

Fetal pulse oximetry   This is one of the newer methods of fetal monitoring to
predict fetal hypoxemia in labour. Arterial oxygen saturation of the fetus is measured with a fetal pulse oximeter. Johnson et al (1991) in their study came to the
conclusion that a single reading during labour is not a useful data. Recently a
preliminary report on 39 cases by Carbonne et al (1994) has been very encouraging.
They have demonstrated that arterial oxygen saturation of the fetus during labour
was significantly correlated to umbilical vein pH and to a one minute Apgar score
when measured continuously. If larger studies also prove this point, then measurement of arterial oxygen saturation of the fetus (SpO_2 value) during labour would
be reassuring especially in cases of abnormal FHR or pH value < 7.20.

It is important to deliver the fetus in optimal condition and failure to do so
leads to hypoxic and/or traumatic damage to the baby and medicolegal problems.
This is more so in the presence of fetal distress as evidenced by ominous FHR
pattern or by scalp blood pH of < 7.20. Temptations to expedite delivery vaginally
should be resisted if the conditions are suboptimal for vaginal delivery.

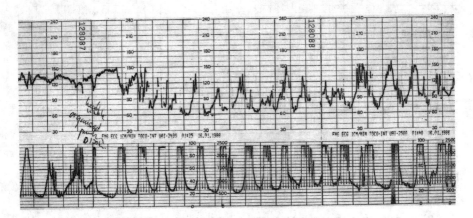

Fig 8.5   Prolonged decelerations where pick-up to original baseline is made with
difficulty and time spent at baseline is minimal compared with the duration of
decelerations. Likely to cause hypoxia if delivery is not expedited. Reason
here appears to be hyperstimulation with contractions every 1½ to 2 mins.

Moulding and caput

The suture lines do not meet each other in early labour. With the descent of the
head into the pelvis there is pressure on the head from all directions (in order to
reduce the presenting diameter) when the suture lines meet - moulding +. Further
descent causes more pressure and the bones override — the occipital and frontal
bones go beneath the parietal bones and one of the latter overlaps the other. When
the overlapping bones can be reduced with gentle pressure it is classified as moulding ++ and when there is difficulty in reducing the overriding bones it is termed as
+++. Excess moulding (+++) is a sign of cephalopelvic disproportion. Caput is
the soft tissue swelling present at the leading part of the head. Estimate of caput
remains subjective and the amount present is dependent on the duration of labour
(Stewart 1977). When there is large caput, it is difficult to assess how much of
the fetal head has gone through the maternal pelvis. Any decision to allow vaginal
delivery should be cautious.

The second stage of labour is the last lap of the journey for the fetus. However
considering the whole duration of the pregnancy it is the most vulnerable period
for the fetus. The attending obstetrician should be very vigilant as complications
can arise any time during the second stage of labour, requiring urgent intervention
the nature of which must be carefully considered, be justified by the circumstances
and executed with care. The delivery of the fetus should result in a healthy neonate
with no hypoxia or traumatic insult.

References

Arulkumaran S, Koh CH, Ingemarsson I, Ratnam
    SS 1987. Augmentation of labour — Mode of
    delivery related to cervimetric progress. *Aust
    NZ J Obstet Gynecol* 27: 304-308.

Arulkumaran S 1994. Poor progress in labour
    including augmentation, malpositions and
    malpresentations. In: James DK, Weiner CP,
    Steer PJ, Gonik B, eds. Higk Risk Pregnancy

Management Options. London (U.K.): W.B. Saunders Company Ltd.

Buchan PC, Nicholls JA 1980. Pain after episiotomy — a comparison of two methods of repair. *J of the Royal College of Gen Prac* 30: 297-301.

Caldeyro-Barcia R 1979. Lecture presented at the First International Meeting of Perinatal Medicine, Berlin.

Carbonne B, Audibert F, Segard L, Sebban E, Cabrol D, Papernik E 1994. Fetal pulse oximetry: correlation between changes in O_2 saturation and neonatal outcome. Preliminary report on 39 cases. *Eur J Obstet Gynecol Reprod Biol* 57(2):73-77.

Chapman MG, Jones M, Spring JE, et al 1986. The use of a birthroom: a randomised controlled trial comparing delivery with that in the labour ward. *Br J Obstet Gynecol* 93: 182-187.

Crawford JS 1972. The second thousand epidural blocks in an obstetric hospital practice. *Br J Anesth* 44: 1277-1287.

Crichton D 1952. The accuracy of X-ray cephalometry in utero. *Proceedings of the Royal Society of Medicine* 45: 535-538.

Derham RJ, Crowhurst J, Crowther C 1991. The second stage of labour: durational dilemmas. *Aust NZ J Obstet Gynecol* 31(1): 31-36.

Ferguson JKW 1941. A study of the motility of the intact uterus at term. *Surgery, Gynecology and Obstetrics.* 73: 359-366.

Gibb D, Arulkumaran S 1992. Control of the fetal heart. In: eds. Fetal Monitoring in Practice. London (Great Britain): Butterworth-Heinemann Ltd., pp 22-39.

Herbst A., Ingemarsson I 1994. Intermittent versus continuous electronic monitoring in labour: a randomised study. *Br J Obstet Gynecol* 101(8): 663-668.

Johnson N, Johnson VA, Bannister J, Lilford RJ 1991. The accuracy of fetal pulse oximetry in the second stage of labour. *J Perinat Med* 19(4): 297-303.

Kadar N, Romero R 1983. Prognosis for future childbearing after midcavity instrumental deliveries in primigravidas. *Obstet Gynecol* 62: 166-170.

Levack ID, Tunstall ME 1984. Systems modification in obstetric analgesia. *Anesthesia* 34: 183-185.

Modanlow H, Hey SY, How EH 1974. Fetal and neonatal acid-base balance in normal and high risk pregnancies during labour and the first hour of life. *Obstet Gynecol* 43: 347-353

Morishima H O, Daniel SS, Richards RT, James LS 1975. The effect of increased maternal paO_2 upon the fetus during labour. *Am J Obstet Gynecol* 123: 257-264

Nicholas Kadar 1985. The second stage. In: John Studd, ed. The Management of Labour, pp 268-285.

Notelovitz M 1972. The graphic monitoring of labour. *South Afr J Obstet Gynecol* 47: 3-7

O'Driscoll K, Meagher D 1975. Active management of labour. *Clin Obstet Gynecol* 2:3-17.

Paintin DB, Vincent F 1980. Forceps delivery: Obstetric outcome. In: Beard RW, Paintin DB, eds. Outcome of Obstetric Intervention in Britain. London: RCOG publication, pp 17-32.

Paterson CM, Saunders NS, Wadsworth J 1993. The characteristics of the second stage of labour in 25,069 singleton deliveries in the North West Thames Health Region 1988. *Br J Obstet Gynecol* 100(12): 1155-1156.

Philpott RH, Castle WM 1972. Cervicograph in the management of labour in primigravidae II. The action line and treatment of abnormal labour. *J Obstet Gynecol Br Cwlth.* 78:599-602.

Philips RD, Freeman M 1974. The management of the persistent occiput posterior position. *Obstet Gynecol* 43: 171-177.

Reading AE, Sledinere CM, Cox DN, Campbells 1982 How women view post episiotomy pain. *Br Med J* 284: 243-252.

Rooth G 1973. The time factor in fetal distress. *J Perinat Med* 1: 7-12.

Russell JGB 1969. Moulding of the pelvic outlet. *J Obst Gynecol of Br Cwlth.* 76: 817-820.

Simons EJ, Philpott RH 1973. The vacuum extractor. *Tropical Doctor* 3: 34-37.

Saunders NS, Paterson CM, Wadsworth J 1992. Neonatal and maternal morbidity in relation to the length of the second stage of labour. *Br J Obstet Gynecol* 99(5): 381-385.

Steel GC 1972. Epidural nerve block in Obstetrics. *Br J Hosp Med* 8: 595-602.

Stefani SJ, Hughes SC, Schnider SM, et al 1982. Neonatal neurobehavioural effects of inhalation analgesia for vaginal delivery. *Anesthesiology* 56: 384-388.

Stewart KS 1977. MD, Thesis. University of Edinburgh.

Stewart KS, Philpott RH 1980. Fetal response to cephalopelvic disproportion. *Br J Obstet and Gynecol* 87: 641-651.

Stewart KS 1984. The second stage. In: John Studd, ed. Progress in Obstetrics and Gynecology. London (Great Britain): Churchill Livingstone, 4: 197-216.

Studd JWW 1973. Partograms and normograms of cervical dilatation. Management of primigravid labour. *Br Med J* 4: 451-456

Studdd JWW, Crawford JS, Duignan NW, Rowbotham CJF, Hughes AO 1980. The effect of lumbar epidural analgesia on the rate of cervical dilatation and the outcome of labour of spontaneous onset. *Br J Obstet Gynecol* 87: 1015-1021.

Thomson AM 1993. Pushing techniques in the second stage of labour. *J Adv Nurs* 18(2): 171-177

Vascika A, Kumaresan P, Han GS, Kumaresan M 1978. Plasma oxytocin in initiation in labour. *Am J Obstet Gynecol* 130: 263-273.

Waldenstrom U 1988. Midwives attitudes to pain relief during labour and delivery. *Midwifery* 4: 48-57.

9

Operative Delivery

Donald M F Gibb

The aim of maternity care is to optimise the health of the mother, the health of the baby and the emotional satisfaction of the mother and her family. In many developing countries the impetus of care must be directed to the survival of the mother. The World Health Organization estimates that fifteen hundred women die every day of childbirth-related complications. The last hundred years have seen a dramatic reduction in maternal mortality as countries have developed. This has been followed by similar reductions in perinatal mortality. These changes can be attributed as much to improvements in socio-economic conditions as to modern medical care. In countries that have achieved low mortality rates the expectations of the community are high. This partly relates to the high media profile of medical achievement and the belief that a living healthy baby is the the only acceptable outcome and indeed the right of every family.

The history of operative delivery is relatively short. The Chamberlen family concealed their secret instrument, the forceps, until about 1720. Before that, devices to deliver a child were available but their purpose was to extract a dead child with a destructive technique in order to save the life of the mother. At that time caesarean section was not an option. This operation did not become safe until developments in surgical techniques, anesthesia and blood transfusion took place in the late nineteenth and twentieth centuries. Then as today new methods were met with initial enthusiasm tempered later by criticism based on experience. The late 18th century saw the overuse and misuse of forceps resulting in a reactionary school of 'leaving to nature' led by William Hunter and Thomas Denman (O'Grady 1988). The 19th century saw the evolution of improved instruments and critical ideas. James Young Simpson introduced his forceps in 1848 and a vacuum device in 1849. His forceps were accepted along with many other designs but the vacuum device was not improved and popularised until the twentieth century.

Birth trauma has declined as a contributor to perinatal mortality in recent decades. The same period has seen an increase in operative delivery. The more complicated manipulative deliveries such as internal version, destructive procedures and symphysiotomy have a very limited place in this country and some obstetricians have no experience of them at all. Abnormal delivery remains a challenge where the easy option is caesarean section. The rate of caesarean section has increased in most countries. This may not be in the best interests of the mother or the child. Conversely the attitude of 'vaginal delivery at all costs' on which the reputation and image of the obstetrician depends may lead to an adverse outcome. Ultimately all parents want a healthy baby as the primary objective. Levels of competence and good practice must be maintained. The focus of this chapter is on forceps delivery, vacuum extraction, breech delivery, twin delivery, shoulder dystocia and caesarean section. Perinatal mortality as a consequence of operative delivery is now rare; however morbidity remains disappointingly prevalent. When a mother complains about her own condition after delivery it most often relates to perineal damage.

Mechanical engineering and obstetrics

Involvement in the care of the woman in labour cannot begin without consideration of the passenger, the passages and the powers. The process of labour and vaginal birth is the most dangerous journey any individual undertakes. It is not the purpose of this text to review the details of this journey in mechanical terms but some critical aspects will be considered. The essence of safe operative delivery is selective tailored assistance rather than extraction. We know a great deal about the passenger and the surveillance of the fetal condition. The development of critical ideas on the active management of labour by O'Driscoll and Meagher (1980), although central to the modern management of labour, has unwittingly resulted in less attention being paid to the elements of the feto-pelvic relationship. Augmentation of labour has become an end in itself without a critical review of the various underlying causes of delay in labour and their inter-relationships. Careful abdominal palpation provides important information about the powers and the passenger. Standard clinical methods of assessing the timing, frequency and subjective strength of contractions are well established. Assessing the size of the baby is controversial, and may not be accurate or precise especially in the obese woman. However a crude estimate of small, average, large or very large is not unreasonable, especially when an operative delivery is anticipated. The level of the presenting part traditionally referred to with respect to the ischial spines is important but an abdominal assessment of engagement or fifths palpable is essential. Although the need for reliability and the relevance of detailed clinical pelvic examination is in doubt, their omission from the assessment of problem labours is imprudent.

Although detailed pelvic assessment is difficult various principles must be established. The normal female pelvic inlet is gynaecoid with the transverse diameter of the inlet being wider than the anteroposterior diameter. At the start of labour the head is therefore constrained in the normal course of events to lie transversely with a left occipito-transverse position being commoner than a right occipito-transverse. As the head enters the brim of the pelvis it undergoes flexion so that the vertex is the leading part (Fig 9.1).

In the mid-cavity the cylindrical shape of the birth canal and the more restricted interspinous diameter leads to the rotation of the head, usually to an occipito-anterior position. The rotating head is accommodated in the curve of the sacrum. Flexion of the head is maintained and increased. At the level of the outlet the occiput passes under the pubic arch with the neck extending and the face emerging over the perineum. This is the mechanism of normal labour and delivery. The anthropoid brim has the widest diameter at the inlet in the anteroposterior direction. Although this may seem unfavourable the mid-cavity and outlet of such a pelvis are usually of good dimensions permitting the rotation of the head or delivery face to pubis. The android brim is so named because of its similarity to that of the

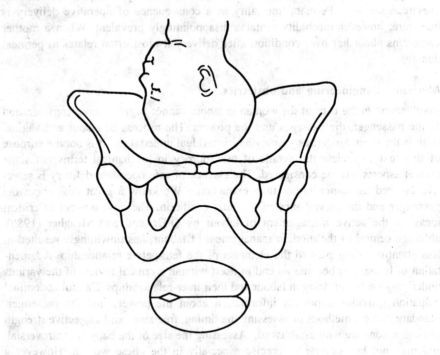

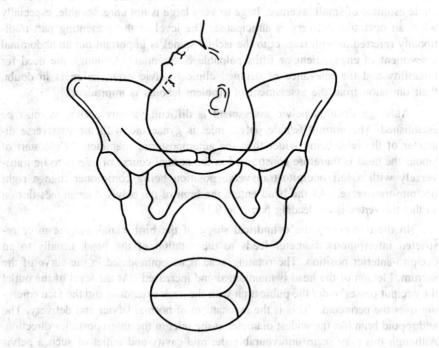

Fig 9.1   Flexion of the fetal head entering the pelvic brim

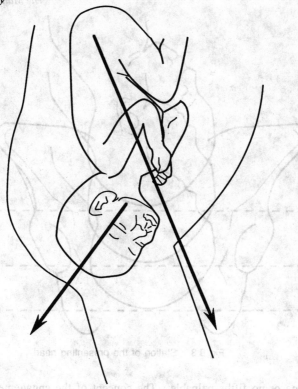

Fig 9.2   Misdirected axis of contraction force in occipito-posterior position

male. In this case the inlet is wedge-shaped with a tendency to engagement in an obliquely posterior position. The mid-cavity and outlet are much less favourable with a greater likelihood of rotational forceps delivery or caesarean section. Determination of the shape of the brim clinically is not possible. However awareness of the association between malposition of the occiput with a differing brim shape is helpful in understanding the mechanisms of the progress of abnormal labour. The main problem with a posterior position of the occiput is that the neck progressively deflexes and the uterine contraction pressure is dissipated in the wrong axis (Fig 9.2). The occiput retreats into the sacral curve. Although progress may continue to a normal delivery there is a substantial chance that secondary uterine inertia will supervene.

The level of the presenting part is critical. Palpated per abdomen, the head is referred to as engaged or not engaged as well as in terms of the number of fifths palpable. Engagement is absolute and occurs when the widest diameter of the presenting part passes through the inlet of the pelvis. This is judged when the examining fingers reach the lower part of the palpable head. If the fingers can lift the head off the pelvis or if they are approaching the midline rather than diverging at this point then the head is not engaged. A head that is not engaged must by definition be three, four or five fifths palpable. Assessment of the fifths palpable, (Fig 9.3) was originally suggested by Crichton (1974) because a greater degree of precision was required than offered by engagement. A head that is engaged must

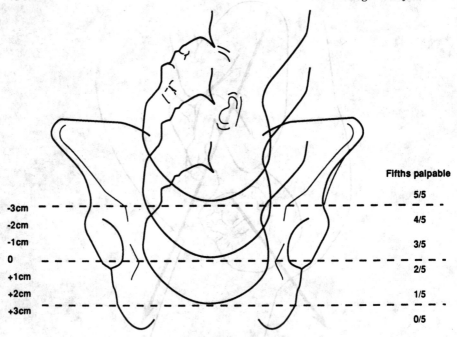

Fifths palpable

5/5

-3cm   4/5

-2cm

-1cm   3/5

0   2/5

+1cm

+2cm   1/5

+3cm

0/5

Fig 9.3   Station of the presenting head

be two, one or no fifths palpable. The concept of the engagement of the breech is problematical. In theory it occurs when the inter-trochanteric diameter enters the pelvic brim. This is a radiological concept. Clinical palpation of the inter-tro-chanteric diameter of the breech is not possible. Obviously there is no useful concept of fifths palpable of the breech. The breech can reasonably be described as being above the brim or in the brim of the pelvis. A free presenting part usually means it is not engaged. However a fixed presenting part may be fixed because of disproportion and therefore not engaged.

Given a fairly constant configuration of the pelvis there is a correlation between the level of the part abdominally and the station judged per vaginum. Although the word station has historically been applied to the vaginal findings it refers to the same phenomenon as the level of the head abdominally; that is, observation of the process of descent of the presenting part. A head that is engaged abdominally and not significantly moulded will have its leading edge at the level of the ischial spines (Fig 9.3). There are two problems with assessing the descent of the head abdominally. Firstly, if the mother is overweight or dis-tressed in the late stages of labour then the abdominal level can be very difficult to define with any precision. Except in very obese women it should be possible to distinguish a five fifths palpable head from a zero fifths palpable head. None-theless the phenomenon of the undiagnosed breech bears witness to the difficulties of this procedure. Observer variability may be quite marked and in abnormal labour the head may be observed to have apparently risen in its level. This is likely to be due to a change in attitude from optimism to pessimism with regard to the prospect of a vaginal birth on account of the clinical situation rather than to a real rise in the head level. It is sometimes a phenomenon seen at the changeover of the duty shifts of midwives and doctors. The second problem with the descent of the head judged abdominally is that the occipito-posterior head feels lower than it really is. This is because the occiput positioned posteriorly sinks into the sacral concavity. The chin and face are asymmetric with respect to the back of the head and less prominent to palpation. It is therefore surprising when vaginal examination finds the head not to be as low as suspected abdominally (Fig 9.4). This is important because of the frequency of difficult labour in a situation where the occiput is posterior.

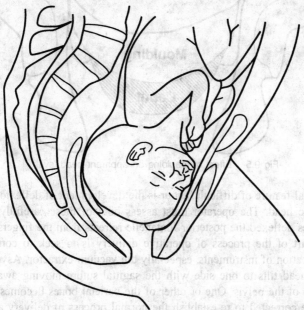

Fig 9.4   Station in occipit-posterior position

Assessment of the station vaginally is not free of problems either. This is because of the phenomena of caput and moulding. Caput appears when the head is pressed very tightly against the cervix for a prolonged length of time. The venous outflow from the scalp is obstructed and there is tissue swelling and edema. This occurs in difficult labour and contributes further to the problem by complicating the detection of the landmarks on the head and the determination of the position of the occiput. Moulding occurs because the skull bones are essentially unfused and mobile. They can move with respect to each other. This occurs to a limited extent during normal birth. If the labour is difficult then it may become very marked in proportion to the degree of obstruction to the passage of the head. Stewart (1977) proposed a method of quantifying moulding to facilitate an objective analysis of the phenomenon, later Vacca (1992) simplified this for easier use. Moulding also renders detection of the landmarks difficult but more importantly, causes the head to appear to be at a lower level vaginally than it really is (Fig 9.5). Thus a head that has a great degree of caput and moulding might nearly appear at the vulva without being engaged.

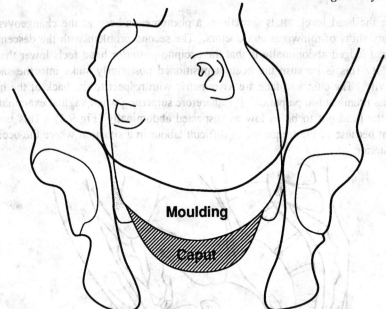

Fig 9.5   Effect of moulding on apparent head level

A critical feature of difficult labour is the development of deflexion and asynclitism of the head. The operator must assess both of these carefully. When the
head becomes deflexed the posterior fontanelle retreats from the fingers examining
vaginally. Part of the process of operative delivery is to seek to correct this by
proper application of instruments, especially the vacuum extractor. Asynclitism occurs as the head tilts to one side with the sagittal suture moving away from the
central plane of the pelvis. One or other of the parietal bones becomes prominent.
This must be corrected to re-establish the normal process of delivery and the correction is an integral part of assisted delivery particularly when it involves a degree
of rotation. The observation of the uterine cervix also provides information about
the ease of the labour process. Slowness of dilatation may indicate a problem and
this is especially so when there is concomitant thickening of the cervix with edema.
Poor application of the cervix to the presenting part particularly during a contraction
is also important. Given these circumstances careful review of the maternal size
and fetal size is appropriate. As contributors to the scenario at operative delivery
they are critical.

Terminology
Proper documentation and comparison of data have been hindered by inconsistent
definitions. These have been clarified by Hibbard (1989) and the American College
of Obstetricians and Gynecologists (1988).

A *high forceps* refers to a delivery situation where the fetal head is not engaged and the lowest part of the fetal skull has not reached the ischial spines. This
procedure is of historical interest only and is never performed now. The baby
used to be extracted through the inlet and the upper strait of the pelvis with the
likelihood of serious mechanical obstruction and damage. It was for these kinds of

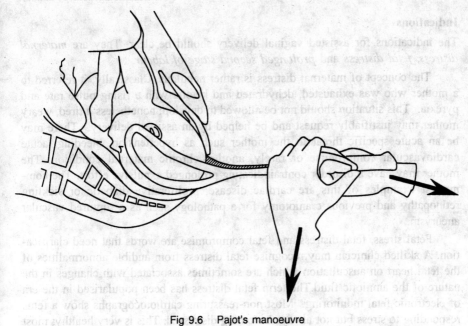

Fig 9.6   Pajot's manoeuvre

deliveries that axis-traction was invented in order to exert a force directed down-wards and backwards. This is still required in some lower forceps procedures but the alternative of Pajot's manoeuvre suffices and limits the force. One hand is placed on the superior aspect of the instruments and pressure applied towards the floor (Fig 9.6). Axis traction equipment is now redundant as is *high forceps delivery*; the equipment should be removed from the labour ward instrument packs.

A *mid forceps* refers to a delivery where the head is engaged but the leading edge of the skull is less than 2 cm below the ischial spines. An unmoulded head is engaged when its leading edge is at the level of the ischial spines. It is important to note that this reference is to the leading bony part of the head and not to the lowest part of caput. In most of these cases the occiput will not be in an anterior position and some degree of rotation will be necessary. This also involves recognition and correction of deflexion and asynclitism. It is this group of deliveries that generates most controversy. The option of caesarean section should be seriously contemplated.

A *low forceps* refers to a delivery where the leading edge of the head is below the ischial spines but is not visible unless the operator parts the labia, and where the head is not distending the perineum with contractions. In this case the sagittal suture will be within 45 degrees of the antero-posterior plane although the occiput may well be in a posterior position.

An *outlet forceps* delivery refers to a situation where the leading edge of the head is seen without parting the labia. The sagittal suture is in the antero-posterior diameter and then the only remaining obstruction to the delivery is the soft tissue of the perineum.

Indications

The indications for assisted vaginal delivery should be clear. They are *maternal distress, fetal distress* and *prolonged second stage of labour*.

The concept of maternal distress is rather nebulous. Classically, it referred to a mother who was exhausted, dehydrated and ketotic with a rising pulse rate and pyrexia. This situation should not be allowed to develop; nonetheless a tired, weary mother may justifiably request and be helped by an assisted delivery. There may be an acute specific threat to the mother such as hypertension, bleeding, acute cardiovascular compromise or rarely, another chronic maternal condition. The mother may have a disorder contraindicating prolonged expulsive effort. The commonest examples of this are cardiac disease, proliferative diabetic or sickling retinopathy and previous craniotomy for a pathology such as a ruptured vascular aneurysm.

Fetal stress, fetal distress and fetal compromise are words that need clarification. A skilled clinician may recognise fetal distress from audible abnormalities of the fetal heart on auscultation which are sometimes associated with changes in the nature of the amniotic fluid. The term fetal distress has been popularised in the era of electronic fetal monitoring. Most non-reassuring cardiotocographs show a fetus responding to stress but not always becoming distressed. This is very healthy; most humans perform well under stress. No fetal heart monitor actually shows distress. It shows a fetal heart rate pattern and it is up to the observer to decide if it represents compromise by skillful interpretation. Fetal compromise is a better term than fetal distress because it demands reflection and careful assessment (Gibb and Arulkumaran 1992). There are various signs of compromise but they hinge on the presence of an abnormal cardiotocograph (CTG) and/or thick meconium staining of the amniotic fluid in a situation suggestive of risk. Meconium passage occurs as a physiological phenomenon with fetal maturation especially as the period of gestation reaches forty weeks. However it may also occur as a response to hypoxic stress. The clinical circumstances at the time are important but the key element is the pattern of the CTG. In the second stage of labour this requires a rather different interpretation from that in the first stage of labour (Arulkumaran et al 1992). Essentially, a progressive bradycardia or a persistent bradycardia below 100 beats per minute or a complicated tachycardia are indications for delivery. Unless the delivery is straightforward, operative delivery risks compound the distress and consideration of the alternative option of caesarean section is indicated. Conversely, unnecessary assisted deliveries should not be performed when evidence for fetal compromise is not convincing.

The concept of a prolonged second stage of labour has evolved in recent years. The older textbooks set arbitrary time limits on the length of labour. These were generally set as two hours for a mother having her first baby and one hour for a second or subsequent delivery. More recently flexibility in allowing a longer second stage has become the norm with due consideration of why it is prolonged, the fetal condition and the progress of descent of the presenting part. The ability to monitor the fetal heart electronically and the use of epidural anesthesia are critical. As long as the fetal heart pattern is reassuring and the progress of descent of the presenting part is being made, a second stage can continue. The second stage is defined as commencing when the woman feels the urge to push. The cervix may have been found to be fully dilated before this especially when epidural anesthesia has been used but it is the pushing phase that represents the particular risk period. Epidural anesthesia has been shown to suppress oxytocin release at this stage of labour (Goodfellow et al 1983) as well as to reduce the strength of the contractions (Bates et al 1985). Although the cervix may be fully dilated, the mother does not have an urge to push. The attendant may find the cervix to be fully dilated under these circumstances but the presenting part is in the mid-cavity and is not seen on parting the labia. Patience is then required and the commencement of active pushing should be deferred until the presenting part is seen or there is an urge to push. There is often an indication to prescribe oxytocin treatment under these circumstances to improve the contractions. In an actuarial analysis of primigravid women who had not had epidural anesthesia Kadar et al (1983) suggested that waiting for up to three hours was worthwhile. With an epidural in situ, slight wearing off of the effect and witholding of the top up dose will allow a more accurate assessment of the dynamics of the labour process. Gaziano et al (1980) have documented a high incidence of variable decelerations and prolonged decelerations in the second stage of labour. The gradual fall in fetal pH that occurs throughout labour is accelerated during the second stage (Jacobson and Rooth 1971; Pearson and Davies 1974). The importance of a reassuring CTG during a long second stage cannot be overstated.

Clinical practice

Every operative delivery should be undertaken by a person who is skilled and practised in the technique or by an operator supervised by such a person. As with any surgical procedure, the operation should be carefully documented in the notes. The name of the procedure, the operation being undertaken should be clear. The indication for the intervention should be stated explicitly. In most operative vaginal deliveries the uterine cervix should be fully dilated. Although the urinary bladder is not a pelvic organ at this stage it may be necessary to pass a urinary catheter. In some cases this may not be necessary; however it is wise to check after the delivery that the urine appears normal. When an epidural anesthetic has been used continuous drainage for about 24 hours may be necessary if there is difficulty in passing urine to obviate the problems of urinary retention with overflow. This procedure should not be used as a substitute for good midwifery care that ensures effective bladder emptying.

In all cases, before embarking on an assisted delivery other options should be considered. These are: to wait and be patient, to improve the strength of the uterine contractions or to perform a caesarean section. In the case of a multiparous woman some gentle but firm massage of the vaginal tissues often leads to increased expulsive effects. Babies are much better born by propulsion than extraction.

It is not the purpose of this text to teach operative delivery. That can only be done by example and experience in the labour ward. However each type of operative delivery will be considered and guiding principles outlined. The key principle is assistance rather than extraction. Assistance is designed to complement the natural process of labour: doctors must understand fully the natural mechanism of labour that is to be complemented. Experience in examining undergraduates and postgraduates suggests that this central concept of our work is poorly taught and poorly understood. In abnormal labour mechanical reasons for delay should be considered and the position of the occiput determined accurately. With adequate pain relief palpation of the fetal ear is useful. The advance of the presenting part with uterine contractions and with a bearing down effort is important. Poor application of the cervix to the presenting part and thickening or edema formation in the cervix are adverse prognostic features. If the uterus is not contracting adequately this should be corrected with an oxytocin infusion. Traction should be exerted only during a contraction. Failure to ensure this makes the delivery more difficult and increases the chance of an atonic post-partum hemorrhage. The lithotomy position is important with a degree of flexion of the hips towards the maternal abdomen. This alters the pelvic configuration analagous to the squatting position. Although there is an advantage in advancing the buttocks beyond the edge of the delivery couch in rotational delivery, breech delivery and situations of expected shoulder dystocia, care should be exercised because of the risk of injury to the lower lumbar spine.

Outlet forceps

In outlet forceps delivery the head is visible without the labia being parted, the sagittal suture is in the antero-posterior diameter and the head is on the perineum and only the soft tissues remain a barrier.

In principle the mother should be in the lithotomy position; however experienced operators may feel comfortable and confident with the mother in a dorsal position for a very low outlet forceps delivery. Having positioned the mother and verified the prerequisites for delivery the operator be comfortably seated facing the perineum. Continuous verbal and intermittent eye to eye contact with the mother should be maintained and each step explained to her. The forceps are assembled in front of the perineum in the position in which they are to be applied. If there is no pre-existing analgesia then the perineum should be infiltrated with a local anesthetic agent. The left blade is applied first followed by the right. The prerequisites are then rechecked before traction is applied. The contraction will then become evident by the woman's response and by the movement of the head. Firm traction is applied, building up with the contraction for the duration of the contraction. In a true outlet forceps delivery the direction of traction, although initially downwards to the floor, soon becomes upwards as the head delivers with extension. Excessive force is a serious risk to the mother and baby. Traction should never be greater than that exerted by the operator flexing the forearm. Placing the index finger between the blades also prevents the use of excessive force. A major degree of rocking movement should not be necessary. The feet of the operator should never be placed on the end of the delivery couch and the woman's buttocks should not rise off the couch. Descent should occur with the first contraction. If it does not, a careful reassessment of the whole situation should be undertaken. The fetal heart is checked before further traction is applied. If the indication is a prophylactic forceps delivery because of a maternal condition and the woman is multiparous then episiotomy may not be necessary. However more commonly, in a primigravida with a prolonged second stage an episiotomy is an integral part of the procedure. A medio-lateral incision is appropriate. After the head has emerged the forceps are removed and the body delivered normally. If the baby is in good condition it should have the oral mucus extracted by the midwife whilst being placed on the mother's abdomen, if that is what she wishes. The vagina and perineum should be examined and carefully sutured at a suitable time after delivery. The operator should then examine the baby with the parents particularly to assess any forceps marks and explain their significance in a reassuring way.

Low forceps

In low forceps delivery the head is at or near the pelvic floor but may not be visible without parting the labia and the perineum does not distend with contractions. The lowest bony part is at least 2 cm below the ischial spines. The sagittal suture may not be in the antero-posterior diameter but will not be more than 45 degrees from it. The head may well be occipito-posterior. The woman should be in the lithotomy position and the operator should be seated facing the perineum. The position of the head should be verified. If an epidural block is in place this will be easier and an attempt may be made to feel the fetal ears or orbital ridges. The sagittal suture and fontanelles may be obscured by caput and moulding. If an epidural has not already been given and if there is no urgency, a regional block (epidural or caudal) can be instituted at this stage. If this is not possible, an effective pudendal nerve block should be established, supplemented with perineal infiltration. If the deviation from the antero-posterior diameter is minimal it might then be possible to ease the head round with digital rotation. Alternatively, less than 45 degrees of rotation can be undertaken with non-rotational forceps (Neville-Barnes, Simpson's). The advantage of these forceps is that traction can subsequently be exerted in the correct direction because of the pelvic curve of the forceps. The left blade is applied before the right. If there is any difficulty in applying the forceps, the situation must be fully reassessed. Before a contraction the head is gently rotated to occipito-anterior. If it does not turn easily the situation should be reassessed. With the following contraction traction is exerted downwards towards the floor. Some operators find it useful at this point to kneel on the floor. Pajot's manoeuvre to exert pressure on the blades from above will also help the head to advance in the correct direction (Fig 9.5).

When the head has reached the perineum, the appropriate upward movement is applied to achieve delivery with extension of the head. An episiotomy is performed when the head distends the perineum. This should not be done too soon. If it is, then the unsatisfactory situation of proceeding to caesarean section after having performed an episiotomy will sometimes arise. Three scars will result: one on the perineum, one on the abdomen and one on the psyche! If during traction the forceps blades adopt a rather more horizontal position, it suggests that the head is in an occipito-posterior position. A large episiotomy is then particularly important because the widest diameter is more posterior and the occiput is exerting greater pressure posteriorly on the perineum with an increased risk of tearing near the anus.

In cases of a recognised occipito-posterior position a decision will be needed on whether to embark on full rotation or deliver face to pubis. If the head is low, it seems sensible to deliver face to pubis as this is closest to the natural resolution. In these circumstances the forceps are applied exactly as if it were occipito-anterior. The pelvic curve of the forceps must always coincide with the actual pelvic curve. A large episiotomy should be performed. The rest of the delivery is conducted as an outlet forceps. Care is taken to examine the genital tract before and after repair. The baby is examined in the presence of the parents and explanation of any minimal trauma is given.

Difficulty in achieving the correct position of the forceps, failure to turn the head with minimal force and failure of descent with the first pull are danger signs that demand full reassessment. This is particularly important in the presence of a major degree of caput and moulding. After every contraction the fetal heart rate must be checked. If after three contractions with bearing down effort and applied traction the head is not delivered then caesarean section should be performed. In doing this the head may have to be dislodged upwards to facilitate delivery. It is important that an assistant remains available and is prepared to place a hand under the drapes to do this from below.

Mid-cavity forceps

In this situation the leading bony part of the head is above the pelvic floor. The head is engaged abdominally with no more than one fifth palpable. The station vaginally shows the leading bony part to be below the ischial spines but not as far as +2 cm. The occiput is unlikely to be anterior and most likely to be transverse. This has been called deep transverse arrest. There is also likely to be asynclitism with the head tilted and one of the parietal bones leading in descent. This is the most controversial form of operative delivery and should only be performed by a highly skilled operator. The most frequently used forceps are Kielland's. Their place and the technique of their use have been comprehensively described by Parry Jones (1952). Chiswick and James (1979) gave a warning of the neonatal morbidity and mortality associated with their use. However Cardozo et al (1983) countered the criticism, highlighting important points of the technique which renders their use safe under proper conditions. Epidural anesthesia is preferred for delivery although an effective pudendal block may suffice. Mid-cavity delay occurs in women in whom an epidural has been used for pain relief during the first stage of labour. This has been shown to be associated with defective oxytocin release and the absence of increase in the power of the contractions seen in normal delivery. Mothers also feel less urge to push. Effective oxytocin treatment should be given first. If there is a normal CTG, spontaneous descent should be awaited. Better contractions and patience may mean that the operative delivery may not be necessary or that it can be done from a lower station.

Before embarking on the procedure the operator must be satisfied that it is appropriate. If there is any doubt at all the most senior person should be consulted before a trial of forceps can be done (see below). If the fetal heart rate is suspicious then a fetal blood sample may be done to confirm fetal health. The appearance of thick meconium at this stage associated with an abnormal fetal heart rate pattern and the possibility of a difficult delivery suggests that caesarean section is the safer option. If the situation is favourable the woman is placed in lithotomy and the prerequisites for delivery checked. The importance of caput, moulding, a palpably big baby and a small pelvis as signs of obstruction have already been highlighted. There must be absolute confidence in recognising the position of the occiput and the presence of asynclitism. The procedure is explained to the woman and the forceps assembled facing the perineum with the operator in a sitting position. The anterior blade is applied first by the classic, direct or wandering method (Hibbard 1989). The posterior blade follows, care being exercised to ease it anterior to the sacrum. The forceps will then lie at different levels reflecting asynclitism. This must be corrected by sliding the blades within the sliding lock to lie at the same level. Between contractions the head is then gently turned using only the force of the forearm. If there is any difficulty or obstruction, the whole situation must be reassessed. If the rotation is successful the next contraction is the signal to exert downward traction. Kielland's forceps do not have a pelvic curve and are not ideal to exert the traction in the correct direction. This must be downwards towards the floor. A kneeling position is most appropriate for the operator. The Kielland's forceps may be removed and a different type with a pelvic curve applied. The fetal heart is assessed throughout and failure of the descent of the head is viewed with concern. The rest of the delivery is conducted as a low forceps procedure. The episiotomy is performed only when the head distends the perineum. If delivery has not occurred in five contractions with bearing down effort then the alternative option of caesarean section should be seriously considered.

Failed forceps

This is a very serious situation, in which the delivery has not been accomplished and the operator has not recognised prospectively that there would be difficulty. The baby may suffer damage during the delay between the conclusion of the failed procedure and the caesarean section to follow. Most cases of failed forceps arise from 'disobeying the ground rules, inexperience and lack of discipline' (Hibbard 1989). Contributory factors may be failure to locate the occiput correctly, unrecognised brow presentation, incomplete dilatation of the cervix and cephalopelvic disproportion. A trial of forceps is acceptable in modern practice, a failed forceps is not. A high incidence of failed forceps that have not been conducted as a trial of forceps should lead to a review of procedures of selection for mode of delivery. Forceps are considered to have failed in two slightly different scenarios. There may have been difficulty in applying, locking or rotating as opposed to failure of traction after successful application. These circumstances are important during an audit when the circumstances as well as the training and skills of the operator should be reviewed.

Trial of forceps

If the operator has any doubt about the outcome of a forceps delivery the procedure should be a trial of forceps. The criteria on which doubt may be judged have been expressed in the preceding paragraphs. Although any forceps might be considered a trial, the term principally applies to mid-cavity and some low procedures. By

definition it is a matter of intent. A trial is performed in the operating theatre with
the theatre staff and the anesthetist ready to perform caesarean section at minutes'
notice. The woman must also be clearly informed and reassured about the situation.
The trial is not seen as a challenge to the skilled operator but as a well-judged
procedure to be abandoned in favour of a caesarean section if any difficulty arises.
There is no need to be ashamed of a failed trial of forceps. The procedure must
be seen as trial of forceps and not a trial by forceps! As Donald said: 'Trial of
forceps is like lion taming. It is not the sort of exercise one would willingly un-
dertake in expectation of failure' (Donald 1969).

Vacuum extraction

The role of the vacuum extractor has been well reviewed by Chalmers (1971) and
Vacca (1992).

In a cephalic presentation most indications for a forceps delivery are also
indications for vacuum extraction. Incomplete dilatation of the cervix has been
sited as a specific indication for the use of vacuum if vaginal delivery is being
pursued. In modern practice this has been questioned (Pearce and Steel 1987;
Chamberlain 1989). A baby compromised by 'true' fetal distress in the first stage
of labour should be delivered by caesarean section. A labour that does not progress
should be treated with oxytocin and patience. The risks of damage to the maternal
tissues by performing vacuum extraction before full dilatation are considerable.
With full dilatation of the cervix, the choice of instrument depends on the experience and skill of the operator. In preterm pregnancies before 34 weeks it is better
not to use the vacuum because of the softer head and wider separation of the
sutures. The vacuum extractor may be superior in the specific circumstances of a
mid-cavity delivery in the presence of a previous caesarean section scar. There is
no supporting published study but the logic is persuasive. Because of improved
equipment and its ease of use the vacuum can be used in situations of fetal compromise. There is no necessity to build up the pressure in stages and extraction
can be done immediately (Vacca et al 1983). The technology of the Silc cup might
have rendered the technique easy to use. The justification for use should not be
that it is easier for a less-skilled operator to use. A problem is that in mid-cavity
procedures the size of the handle of the vaccum extractor makes it difficult to
manoeuvre it to the necessary position over the occiput. This is critically important
and the older metal cups, and in particular the occipito-posterior cup, are superior.
This is reflected in the higher rate of failure to deliver with the mid-cavity vacuum
extractor when compared to the forceps (Johanson 1991). Vacca and Keirse (1989)
correlated the failure of vacuum delivery with the failure to place the cup in the
correct position towards the occiput.

The mother should be warned of the nature of the technique before it is used.
Increasing numbers of informed women with birth plans have indicated a preference
for vacuum extraction to forceps. The patient should be informed of the sounds
that may accompany the procedure and the chignon to be expected on the baby's
head at birth. This can be unsightly but can easily be covered with a towel. The
preparations are the same as for the equivalent category of forceps delivery. Anesthesia is important, but because in mid-cavity procedures instruments are not

being pushed as far in to the genital tract, pudendal nerve block may suffice. Locating the occiput is crucial. With good analgesia, feeling the ears and orbital ridges may provide guidance. The cup must be directed to the occiput in the midline of the head with due allowance for deflexion of the head and asynclitism. The vacuum is applied and the cup checked carefully to ensure that the mother's tissues have not been caught in it. With the next contraction traction is applied downward and backwards towards the woman's anus with one hand. The other hand must be applied to steady the cup on the head and feel for any sign of it coming off. The operator must think of how the natural process is being complemented. The head should show a tendency to rotate on its own as descent occurs. The cup should be used to encourage flexion of the head, drawing it in the direction of the curve of the birth canal. An episiotomy will usually be appropriate but might not be necessary. The use of an episiotomy encourages traction in the correct direction. Incorrect application of the cup and pulling in the wrong direction are two causes of failed vacuum delivery. Each contraction and episode of traction should lead to a change in the level of the head. The fetal heart must be observed between contractions. The fetal head should be delivered within 15 minutes of applying the cup. In case of delay a critical review of the situation should be undertaken and caesarean section considered. The cup may come off due to faulty equipment or mechanical obstruction. If the head has advanced in an occipito-anterior position and obstruction has been excluded forceps can be appropriately applied. As vacuum extraction is more likely to fail than forceps it is logical to attempt forceps after vacuum in selected cases but not vacuum after forceps. The role of a trial of vacuum delivery is the same as a trial of forceps. The mother should be shown the baby and its chignon by the operator. Cephalhematoma and subgaleal hemorrhage are commoner after vacuum extraction than after forceps delivery. Facial injuries and bruising are equal in both cases. Retinal hemorrhage might be common and neonatal jaundice is more common. Although maternal trauma occurs less after vacuum extraction than after the equivalent forceps procedure the operator must examine the genital tract very carefully after delivery. Shoulder dystocia probably relates to mid-cavity assisted delivery of a large baby, irrespective of which instrument is used (McFarland et al 1986). However its relationship to the vaccum extractor should engender caution in performing these deliveries without an episiotomy.

Shoulder dystocia

Shoulder dystocia is the most frightening and threatening obstetric emergency because of the desperate need to act quickly to prevent morbidity and mortality. The greatest requirement is to be prepared both in anticipation and practice. The antecedents of shoulder dystocia have been clearly documented: maternal obesity, diabetes mellitus, gestational age of greater than 41 weeks, previous shoulder dystocia or a big baby, recognised macrosomia of present pregnancy (Boyd et al 1983; Parks and Ziel 1978), prolongation of the late first stage of labour (Hopwood 1982), prolongation of the second stage of labour and operative delivery (Benedetti and Gabbe 1978). Unusual circumstances like a microcephalic fetus or hydropic fetus should be recognised. The emergency can therefore be anticipated in a number of cases. The special features box on the partogram or labour record in such cases should be marked 'BEWARE SHOULDER DYSTOCIA'. In these cases a doctor with appropriate experience in the management of this emergency should be in the room during the delivery. In most cases such assistance will not be necessary. If it is, then a clear plan of action, a 'SHOULDER DYSTOCIA' drill must be implemented (Gibb 1988). All units should have this written down in the labour ward protocol.

1. Help should be summoned in the form of the most experienced obstetric doctor and an anesthetist.

2. The woman should be placed in the lithotomy position or turned on her side. This is not only to make space for manipulation at the perineum but to facilitate flexion of the hips on to the woman's abdomen (McRobert's manoeuvre).

3. McRobert's manoeuvre: the hip joints are fully abducted, rotated outwards and flexed with the thighs touching the mother's abdomen. This involves removing the legs from the lithotomy poles. This manoeuvre was described by Gonik et al (1983). Although it does not alter the dimensions of the pelvis it changes the angle of inclination of the pelvic inlet, possibly also opening the outlet (O'Leary and Pollack 1991; Seeds 1986). Many experienced midwives encountering shoulder dystocia during mome confinement recommend rolling the mother into a knee chest position. This may be useful in stopping the mother pushing and in rotating the pelvic girdle although anterior pressure is then difficult (Seeds 1986).

4. An episiotomy must be done or liberally extended if it has already been done.

5. Pressure is exerted suprapubically to try to dislodge the anterior shoulder. Firm but gentle pressure is applied posteriorly within the pelvis towards the anus. This pressure must not be aggressively outwards.

6. If analgesia is adequate then manipulation should be undertaken to dislodge the posterior shoulder. This involves passing the hand into the pelvis and attempting rotation (Rubin 1964) or pushing the posterior arm forwards past the trunk and pulling it down thereby reducing the shoulder diameters and allowing the anterior shoulder to pass behind the symphysis pubis.

These manouevres are usually successful. Deliberate fracture of the clavicle should never be performed with a living baby. The Zavanelli manoeuvre (Sandberg 1985) might be attempted in exceptional circumstances; however it has never been reported in the United Kingdom. This involves replacement of the head under anesthesia and delivery by caesarean section. Its role is controversial and all vaginal manoeuvres must have been first attempted. Many of the more complicated manipulations cannot be undertaken without general anesthesia. Careful examination of the genital tract must be undertaken after delivery to assess and repair traumatic damage. Should all large babies be delivered by caesarean section to avoid this problem? The answer is not so simple because a significant proportion of deliveries with shoulder dystocia do not result in big babies (Acker et al 1986). Such a policy would also result in a great increase in the number of caesarean sections in order to prevent a few cases of shoulder dystocia. (Hofmeyr 1989). In a few cases the caesarean section itself may be complicated because of the same factors. Shoulder dystocia remains an important cause of morbidity and mortality. Anticipation and appropriate action are critical.

Breech delivery

Babies presenting by the breech have a much higher morbidity and mortality than those presenting by the vertex. Important associates are prematurity and congenital malformations. Nonetheless the delivery process itself is more hazardous. The main mechanical reasons are the failure of the presenting part to plug the birth canal, increasing the possibility of umbilical cord prolapse and the more rapid passage of the head through the birth canal, compared to cephalic delivery. In cephalic delivery the cervical spine, the base of the skull and intracranial contents are protected by the slow steady process of expulsion with an appropriate degree of moulding of the head. The expulsion of the head takes hours in a cephalic presentation but minutes in a breech.

A previous chapter has considered the assessment of the woman with a breech presentation antenatally. Problems may occur with breech delivery when there has not been adequate opportunity for antenatal assessment. Clinical and imaging assessment must be comprehensive. Experienced obstetricians can grossly estimate fetal weight; however an ultrasound scan is required for several reasons. It is important to educate radiographers about the detail required from such a scan. Ideally it is performed by an obstetrician to minimise confusion. The scan confirms breech presentation providing measurements of the bi-parietal diameter, head circumference, abdominal circumference and femur length. The absence of fetal malformation and placenta previa, both associated with breech presentation, is reconfirmed. The volume of amniotic fluid is observed. Finally and critically the attitude of the legs and head is documented. Extended legs are reassuring to the obstetrician for the delivery process because of a reduced risk of umbilical cord prolapse (Collea et al 1978). Extension of the fetal head is associated with a high risk of injury to the cervical spine and the base of the skull if the baby is delivered vaginally (Daw 1974; Caterini et al 1975). The estimated fetal weight is provided bearing in mind a potential 10% margin of error. In an average sized mother the optimum fetal weight for breech delivery is 2.0–3.5 kg. If the option of vaginal birth is being pursued, after initial discussions with the woman the physical characteristics of the maternal pelvis should be considered. A simple observation of the woman's stature is the first guide. Women of small stature tend to have a small pelvis. If the mother is multiparous then the size of previous babies delivered vaginally is relevant. Clinical, digital examination of the pelvis is generally considered inaccurate but might be performed. The presence of a prominent sacral promontory, a flat sacrum or an acutely hooked coccyx are adverse factors. The role of radiological pelvimetry is unclear. Those who do not do it believe that the evidence suggesting a caesarean section will come from the nature of progress in labour on the grounds that poor progress reflects a mechanical problem. The counter view is that good radiological measurements permit the confident use of oxytocin treatment in abnormal labour associated with poor contractions. The underlying principle is that a breech selected carefully for vaginal delivery is also selected for oxytocin use. The erect lateral x-ray should always be seen and should be available to the obstetrician responsible for and conducting the delivery. It should confirm breech presentation and provide a measurement of the antero-posterior diameter of the inlet and the outlet of the pelvis. These should be at least 11.5 cm. The arc of the sacral curve is also documented. It is unfavourable if it is quite flat or if the terminal part is hooked. The woman should be reassured that a skilled obstetrician, a skilled midwife, a skilled pediatrician, a skilled anesthetist and an electronic fetal monitor will all be available in the labour ward when she presents in spontaneous labour. It is important that she agrees to vaginal delivery. It is unwise to pursue a line of management in which the woman and her partner do not have total confidence. Induction of labour is not indicated because of breech presentation alone. Given another standard indication it is acceptable, but only with other factors such as the cervical condition being particularly favourable.

Term breech delivery

Whilst epidural anesthesia administered for pain relief in the first stage of labour will provide cover for a manipulative delivery it may interfere with the second stage and the expulsive phase. An epidural should not be given primarily to cover the delivery. The alternative is that an anesthetist should be present in the delivery room with equipment to hand for the immediate administration of sedation and general anesthesia should there be any acute complication. During labour with a breech presentation, variable decelerations of the fetal heart are common due to umbilical cord compression and pressure of the fundus of the uterus over the head. These decelerations can be tolerated as long as there are no changes in baseline rate and baseline variability suggesting asphyxia.

The essence of safe breech delivery is minimal assistance from the operator. Breech extraction is only rarely indicated in situations such as acute fetal compromise or delivery of a second twin. Under these circumstances the operator must be highly skilled and the pelvis capacious. The procedure may do more damage than was present in the original condition. During assisted breech delivery the baby is delivered as far as the lower trunk by maternal effort. The only interference until this stage is an episiotomy. The operator should then grasp the buttocks with a towel encouraging the sacrum to turn anteriorly. If the legs are extended, they are gently manipulated with a finger behind the knee to induce flexion and delivery of the legs. The umbilical cord should be loosened if it is tight but the temptation to fiddle with it and feel for fetal heart pulsations should be resisted. Patience and maternal pushing is of the essence and the obstetrician should not feel distressed. As the upper half of the trunk emerges a finger can be passed up over the scapula to bring the arms down if they are not already visible. If the arms are persistently extended, then Lovset's manoeuvre may be applied. When the body has been delivered it should not be allowed to hang (Clinch 1989). This encourages the extension of the head which is undesirable and may also trap an anterior rim of the cervix. The body is supported in a towel and when the nape of the neck descends under the symphysis pubis, preparations are made for delivery of the head. The body is lifted up above the horizontal level by an assistant and forceps are applied to protect the head, which follows (Milner 1975). Piper forceps are ideal for this because they do not have a pelvic curve; however in most hospitals the Neville-Barnes forceps prove satisfactory. The forceps should have a long handle. The Mauriceau-Smellie-Veit manoeuvre is an inferior choice because traction is exerted through the cervical spine. The mechanism of delivery of the head must focus on the need for its flexion. This is another reason not to pull on the breech but to allow the woman and the uterus to push it down maintaining a good degree of flexion. If manipulations become necessary, then flexing the head with a finger in the mouth and turning it laterally if it remains high is important.

Fetal blood sampling for an abnormal CTG in breech presentation is inappropriate as is instrumental delivery of the buttocks themselves. The obvious alternative of caesarean section should be selected. Failure of descent in the second stage is a cause for concern.

Preterm breech delivery

The mode of delivery for preterm breech is a very controversial subject. In spite of several attempts it has not proved possible to conduct a randomised controlled trial. There are several reasons for this. A preterm breech in established labour is likely to labour very quickly and preempt the decision to intervene by having a vaginal delivery. Those not in established labour may present with premature rupture of the membranes. This pathology in itself may be the important factor in making a decision on the mode of delivery. Most specialists advocate selective caesarean section for preterm breech delivery. Factors such as fetal weight 1.0–1.5 kg, footling presentation, maternal age, previous infertility and other medical or obstetric complications affect the decision. A preterm breech that presents as a footling is a special problem particularly in a multiparous woman. This is a typical scenario for the entrapment of the aftercoming head. Epidural block is a wise option in labour under these circumstances because of the likelihood of the woman pushing against an incompletely dilated cervix.

Twin delivery

Multiple pregnancy has a much higher complication rate than singleton. The principal complication leading to the loss of a baby is prematurity. Delivery problems are now less common but staff should be alert to danger signals in the antenatal period. Most multiple pregnancies are now advised serial ultrasound scans. An aspect often not documented is the presence or absence of a dividing membrane. Mono amniotic twins are rare but susceptible to specific complications in late pregnancy and during delivery. These are cord entanglement during the later part of pregnancy (Tessen and Zlatnik 1991; Carr et al 1990; Bryan 1992) and malpresentation of the second twin after delivery of the first due to the absence of the protective second sac. Immediate facilities for caesarean section must be available. Some consider elective caesarean section to be the better option. The potential complications during delivery of the even rarer conjoined twins are obvious. Even if their survival is not anticipated caesarean section should be undertaken because of the clear hazards to the mother.

The mode of delivery of twins should be individualised according to certain principles (Gibb and Greenough 1991). If the first twin is presenting by the vertex most consider vaginal birth to be advisable in the absence of other complications. Care should be exercised when there is discordant growth of twins especially when it is the second one that is bigger and that may deliver as a breech. With discordant growth and the difference estimated fetal weights on ultrasound greater than 25%, the chance of asphyxial complications in the second twin is high. If the first twin presents by the breech the conditions necessary to satisfy safe singleton breech delivery should be fulfilled. If the second twin is cephalic there is only a very small chance of the rare complication of locked twins arising although the possibility may be higher if the twins are monoamniotic.

The woman should be reassured that skilled staff will be available in the labour ward when she presents in spontaneous labour. Electronic fetal monitors with twin minitoring facilities should be available. If staffing levels and facilities do not offer the patient the confidence that these will be available round the clock, induction of labour as a planned procedure in the daytime should be considered. Multiple pregnancies frequently deliver before term and the cervix is often found to be favourable. The importance of monitoring the second twin is clear and can often be difficult. It is important that the mother be informed of the situation and that she agrees to vaginal delivery.

Epidural anesthesia given for pain relief in the first stage of labour will cover manipulative delivery. If it does not, an anesthetist must be present in the delivery room during delivery. If the first twin advances by the vertex the midwife should proceed towards delivery as a normal singleton. The doctor supervising the delivery should be in the room and positioned above the perineum rather than below it. The role of the doctor is to palpate the abdomen immediately after the first twin has emerged. In doing so, the lie of the second twin can be determined and converted to longitudinal, preferably vertex. An ultrasound machine should be in the room but need not be used until this simple clinical procedure is complete. Any difficulty with this procedure requires the use of the ultrasound to determine the lie of the second baby to aid further manipulation. This will also localise the fetal heart to aid the placement of the external transducer of the fetal monitor. When the second twin is in a longitudinal lie a uterine contraction should be awaited. In primigravidae this is often delayed and an oxytocin infusion may be used prophylactically. A higher dose than that used for the standard augmentation of the first stage of labour is required and 10 milliunits per minute is appropriate. The fetal heart is then monitored continuously and patience exercised. The second sac of membranes should not be ruptured too early, since this generates anxiety and contributes to unnecessary manipulation sometimes resulting in the need for caesarean section for the second twin. The presenting part should be allowed to descend and the membranes ruptured artificially only if they remain intact with the presenting part well into the pelvis. If the fetal heart is normal there is no reason to rupture the membranes until the presenting part is expelled. Indeed this is a highly desirable manoeuvre with a breech presentation. If the fetal heart poses a problem with the presenting part high up, then breech extraction or a high vacuum extraction for a cephalic presentation performed by a skilled operator may be appropriate.

Caesarean section is the other option. Before electronic fetal monitors became available limits were set on the time allowed for the twin delivery interval. Such arbitrary limits are no longer applicable as long as the fetal condition is good.

The chance of postpartum hemorrhage in multiple pregnancy is much greater because of atony of the uterus and because of the possibility of genital tract trauma. This must be recognised and appropriate steps taken. The genital tract must be examined for trauma both before and after repair of the episiotomy. An oxytocin infusion in high dosage (50-100 milliunits per minute) should be maintained for a few hours after delivery.

The delivery of higher multiple pregnancies is controversial. Electronic fetal monitoring is problematical for three babies and mechanical problems are more likely. These are often pregnancies after a period of infertility and the logistics in the delivery room are difficult. There is compelling logic in delivering these cases by planned elective caesarean section. This has to be planned before term because of the high incidence of preterm birth (Botting et al 1990).

Perineal trauma

Normal delivery may lead to perineal trauma with the typical face to pubis delivery of a big baby. However perineal trauma is characteristically associated with operative vaginal delivery. A timely and relatively large episiotomy under these circumstances may prevent an irregular problematical tear. It is not the purpose of this text to describe the techniques and materials used but rather to clarify the principles.

Any woman with known or suspected perineal trauma must be examied by a skilled doctor, in the lithotomy position, with a good light and proper anesthesia. When a third degree tear is immediately recognised and repaired in optimum circumstances the prognosis for complete recovery is excellent. Poorer results follow interval repair when the injury has been undiagnosed or has been inadequately repaired. For anything other than minor tears nitrous oxide inhalation and local anesthesia are inadequate. For examination of the upper genital tract epidural or general anesthesia is mandatory. Damage to the ano-rectal structures must be meticulously repaired by an expert. The rectal mucosa is first closed and the retracted ends of the anal sphincter drawn together and secured. The deep perineal tissues are closed with interrupted sutures. The vaginal skin and perineal skin are then closed. Great care must be taken to achieve anatomical approximation. Although damage may be extensive avoiding overuse of suture material is important. Individual bleeding points should be secured. During repair, care should be taken to ensure that the uterus has contracted properly or bleeding from above will confuse the picture and hinder the process. A swab on a piece of string is often placed in the upper vagina. Removal of this swab and a detailed swab count at the end of the procedure are critical. Patience is required at the end of any repair. It is important to ensure that there is no untoward bleeding before the legs are lowered and the procedure considered complete. Ice packs are helpful but proprietary medicines applied to the perineum have not been shown to be useful. The woman should be advised to keep her stools soft by generous fluid intake and an appropriate diet. Bulk laxatives may sometimes be prescribed. Where a third degree tear breaks down it is imperative that no attempt be made to effect a secondary repair whilst the wound remains infected. Proper follow up should be arranged by the person involved in the repair or by the consultant. Further corrective repairs must be undertaken by senior experienced staff after the necessary delay to ensure healthier tissues. For such repairs non-absorbable material such as silk should be used which is then removed. If subsequent repair is unsuccessful then a second opinion should be sought.

Caesarean section

Used as a method to avoid traumatic delivery caesarean section in itself may prove traumatic. The documentation in the notes should be as for other operative deliveries. Often caesarean section notes are less informative than they might be. Unusually the incision on the lower segment may not be transverse. A longitudinal, sometimes classical, incision in the uterus may be done to minimise trauma to the preterm breech. The skin incision does not parallel the uterine incision under these circumstances and should be transverse.

Elective caesarean section is safer than emergency caesarean section. Emergency caesarean section should be classified into immediate and emergency depending on the degree of urgency. Immediate is a better word than 'crash' especially when used in the presence of the mother or the family. Corners may be cut when there is a great degree of urgency and this compromises safety. The real emergency, 'immediate' caesarean sections are done for abruption of the placenta, fetal bradycardia and possibly umbilical cord prolapse although first aid measures will take the urgency out of this situation. The decision to delivery interval for immediate caesarean section should be less than 20 minutes. Dunphy et al (1991) showed that the relative risk of admission to the special care baby unit for neonatal asphyxia doubled between the interval of 10 and 35 minutes. They advocate protocols to minimise this decision to delivery interval. These should be audited and if acceptable results are not achieved procedures should be altered. If an emergency caesarean section is undertaken in abnormal labour, the recording of the level of the head, the position of the occiput and the presence of caput and moulding are all important. The condition of the baby at birth and the umbilical cord blood pH value are important especially if the procedure was done for suspected fetal compromise. After a failed trial of forceps an assistant must be available to push the presenting part up by placing a hand under the drapes. At the end of a long augmented labour the lower segment may be bruised and edematous. It should be incised and opened in a steady controlled fashion. Tearing of the lower uterine segment is not uncommon under these circumstances. Good surgical technique, skilled anesthesia, blood transfusion and the appropriate use of antiobiotics minimise complications. Caesarean section is more traumatic than easy vaginal delivery; however, elective caesarean section is much to be preferred to difficult operative vaginal delivery with consequent fetal and maternal trauma. A caesarean section rate should neither be high or low; it should be appropriate for the community in question. Each case should be fully justified and the indication able to stand the scrutiny of colleagues in a local audit.

The nature of our work in reproduction generates high expectations from women and families. In childbirth everyone hopes for the very best outcome. Birth trauma has become less frequent in recent years. Doctors have become more circumspect about performing complicated vaginal deliveries and caesarean section has inevitably become more frequent. There should be protocols and guidelines of good practice. During operative delivery the mother must be fully informed about the procedure. The doctor who has conducted the delivery must look at the baby with the mother and explain any superficial marks that may relate to the instruments. Explanation of the chignon seen after vacuum extraction is important. If the baby is transferred to the special care baby unit then the labour ward staff should visit it and retain an interest. The doctor who has conducted the delivery must visit the postnatal ward to discuss important issues with the mother and supervise blood transfusion, antibiotic therapy and other management. In the case of unfavourable outcomes senior staff must be involved and an appropriate follow up arranged. This principle is also applied to the damaged perineum. It is often useful to call the mother back to the postnatal ward for subsequent checks. Full and frank discussion is required at every level. Doctors should not complain about the interest of lawyers in their work but improve standards and communication to such an extent that the lawyer becomes redundant.

References

Acker DB, Sachs BP, Friedmann EA 1986. Risk factors for shoulder dystocia in the average weight infant. *Obstet Gynecol* 67:614-618

Arulkumaran S, Ingemarsson I, Montan S et al 1992. Guidelines for Interpretation of Antepartum and Intrapartum Cardiotocography. Singapore: Hewlett-Packard.

Bates RG, Helm CW, Duncan A, Edmonds DK 1985. Uterine activity in the second stage of labour and the effect of epidural analgesia. *Br J Obstet Gynecol* 92: 1246-1250.

Benedetti TJ, Gabbe S 1978. Shoulder dystocia: A complication of fetal macrosomia and prolonged second stage of labour with midpelvic delivery. *Obstet Gynecol* 52: 526.

Botting BJ, MacFarlane AJ, Price FV, Richards HAM 1990. Background. In: Botting BJ, MacFarlane AJ, Price FV, eds. Three, four or more—A study of triplets and other higher order births. London: HMSO, pp 15-27.

Boyd ME, Usher RH, McLean FH 1983. Fetal Macrosomia - Prediction, risks and proposed management. *Obstet Gynecol* 67:715.

Bryan E 1992. Twins and higher order multiple births. A guide to their nature and nurture. London: Edward Arnold, pp 78-79.

Cardozo LD, Gibb DMF, Studd JWW, Cooper DJ 1983. Should we abandon Kielland's Forceps? *Br Med J* 287:315-317.

Carr SR, Aronson MP, Coustan DR 1990. Survival rates of monoamniotic twins do not decrease after 30 weeks gestation *Am J Obstet Gynecol* 163:719-722.

Caterini H, Langer A, Sama JC, et al 1975. Fetal risk in hyperextension of the fetal head in breech presentation. *Am J Obstet Gynecol* 123: 632.

Chalmers JA 1971. The Ventouse: The Obstetric Vacuum Extractor. London: Lloyd-Luke.

Chamberlain G 1989. The Vacuum Extractor. In: Turnbull A, Chamberlain G, eds. Obstetrics. Edinburgh: Churchill Livingstone, pp 849-856.

Chiswick ML, James DK 1979. Kielland's forceps: association with neonatal morbidity and mortality. *Br Med J* 1:7-9.

Clinch J 1989. Abnormal fetal presentations and positions. In: Turnbull A, Chamberlain G, eds. Obstetrics. Edindurgh: Churchill Livingstone, pp 793-812.

Crichton D 1974. A reliable method of establishing the level of the fetal head in obstetrics. *S Afr Med J* 48:784-787.

Collea JV, Rabin SC, Weghorst GR et al 1978. The randomised management of term frank breech presentation—Vaginal delivery versus caesarean section. *Am J Obstet Gynecol* 131:186.

Daw E 1974. Hyperextension of the head in breech presentation. *Am J Obstet Gynecol* 119:564.

Dunphy BC, Robinson JN, Shiel OM, Nicholls JSD, Gillmer MDG 1991. Caesarean section for fetal distress, the interval from decision to delivery, and the relative risk of poor neonatal condition. *J Obstet Gynecol* 11:241-244.

Gaziano EP, Freeman DW, Bendel RP 1980. Fetal Heart Rate variability and other heart rate observations during the second stage of labour. *Obstet Gynecol* 56:42-50.

Gibb D 1988. A Practical Guide to Labour Management. Oxford: Blackwell Scientific Publications.

Gibb D, Arulkumaran S 1992. Fetal Monitoring in Practice. Oxford: Butterworth-Heinemann.

Gibb D, Greenough A 1991. Problems of multiple pregnancy *Br J Hosp Med* 46:367-370.

Gonik B, Stringer C, Held B 1983. An alternative manoeuvre for the management of shoulder dystocia. *Am J Obstet Gynecol* 145:882.

Goodfellow CF, Hull MGR, Swaab DF, Dogterom J, Buijs RM 1983. Oxytocin deficiency at delivery with epidural analgesia. *Br J Obstet Gynecol* 90: 214-219.

Hibbard BM 1989. Forceps Delivery. In: Turnbull A, Chamberlain G, eds. Obstetrics, Edinburgh: Churchill Livingstone, pp 833-848.

Hofmeyr GJ 1989. Suspected fetopelvic disproportion. In: Chalmers I, Enkin M, Keirse MJNC, eds. Effective Care in Pregnancy and Childbirth. Oxford: Oxford University Press, pp 493-498.

Hopwood HG 1982. Shoulder Dystocia - Fifteen years experience in a community hospital. *Am J Obstet Gynecol* 144:162.

How to Avoid Medico-Legal Problems in Obstetrics and Gynaecology 1990. London: Royal College of Obstericians and Gynaecologists.

Indications for Forceps Operations 1988 Committee on Obstetrics: Maternal and Fetal Medicine 59: Obstetric Forceps. Washington DC: American College of Obstetricians and Gynaecologists.

Jacobson L, Rooth G 1971. Interpretative aspects on the acid base composition and its variation in fetal scalp blood and maternal blood during labour. *J Obstet Gynecol Br Cwlth* 78: 971-980.

Johanson R 1991. Vacuum extraction versus forceps delivery. In: Chalmers I, ed. Oxford Database of Perinatal Trials. Version 1.2, Disc Issue 5.

Liu DTY, Fairweather DVI 1985. Labour Ward Manual, London: Butterworth.

Milner RDG 1975. Neonatal mortality of breech deliveries with and without forceps to the aftercoming head. *Br J Obstet Gynecol* 82:783.

McFarland LV, Raskin M, Daling JR, Benedetti TJ 1986. Erb/Duchenne palsy: a consequence of fetal macrosomia and method of delivery. *Obstet Gynecol* 68: 784-788.

O'Driscoll K, Meagher P 1980. Active Management of Labour, London: WB Saunders.

O'Grady JP 1988. Modern Instrumental Delivery. Baltimore: Williams and Wilkins.

O'Leary JA, Pollack NB 1991. McRobert's manoeuvre for shoulder dystocia: a survey. *Int J Gynecol Obstet* 35: 129-131.

Parks DG, Ziel HK 1978. Macrosomia - A proposed indication for primary caesarean section. *Obstet Gynaecol* 52:407.

Parry Jones E 1952. Kielland's Forceps. London: Butterworth.

Pearce JM, Steel SA 1987. A Manual of Labour Ward Practice. Chichester: Wiley.

Pearson JF, Davies P 1974. The effect of continuous lumbar epidural analgesia upon fetal acid base status during the second stage of labour. *J Obstet Gynecol Br Cwlth* 81:975-979.

Rubin A 1964. Management of Shoulder Dystocia. *JAMA* 189:11:835-837.

Sandberg EC 1985. The Zavanelli manoeuvre: A potentially revolutionary method for the resolution of shoulder dystocia. *Am J Obstet Gynecol* 152:479-484.

Seeds JW 1986. Malpresentations. In: Gabbe SG, Niebyl JR, Simpson JL, eds. Obstetrics, Normal and Problem Pregnancies. Edinburgh: Churchill Livingstone, pp 476-484.

Stewart KS 1977. MD Thesis, University of Edinburgh. Cited in: Myerscough PR, ed. Munro Kerr's Operative Obstetrics, London: Bailliere Tindall, p 32.

Tessen JA, Zlatnik FJ 1991. Monoamniotic Twins: A retrospective controlled study. *Obstet Gynecol* 77:832- 834.

Vacca A 1992. Handbook of Vacuum Extraction in Obstetric Practice, London: Edward Arnold.

Vacca A, Grant A, Wyatt G, Chalmers I 1983. Portsmouth Operative Delivery Trial: a comparison of vacuum and forceps delivery. *Br J Obstet Gynecol* 90: 1107-1112.

Vacca A, Keirse MJNC 1989. In: Chalmers I, Enkin M, Keirse MJNC, eds. Effective Care in Pregnancy and Childbirth. Oxford: Oxford University Press, pp 1216-1233.

10

Antepartum Hemorrhage

Kuldip Singh
S Arulkumaran

Antepartum hemorrhage (APH) has been defined as any bleeding from the female genital tract between fetal viability (usually > 22 weeks of pregnancy) and delivery of the fetus. In the past, 28 weeks was the cut-off point, but because of improved neonatal intensive care facilities, fetal survival can occur as early as 22 weeks. For this reason, the World Health Organisation redefined any perinatal death as that of any fetus born after 22 weeks or weighing 500 g or more. APH complicates 2–5% of all pregnancies (Chamberlain et al 1978; Hibbard 1989).

Causes

Table 1 shows the various causes of antepartum hemorrhage. The major, although not the most common, causes of APH are placenta previa and abruptio placenta. In the majority of cases, the bleeding is of undetermined origin. In a small but important minority, the bleeding indicates a local cause in the lower genital tract.

Table 1: Causes of antepartum hemorrhage

Cause	Incidence (%)
placenta previa	31
abruptio placenta	22
local causes	5
undetermined	42

Maternal mortality

This has dropped from 5% when Macafee (1945) began his pioneering work on the management of placenta praevia to less than 0.1% in developed countries with the introduction of improved medical care and facilities (Hibbard 1988). However in developing countries, widespread pre-existing anemia, difficulties with transport and restricted medical facilities ensure that APH continues to be responsible for a large number of maternal deaths (Harrison and Rossiter 1985).

Fetal loss

Fetal loss is much more common than maternal death. Whitfield et al (1986) showed that 21 out of 155 losses (14%) in Scotland during 1989–1990 were associated with APH : 10 from abruptio placenta, none from placenta previa and three associated with bleeding of undetermined origin. Neonatal deaths with abruptio placenta are principally related to the complications of preterm delivery and perinatal mortality varies from 144 to 673 per 1,000. Over 50% of the perinatal deaths are stillbirths (Chamberlain et al 1978; Okonofua and Olatubosum 1985). Amongst surviving infants, rates of respiratory distress, patent ductus arteriosus, low apgar scores and anemia are more common than in unselected hospital cases (Hibbard, 1985). For placenta previa, conservative management and effective treatment of hemorrhage has reduced the gravity of the condition and perinatal mortality has dropped from 126 per 1,000 (Cotton et al 1980) to 42 per 1,000 (McShane et al 1985).

Principles of management

Antepartum hemorrhage is unpredictable and at any time before, during or after presentation, the patient's condition may deteriorate abruptly. The management must therefore aim to treat or prevent such a deterioration. It is only after this has been achieved that specific measures can be instituted. The general measures discussed below will apply to all cases of APH, although modifications would have to be made depending on the severity of bleeding.

Specific measures implemented once the diagnosis is made will be discussed under the various causes of APH.

Initial assessment and general measures

Management of any patient with APH should be in the hospital with adequate facilities for transfusion, delivery by caesarean section, neonatal resuscitation and intensive care. Immediate transfer to the hospital via an ambulance or by the fastest means available is recommended if the emergency occurs at home. Initial management must include a brief history, evaluation of the patient's general condition and initiation of various laboratory tests and treatment.

History

This must ascertain any initiating factors such as trauma or coitus, the amount and character of bleeding, association of abdominal pain or regular uterine contractions, a history of ruptured membranes or previous vaginal bleeding, known gestational age either by the last menstrual period or a previous ultrasound scan, information about the placental site from previous scans and perception of fetal movements.

Physical examination

This is aimed at assessing both maternal and fetal conditions and should include:
- measuring the maternal pulse, blood pressure and respiratory rate.
- looking for clinical evidence of shock: restlessness, pallor, cold and clammy extremities.
- abdominal examination to ascertain whether the uterine fundus is compatible with the gestational age, the presence of tenderness, irritability and the

presence of uterine contractions. Auscultation of the fetal heart rate to check whether fetus is alive, distressed or dead.

- vaginal examination. Unless placenta previa has been excluded, this is usually confined to inspection only in order to assess quickly the amount of blood loss and to determine whether bleeding has stopped or is continuing. Speculum examination should be performed to exclude any local lesions and if bleeding is suspected to be fetal, the Apt test can be performed. This test is based on the principle that fetal hemoglobin is alkaline stable when mixed with 1% sodium hydroxide whereas adult hemoglobin is not. It is thus designed to distinguish fetal from maternal blood passed per vaginum.

Investigations and immediate management

As a general rule, all patients presenting with APH should initially be investigated and managed as outlined below. Subsequent management should be determined by the severity and type of bleeding and the gestational age of the pregnancy. The initial management should include the following:

- an intravenous line with a wide bore cannula (preferably size 14–16 French gauge) should be established.
- blood must be obtained for immediate hemoglobin estimation, a full blood count done and grouping and crossmatching of at least 4 units of blood.
- where abruptio placenta is suspected, a coagulation profile, urea and electrolytes and liver function tests should be performed. Other tests that may be performed are the Kleihauer test on maternal blood and the Apt test on vaginal blood if fetal bleeding is suspected.
- intravenous fluids in the form of colloids should be given if the bleeding continues or is severe causing hemodynamic changes while the crossmatched blood is being awaited.
- ultrasound scan to exclude placenta previa if this has not been done. It is difficult to exclude placental abruption by ultrasound but rarely, retroplacental clots and lifting of the membranes may be noted. This should only be performed if and when maternal and fetal condition are stable.

After the initial management, the patient may fall into one of the following categories where:

- the bleeding has stopped.
- the bleeding is continuing but remains mild or moderate and is not life threatening.
- the bleeding is continuing and is severe and life threatening.
- the fetus is in distress irrespective of the bleeding pattern.
- the fetus is dead.

Subsequent management will be determined by the above circumstances. It can be divided into (a) immediate delivery or (b) expectant management. These will be discussed under the various types of APH.

Specific measures : Placenta previa

This is a placenta that is implanted entirely or in part in the lower uterine segment. Hemorrhage is especially likely to occur when uterine contractions dilate the cervix. Placenta previa may be divided into four types as shown in Table 2.

Table 2 : Types of placenta praevia

Types	Description
I	Placenta is in the lower uterine segment but the lower edge does not reach the internal os
II	Lower edge of the placenta reaches internal os but does not cover it
III	Placenta covers the internal os asymmetrically
IV	Placenta covers the os symmetrically

The most important distinction is between the major (types 3, 4, and 2 posterior) and minor types (types 1 and 2 anterior) of previa. As will be discussed, placentas which appear to be previa but of minor degree may get shifted upwards to become normally sited as the lower uterine segment develops; placentas which are genuinely implanted across the cervical os will remain previa. The distinction should not engender clinical complacency as profuse hemorrhage can occur from either major or minor placenta previa.

Clinical presentation

The two classical presentations of placenta previa are a painless APH or fetal malpresentation in late pregnancy. The first hemorrhage is usually not severe, although this is not invariable and may on occasion be considerable. The hemorrhage is typically painless, although again this is not invariable. In some cases, hemorrhage has been precipitated by a burst of Braxton Hicks' contractions causing some dilatation and stretching of the lower uterine segment. In others, the effect of blood lifting the placental membranes may produce uterine activity with the consequent experience of pain. Moreover 10% of women with placenta previa have a co-existing abruption (Hibbard 1988).

Abdominal examination shows the uterus to be soft and non-tender. There is typically an unusually high head presenting or a fetal malpresentation. This may be a breech presentation or a transverse or an oblique lie. The fetal heart rate is usually normal.

In current obstetric practice, the diagnosis of asymptomatic placenta previa is made on routine ultrasound examination.

Diagnosis

Vaginal Examination   There is no place for routine digital vaginal examination in the diagnosis of placenta previa. The practice of speculum examination is justified because it excludes local causes of vaginal bleeding and the speculum does not enter the cervix to cause placental separation. The speculum examination is best done at the time of bleeding to identify local causes or to confirm that bleeding is from the os, unless it is severe when it is more likely to be from the placental site. Vaginal examination is only indicated during examination in the theatre with full preparation for caesarean section.

Ultrasound   This is safe, accurate and non-invasive. However the earlier the scan is performed, the more likely is an over-diagnosis of placenta previa. For example, about 28% of placentas of women scanned before 24 weeks were found to be low lying but by 24 weeks they had dropped to 18% and only 3% were low lying by term (Chapman et al 1989). The apparent change of placental position results from the formation of the lower uterine segment and the enlargement of the upper segment. Thus all women with a low placenta on an early scan should be rescanned at about 34 weeks.

Magnetic Resonance Imaging   This is a new but expensive method of tissue imaging available at present in only a few centres. Localisation of the placenta is excellent since both the placental edge and the cervical canal can be readily identified (Powell et al 1986). This may be the most precise method of diagnosing placenta previa though ultrasound gives fairly accurate results. The equipment required for Magnetic Resonance Imaging is extremely expensive and thus it is very unlikely that this technique will play a major role in practical placentography in routine clinical practice.

Management options: Placenta previa

Specific measures will be either immediate delivery or expectant management.

Immediate delivery

Bleeding that is severe and continuous and which has caused or is likely to cause hemodynamic changes is an indication for immediate operative delivery. If bleeding continues but is neither profuse nor life-threatening and fetal maturity is more than 36 weeks, delivery will be preferred. In such patients the mode of delivery will depend on the type of placenta previa based on earlier placental localisation. The options available in this situation are immediate caesarean section for major types and examination in the theatre with the view to induction of labour in minor types.

Examination in the theatre is indicated in patients who are bleeding actively but is unlikely to cause hemodynamic changes to the mother especially where ultrasonography is not available. It should also be considered when ultrasound evidence is inconclusive or when dealing with a minor degree of placenta previa in patients with repeated bleeding. This is more important with posterior placenta previa where at times the limits of the lower uterine segment cannot be identified with absolute precision.

Opinions vary as to whether or not the patient should be anesthetised at the time of examination in the theatre. The advantages of general anesthesia include proper relaxation of the patient thereby making examination easier and facilitating a quicker progression to caesarean section should the need arise. The main disadvantage is that the patient has to be woken up from anesthesia after inducing labour if vaginal delivery is considered to be possible. In these cases, if caesarean section eventually becomes necessary, a second anesthetic will increase the risk. A compromise is to have the drugs for induction of general anesthesia and the anesthetic equipment well prepared and the anesthetist in attendance. With such precautions, the interval between the examination and delivering the fetus can be shortened.

At vaginal examination, the obstetrician's finger should first explore the vaginal fornices, the objective being to feel whether there is a placenta between the presenting part and the finger. If there is no sensation of 'bogginess' and if the presenting part (preferably the head) can be felt through the four fornices, the index finger is then gently introduced into the cervical os and the surroundings explored for the placental edge. If this proves negative, induction of labour is carried out by amniotomy and oxytocin infusion started to induce labour.

Expectant management

Management depends on the stage of the pregnancy and the extent of the hemorrhage. It is preferable to allow the pregnancy to continue with the aim of achieving maximum fetal maturity while minimising the risks to both mother and fetus, the overall objective being to reduce perinatal mortality while at the same time reducing maternal mortality (Macafee 1945). The Macafee regime required adherence to several principles. The patient was required to remain in a fully equipped and fully staffed maternity hospital from the time of initial diagnosis to delivery. Facilities had to be available for immediate caesarean section. Anemia was to be identified and corrected, if necessary by repeated blood transfusion because of the likelihood of further hemorrhage.

This scheme still forms the essence of management but it can tax to the limit the combined resources of obstetricians, midwives and social services and encourage women to remain in hospital when they feel perfectly well and their families are missing their presence. Various researchers have advocated a policy of permitting selected women to return home as part of expectant management (Hibbard 1989; Silver et al 1984). Cotton et al (1980) reported no difference in the perinatal and maternal mortality rates between those sent home and those managed in hospital. This line of management remains controversial as reports from different units are conflicting. The continued value of in-patient management has been confirmed even in recent years by D'Angelo and Irwin (1984).

In patients in whom a low placenta has been noticed incidentally by ultrasound, it would be prudent to repeat another scan at 34 weeks and interpret the findings, as there is a possibility of the placenta shifting upwards. As far as management is concerned, it would be reasonable to admit women with asymptomatic major placenta previa from 34 weeks gestation. Those with asymptomatic minor placenta previa can be managed on an outpatient basis unless they stay far from the hospital. They should be warned to avoid coitus, travel and being in crowded places. Communication and transport should be readily available to enable the patient to reach the hospital within 30 minutes.

During expectant management, preterm labour remains a problem. Sampson et al (1984) advocate the use of tocolytic drugs in cases of placenta previa with uterine contractions and have claimed a reduction in perinatal mortality. However in general these have been beneficial and their actions on the maternal cardiovascular function could be positively unhelpful. The frequently associated tachycardia can make the assessment of the maternal condition difficult. Further bleeding needs a maternal cardiovascular response to acute hypovolemia which may be impaired due to vasodilatation caused by the betamimetic drug. Furthermore betamimetic infusion therapy causes hypokalemia. Should surgery be needed due to acute bleeding, the patient may be at a risk of cardiac arrest or arrhythmia with anesthetic drugs because of hypokalemia. The antiprostaglandin drug, indomethacin, does not carry these disadvantages but there have been reports of constriction of the fetal ductus arteriosus associated with its use and it has yet to be shown to be effective in practice in situations of antepartum hemorrhage (Moise et al 1988).

Delivery

Where the degree of placenta previa is minor (types I and II anterior) and the fetal head is engaged, pregnancy may be allowed to continue with induction after 38 weeks and vaginal delivery anticipated. In those with more major grades of placenta previa, delivery by caesarean section is indicated at 38 weeks.

Caesarean section for placenta previa can be difficult and should be done by senior obstetricians or under their supervision. The incision on the uterus is commonly a transverse lower segment incision. It is only very rarely that a midline vertical incision on the uterus is required, although large blood vessels are usually encountered over the lower uterine segment. If the incision on the uterus is transverse and the placenta is anterior, two approaches are available; in the first case, the placental edge is defined and the membranes above or below the placenta gone through, to reach the presenting part. The ultrasound placental localisation done previously will help to identify the best direction to reach the membranes. In the second approach, the placenta is incised and this is preferably avoided as there is often significant fetal blood loss and exsanguination may occur (Myerscough 1982).

As the lower uterine segment is less muscular, contraction and retraction which result in the closure of the sinuses of the placental bed are inadequate and intra-operative hemorrhage is therefore not uncommon. When hemostasis is difficult to achieve, bleeding sinuses can be oversewn with atraumatic sutures (Neilson 1995). If this is unsuccessful, direct pressure with warm packs, administration of intravenous oxytocics and intramyometrial injection of prostaglandin $F_{2\alpha}$ have been shown to be useful in some cases (Bigrigg et al 1991). When the bleeding remains uncontrollable, ligation of the internal iliac artery or even hysterectomy may be necessary to save the woman's life.

Specific measures : Abruptio placenta

In abruptio placenta, there is bleeding following premature separation of a normally sited placenta. The basic cause is unknown. It is a self extending process with the accumulating blood causing more separation and thus more hemorrhage until the edge of the placenta is reached and this blood escapes between the chorion and decidua until it reaches the cervix. Blood can also reach the amniotic cavity by disrupting the placenta and membranes, producing bloodstained liquor. It can seep into the myometrium causing Couvelaire uterus. There is inevitably great risk of fetal hypoxia because of the tetanic contraction brought about by blood seeping into the myometrium or severe placental separation. In such cases sudden fetal death is common. A case with minimal bleeding and placental separation which however causes fetal compromise due to irritable polysystolic (> 6 in 15 min) or too frequent contractions are shown in Fig 10.1. The major immediate maternal risk is hemorrhagic shock; renal damage may ensue later in the form of either acute tubular or cortical necrosis. There may also be clinical and hematological evidence of coagulopathy as thromboplastins are released by placental damage and coagulation factors are consumed in the enlarging retroplacental clot as well as in the process of disseminated intravascular coagulation.

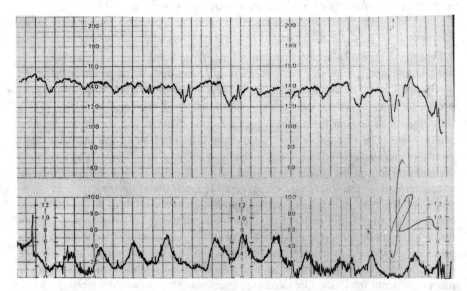

Fig 10.1 A cardiotocograph showing frequent contractions with an abnormal fetal heart rate pattern. The cervix was closed and 2 cm long and intrauterine death occurred within a short time of the trace.

Abruptio placenta is concealed in 20–35% and revealed in 65–80% of cases (Fraser and Watson 1989). The concealed type is the most dangerous with very much more severe complications.

Clinical presentation

The patient typically presents with pain over the uterus and this increases in severity. There is usually no periodicity until uterine contractions start and superimpose additional intermittent pain in addition to the continuous pain. The presence of uterine contractions may be difficult to distinguish from the abdominal pain of abruption. Where this distinction is possible, the contractions are characteristically of high frequency.

Placental abruption may not be associated with apparent bleeding at the outset, and may be first concealed and revealed subsequently. Vaginal bleeding is a symptom only in 70–80% of cases (Green 1989). Faintness and collapse may occur while some patients may complain of absent fetal movements.

On examination there may be signs of shock: tachycardia with a weak and thready pulse, pallor, cyanosis and cold and clammy skin. The uterus is extremely hard and tender and is typically described as 'woody' hard. It does not relax, the fetal parts are difficult to palpate and the fetal heart may be inaudible. In severe cases complicated by disseminated intravascular coagulation, there may be absence of clotting as observed in the vaginal blood loss which may be dark coloured.

Diagnosis

This is usually made on clinical grounds. The symptoms and signs presented above will be diagnostic in moderate to severe cases. In the mild form, the diagnosis may not be quite obvious until after delivery when a retroplacental clot is identified.

Ultrasound imaging has a much smaller role than in the diagnosis of placenta previa. In acute severe abruption, the ultrasound appearances are often unimpressive because the fresh retroplacental hematoma has acoustic characteristics which are very similar to the placenta itself. What appears therefore is a thick heaped up placenta. In less severe cases, in which the pregnancy continues, the clots become hyperechogenic within one week and sonoluscent within two weeks and therefore more obvious to the ultrasonographer (Nyberg et al 1987). Thus ultrasound is not an accurate diagnostic tool but may be useful in monitoring the cases managed expectantly.

Management options : Abruptio placenta

For the purpose of management, Sher and Statland (1985) divide abruptio placenta into three grades of severity. These are: Grade I, which is not recognised clinically before delivery and is usually diagnosed by the presence of a retroplacental clot at delivery; in Grade II, the classical signs of abruption are present but the fetus is still alive; in Grade III the fetus is dead and coagulopathy may be present. The principles of management in the obvious case of placental abruption are:

- immediate delivery
- adequate blood transfusion
- adequate analgesia
- detailed monitoring of maternal condition
- assessment of the fetal condition

Immediate delivery

This is vital in the obvious case of abruption. If the fetus is dead, as is often the case, vaginal delivery is the goal. Amniotomy should be performed to hasten delivery and is also believed to reduce the incidence of coagulopathy as the intra-amniotic pressure is lowered, thus preventing tissue thromboplastin entering the maternal circulation. Amniotomy is effective in most cases but in a few, augmentation with oxytocin may be necessary.

When the fetus is alive, the decision on how best to achieve delivery is not always easy. This is compounded by the fact that the outlook for the fetus is poor, not only in terms of immediate survival but also because studies have shown that as many as 15.4% of live-born infants do not survive (Abdella et al 1984). However when the perinatal mortality of vaginal delivery is compared with that of caesarean section: 52 versus 16% (Okonofua and Olatubosum 1985), 20 versus 15% (Hurd et al 1983), it is clear that delivery by caesarean section is associated with better survival rates. Where abruption is severe, many advocate that caesarean section must be considered in all cases where the fetus is alive, particularly if there is evidence even transiently of fetal distress and vaginal delivery is not imminent. The presence of coagulopathy adds considerable risk to the mother and could be increased by surgery. Nevertheless caesarean section must be performed once resuscitation and correction of the coagulopathy is commenced. Correction of co-agulopathy in abruptio placenta is discussed in the chapter on eclampsia.

In mild to moderate cases of abruption, the mode of delivery will be deter-mined by the state of the baby, its presentation and the state of the cervix. Fetal distress will be an indication for immediate delivery by caesarean section. However if the decision is to deliver vaginally, continuous fetal monitoring must be available in order to identify early fetal distress. Artificial rupture of the membranes and oxytocin infusion may be used to hasten the delivery of the fetus. Generally, with a non-irritable uterus and revealed abruption, vaginal delivery of a healthy fetus can be expected if the fetal heart rate is normal. The fetal condition can suddenly deteriorate when the uterus is irritable. This is common in concealed or mixed abruption. In these cases and where the fetal heart rate is suspicious or abnormal, immediate caesarean section is advisable.

Prompt treatment and monitoring of the mother are vital. Since most of the blood loss from placental abruption is not revealed, an abruption of sufficient se-verity to produce fetal death may require blood transfusion because of the quantity of blood lost. If minimal loss and death were due to uterine irritability and hypoxia, it may be associated with DIVC and potential blood loss. Evidence of coagulopathy by decreased fibrinogen levels, decreased platelet concentrations and raised levels of fibrin degradation products indicate the need to maintain a hemotherapy chart (see chapter on eclampsia) and obtain an expert hematological opinion. The third stage is treacherous with the lurking hazard of postpartum hemorrhage. It must be managed aggressively with the appropriate use of oxytocics, coagulation factors, fibrinogen or fresh blood as indicated.

Expectant management

Expectant management is aimed at prolonging pregnancy with the hope of improv-ing fetal maturity and survival. It should only be considered in cases of mild abrup-tio placenta occurring before 36–37 weeks where the vaginal bleeding is slight, the abdominal pain is mild and usually localised, the uterus is not irritable, the fetal heart rate pattern is normal and the patients are cardiovascularly stable. In such cases the fetal condition must be monitored closely in hospital as indicated with cardiotocography, a biophysical profile and umbilical artery Doppler velo-cimetry recordings. If the bleeding episodes are recurrent or there is deterioration of the fetal condition, then delivery must be considered.

Other causes of antepartum hemorrhage

The exact cause of APH is unknown in 47% of cases (Chamberlain et al 1978). The cause of bleeding may later become apparent but in the majority of cases, no cause can be demonstrated (Fraser and Watson 1989). Where causes have been identified, they include marginal sinus rupture, 'show', cervicitis, trauma, vulval varicosities, genital tumours, genital infections and vasa previa. This group will invariably include unrecognised cases of minor abruption or placenta previa. Marginal sinus rupture is the most common source of bleeding in APH of unknown cause (Cotton et al 1980).

Clinical presentation

The patient presents with painless vaginal bleeding of unknown origin. There are usually no symptoms and signs diagnostic of either placenta previa or abruption. In the majority of cases the bleeding is mild and settles spontaneously (Neilson 1995).

Diagnosis

This is often made after excluding abruptio placenta and placenta previa. An ultrasound scan is therefore necessary to exclude placenta previa as minor grades may present in a similar manner.

Speculum examination should be routinely performed in patients with APH at the time of bleeding so that the cause if local can be identified and treated, and if not the bleeding from within the uterus via the os can be confirmed. Even in the presence of a local cause, a digital examination should be performed only after excluding placenta previa by a scan. If the blood is mucoid and there is a suspicion of labour, uterine contractions should be monitored. A polyp from the external cervix, if small, can be avulsed and the base cauterised. Bleeding from the cervix needs a PAP smear (or a biopsy) to be taken and infection excluded by taking a high vaginal swab. To exclude fetal bleeding as the cause of APH, an Apt test is performed.

Management options : Other causes of bleeding

If placenta previa and abruption have been excluded, further management will depend on gestational age, the nature of bleeding, and whether it is persistent or recurrent, severity of bleeding, the state of the fetus, the absence or presence of fetal distress and the presumed cause.

Further management will either be expectant or delivery. When the pregnancy is 37 weeks or more and the bleeding is recurrent, significant or there are associated fetal factors such as growth retardation or distress, then delivery is the management of choice. There is no contraindication to vaginal delivery provided there is no fetal compromise. In those presenting before 37 weeks, if episodes of bleeding are recurrent and significant, there may be need for immediate delivery. The mode of delivery will be determined by the state of the fetus, its lie, presentation and other associated factors like the state of the cervix.

Presently most units tend to monitor the patients in hospital until bleeding has stopped for at least 24 hours before discharging them. Thereafter the patients may either be monitored at home or in the hospital. In a retrospective review, Watson (1982) showed that there was no significant advantage in managing such patients in the hospital. Irrespective of where the patient is being managed, fetal surveillance must be provided. Unless there is fetal compromise, the practice is to await the spontaneous onset of labour up to 40 weeks. Induction at 40 weeks is based on the fact that placental function is damaged by bleeding (Neilson 1995).

One of the potential hazards of vaginal bleeding in later pregnancy is fetal exsanguination from vasa previa. Classically, profuse vaginal bleeding follows amniotomy with subsequent fetal tachy or bradycardia. The diagnosis of this condition before these events is difficult, but the experienced observer may be able to feel vessels coursing over the membranes. A speculum examination may also show these vessels. In some cases where there is mild bleeding after amniotomy, but a normal fetal heart rate, this diagnosis cannot be excluded. An Apt test will therefore have to be performed. If fetal blood is documented, the baby should be delivered immediately by caesarean section. When there is doubt, the labour should be allowed with continuous fetal heart rate monitoring and normal vaginal delivery anticipated.

Antepartum hemorrhage is an important cause of maternal morbidity and mortality. The etiology of the various types is poorly understood. Various management options are, however, available. Initial assessment of patients with subsequent planned management aimed at resuscitation and prolongation of pregnancy if possible, or immediate delivery either for fetal or maternal indications, is associated with a better outcome.

References

Abdella TN, Sibai BM, Hays JM, Anderson GD 1984. Relationship of hypertensive diseases to abruptio placentae. *Obstet Gynecol* 63:365-370.

Bigrigg A, Chui D, Chissell S, Read MD 1991. Use of intramyometrial 15-methyl prostaglandin F_2 to control atonic postpartum hemorrhage following vaginal delivery and failure of conventional therapy. *Br J Obstet Gynecol* 98:734-737.

Chamberlain GVP, Philipp E, Howlett B, Masters K 1978. British Births 1970. London: Heinemann.

Chapman MG, Furness ET, Jones WR, Sheat JH 1989. Significance of the location of placenta site in early pregnancy. *Br J Obstet Gynecol* 86:846-848.

Cotton DB, Read JA, Paul RH, Quilligan EJ 1980. The conservative aggressive management of placenta previa. *Am J Obstet Gynecol* 137:687-695.

D'Angelo LJ, Irwin LF 1984. Conservative management of placenta previa: A cost benefit analysis. *Am J Obstet Gynecol* 149:320-323.

Fraser R, Watson R 1989. Bleeding during the latter half of pregnancy. In: Chalmers I, ed. Effective Care in Pregnancy and Childbirth. Oxford: Oxford University Press.

Green JR 1989. Placenta abnormalities: placenta previa and abruptio placenta. In: Creasy RK, Resnik R, eds. Maternal Fetal Medicine : Principles and Practice. Philadelphia, PA:WB Saunders.

Harrison KA, Rossiter CE 1985. Maternal mortality. *Br J Obstet Gynecol (suppl)* 5:100-115.

Hibbard LT 1969. Placenta previa. *Am J Obstet Gynecol* 104:172-184.

Hibbard BM 1988. Bleeding in late pregnancy. In: Hibbard BM, ed. Principles of Obstetrics. London: Butterworth.

Hurd WW, Miodovnik M, Lavin JP 1983. Selective management of abruptio placenta: A prospective study. *Obstet Gynecol* 61:467-473.

Macafee CHG 1945. Placenta previa : A study of 174 cases. *J Obstet Gynecol Br Emp* 52:313-324.

McShane PM, Heye PS, Epstein MF 1985. Maternal and perinatal mortality resulting from placenta praevia. *Obstet Gynecol* 65:176-182.

Moise KJ, Huhta JC, Sharif DS 1988. Indomethacin in the treatment of premature labour. Effect on the ductus arteriosus. *N Engl J Med* 319:327-331.

Myerscough PR 1982. Munro Kerr's Operative Obstetrics, 10th edition. London: Bailliere Tindall.

Neilson JP 1995. Antepartum hemorrhage. In: Whitfield CR, ed. Dewhurst's Textbook of Obstetrics and Gynecology for Postgraduates. London: pp 164-174.

Nyberg DA, Cyr DR, Mack LA, Wilson DA, Shuman WP 1987. Sonographic spectrum of placental abruption. *Am J Roentgenol* 148:161-164.

Okonofua FE, Olatubosum OA 1985. Caesarean versus vaginal delivery in abruptio placentae associated with live fetuses. *Intl J Gynecol Obstet* 23:471-474.

Powell MC, Buckley J, Price H, Worthington BS, Symonds EM 1986. Magnetic resonance imaging and placenta previa. *Am J Obstet Gynecol* 154:565-569.

Sampson MB, Lastres O, Thomasi AM, Thomason JL, Work BA 1984. Tocolysis with

terbutaline sulphate in patients with placenta previa complicated by premature labour. *J Reprod Med* 45:415-440.

Sher G, Statland BE 1985. Abruptio placentae with coagulopathy: A rational basis for management. *Clin Obstet Gynecol* 28: 15-23.

Silver R, Depp R, Sabbagha RE, Dooley SL, Socol MI, Tamura RK 1984. Placentae praevia: Aggressive expectant management. *Am J Obstet Gynecol* 150:15-22.

Watson R 1982. Antepartum hemorrhage of uncertain origin. *Br J Clin Pract* 38:222-226.

Whitfield C.R., Smith NC, Cockburn F, Gibson AAM 1986. Perinatally related wastage - A proposed classification of primary obstetric factors. *Br J Obstet Gynecol* 93:694-703.

11

The Third Stage of Labour

Kuldip Singh
S Arulkumaran

The third stage of labour commences with the delivery of the infant and ends with the delivery of the placenta. It is thus an event related to the process of labour. After the excitement of the birth of a baby, the delivery of the placenta (that is, the third stage of labour) may be a time of great potential hazard. The main complication of the third stage is blood loss and this may be excessive before the delivery of the placenta and for a period of time after that. Postpartum hemorrhage remains an important cause of both maternal mortality and morbidity and is discussed in another chapter. A retained placenta may necessitate manual removal, and inversion of the uterus, while rare, can be frightening and life-threatening. Abnormal events in the third stage of labour can have important consequences.

Physiological mechanisms in the delivery of the placenta

Uterine contractions continue after the birth of the infant and the intrauterine pressure continues to be rhythmically raised. After delivery of the infant, the uterine muscles contract and retract, with a resultant reduction in the size of the upper segment. This shortening reduces the area of the uterine surface to which the relatively incompressible placenta is attached. Separation of the placenta occurs as a result of this retraction and the consequent reduction in intrauterine volume tends to force the placenta into the relaxed lower segment (Macpherson and Wilson 1965).

When placental separation is complete and the placenta is forced into the lower uterine segment and vagina, it may be delivered spontaneously by maternal effort, the lower edge presenting first at the vulva (the Matthews–Duncan method of expulsion). If traction is exerted on the umbilical cord or the uterine fundus is forcibly compressed, the fetal surface may appear first, with the membranes covering the maternal surface (the Schultz method).

The continued retraction of the uterine muscle is of paramount importance in minimising blood loss during and after this stage. The blood vessels supplying the placental site are compressed by the oblique fibres of the middle layer of the myometrium. This mechanism of controlling bleeding is effective only if the uterine muscle is capable of effective contraction and retraction and any impairment of this will predispose to hemorrhage.

Most patients can be delivered without undue blood loss, but because the consequences of severe hemorrhage are very serious, active management of the third stage is recommended.

Active management of the third stage

Active management of the third stage of labour, including prophylactic use of oxytocic drugs and controlled cord traction for delivery of the placenta has been widely adopted as a measure to prevent postpartum hemorrhage and retained placenta.

The report on Confidential Enquiries into Maternal Deaths in England and Wales (1972) indicated that between 1967 and 1969, there were 16 maternal deaths directly due to postpartum hemorrhage and in nine others this was an important factor. Little or no improvement was seen in the 1973-75 report (1979) in which 13 deaths were directly due to postpartum hemorrhage, and this was also a contributory factor in another 13. The active management of the third stage subsequently saw a reduction by 1982-84 (1989) with only three deaths from postpartum haemorrhage. There were 10 deaths due to postpartum hemorrhage in the all-UK report for 1988-90 (1994).

Action of oxytocic drugs   The drugs used in the management of the third stage are oxytocin and ergometrine, given alone or in combination. They may be given intravenously or intramuscularly and the injection may be administered with the crowning of the head, with the delivery of the anterior shoulder, after delivery of the infant or after delivery of the placenta. Oxytocin produces rhythmical contractions of the uterus augmenting retraction, and its effect is noticeable about three minutes after an intramuscular injection (Embrey 1961). Ergometrine by intramuscular injection results in a more prolonged contraction with retraction and its effect is noticeable about seven minutes after an intramuscular injection. When either drug is given intravenously, the uterine contraction commences in 30–40 seconds.

From trials in which oxytocin has been compared with ergot alkaloids, there is no evidence that these two kinds of oxytocics differ greatly in their effects on the incidence of postpartum hemorrhage. The use of oxytocin was associated with a trend towards less postpartum hemorrhage and was shown to be less likely than ergot alkaloids to lead to a delay in placental delivery or to a rise in blood pressure. None of these differences achieved statistical significance (Enkin et al 1989).

There is no suggestion of a difference in the effect of syntometrine and ergot alkaloids on the rate of postpartum hemorrhage. Syntometrine is somewhat less likely than ergot alkaloids to be associated with a prolonged third stage. In the only trial that considered effects on blood pressure, syntometrine was less likely than ergometrine to be associated with a 20 mm Hg elevation of diastolic blood pressure. The comparison of syntometrine with oxytocin suggests that syntometrine reduces the risk of postpartum hemorrhage more effectively than oxytocin used alone (Enkin et al 1989). However, the use of oxytocin was associated with a lower mean blood pressure than that of syntometrine (Enkin et al 1989). More recently it has been shown that the use of intramuscular syntometrine as compared to intramuscular syntocinon during the third stage of labour is associated with a significantly lower blood loss, a lower risk of primary postpartum hemorrhage and minimal maternal side effects (Yuen et al 1995). Moreover, hypertension did not appear to be a significant problem with the use of syntometrine in this study.

The advantages of prophylactic oxytocics must be weighed against the rare but serious morbidity that has sometimes been associated with their administering.

Maternal deaths from cardiac arrest and intracerebral hemorrhage have been attributed to ergometrine as have non-fatal instances of cardiac arrest, myocardial infarction, postpartum eclampsia and pulmonary edema. Because of the rarity of these events, the available randomised trials cannot provide useful estimates of the extent to which they may be attributed to oxytocin administration. Other rare but definite adverse consequences of routine oxytocic administration include intrauterine asphyxia of an undiagnosed second twin. In principle, randomised trials should be able to provide useful information about adverse effects which are less serious but more commonly encountered, such as nausea, vomiting and headache. However little information is available from these trials.

On balance, however the evidence suggests that the benefits of routine oxytocic administration outweigh the likely risks.

Use of oxytocic drugs in management   Although the prophylactic use of oxytocic drugs is now well established, differences exist in the technique of administration and selection of the drug. The theoretical objective of prophylactic oxytocics is to ensure efficient contractions of the uterus after the delivery of the infant, thus minimising the amount of blood loss. This is achieved by promoting rapid and complete separation and the descent of the placenta and occlusion of the vessels and capillaries in the placental site. If an oxytocic drug is given before the delivery of the placenta, the procedure of controlled cord traction should be applied for its subsequent delivery. Otherwise the placenta may be retained, leading to excessive blood loss that could have been prevented.

If the injection of syntometrine is given intramuscularly, delivery of the placenta can be achieved only by administering the drug at the crowning of the head or after its delivery and allowing an interval of about two minutes before completing the delivery of the infant. If syntometrine is given with the delivery of the anterior shoulder, it is comparable to administering the injection after the infant is delivered. Time must then be allowed for the uterus to respond to the preparation and for the delivery of the placenta to be accomplished. Intravenous oxytocics are given with the delivery of the anterior shoulder, and the resulting contraction should follow very soon after the one which delivers the infant. If the placenta is partially or completely sheared off the uterine wall at the time of the delivery of the infant, a further contraction should complete its separation and encourage its descent into the lower segment of the vagina. It is necessary to anticipate this process by assisting the delivery of the placenta immediately after the delivery of the infant and before further uterine contractions prevent the complete descent of the placenta. After the umbilical cord has been clamped and separated from the infant, controlled cord traction is applied and the placenta is delivered.

When oxytocic is not given until after the delivery of the placenta, it is necessary to rely on uterine contractions to separate the placenta completely from its attachment and to then expel it into the vagina. Uterine contractions are sometimes inefficient and ineffective, hence there is a greater risk of hemorrhage with partial separation of the placenta. To avoid this situation, it is preferable to give the woman the injection before placental separation.

Clamping of the cord   Active management of the third stage of labour usually entails the clamping and dividing of the umbilical cord relatively early before beginning controlled cord traction. The necessity of clamping and dividing the cord has been questioned. Botha (1968) reported a reduction in the incidence of retained placenta and postpartum blood loss in women who delivered their infants and later delivered the placenta without separating the child from it. This results in an increase in the blood volume of the infant. The exsanguinated placenta is thought to separate more readily and to be more readily delivered. If the infant is separated from the placenta soon after delivery, the blood in the placenta may be allowed to flow into a receptacle while a uterine contraction and the delivery of the placenta are awaited.

Yao and Lind (1969) have shown the effect of gravity on the volume of placental transfusions. When the infant was 40 cm below the introitus, the placental transfusion was completed in 30 seconds. If the infant was held above the introitus, placental transfusion was lessened or prevented. Yao et al (1969) also showed that the distribution of infant–placental blood volume at birth was 67–33%, at one minute 80–20% and at three minutes 87–13%. Yao et al (1968) demonstrated that the postnatal transfer of blood was rapid and amounted to 55% of the infant's blood volume at birth. More than one quarter of the blood was transferred with the contraction, resulting in delivery, while the remainder of the blood was transferred at one minute after a contraction if ergometrine had been given. If no oxytocin was given, the transfer took three minutes. No significant change in distribution was achieved by delaying clamping longer than this.

Thus, in general, if there has been fetal distress, meconium staining of the amniotic fluid or evidence of an unreactive baby likely to have a low Apgar score, the cord should be clamped immediately and the baby resuscitated. If the baby is active and cries immediately on delivery, clamping of the cord can be deferred to allow blood flow from the placenta to the fetus, which should be held below the level of the introitus. Prolonged deferment of cord clamping beyond three minutes provides no great advantage to the newborn and does not hasten the expulsion of the placenta. In practical terms, the uterine arteries go into spasm from the fetal umbilical end and the spasm gradually progresses towards the placenta. So there is no blood leaving the fetus whilst it is entering via the umbilical vein. An alternative method of cutting the cord would be to clamp and divide when pulsations are not felt in the cord.

Delivery of the placenta   After the baby has been treated by oropharyngeal aspiration, he/she is wrapped up and presented to the mother, whilst the obstetrician or midwife is preparing for the delivery of the placenta. The border of the left hand is placed on the abdominal wall at the level of the fundus, the umbilical cord grasped with the right hand and kept under gentle tension. Placental separation is indicated when the uterus contracts, the fundus becomes globular, a small amount of blood flows from the vagina and the umbilical cord lengthens. Once these signs are recognised, the hand should be placed just below the fundus of the uterus. Gentle but steady traction is applied to the umbilical cord directed downwards and posteriorly while the uterus is pushed upwards by the other hand to aid delivery of the placenta and its membranes (Fliegner and Hibbard 1966). The uterus can then be massaged to stimulate contraction and reduce bleeding. It is essential that the uterus is contracted whenever cord traction is practised. Energetic traction of the cord with a relaxed uterus may snap the cord leading to an inevitable manual removal, or may invert the uterus.

Examination of the placenta   The placenta should be examined after it has been delivered to ensure that the cotyledons are all present and that the placenta is complete. Immediate exploration of the uterus is required if it is certain that placental tissue is missing or if the nature of the delivery of the placenta makes it likely that a cotyledon is retained. The completeness of the membranes is less easy to assess but a careful examination will give some indication. A fragment may be detected on vaginal examination and can be removed with long artery forceps. Exploration of the uterus is not a usual practice for suspected retained membranes. The amniotic surface should be examined to make sure that there are no blood vessels leaving the periphery of the main placental mass. A sieve of blood vessels from the periphery ending in another area of the membrane without corresponding placental tissue in that area indicates the possibility of retained succenturiate lobe. The inspection of the chorionic surface will indicate missing cotyledons. Inspection of the corresponding amniotic surface will make it easy to identify a missing cotyledon.

The vessels of the umbilical cord should also be inspected for any anomaly, including the absence of an umbilical artery. If an artery is absent, the incidence of congenital abnormalities in the child is about 30%, especially those involving the renal and cardiovascular systems (Benirschke 1965).

Assessment of trauma to the genitalia   Following delivery of the placenta, the vagina, introitus and perineum should be carefully inspected to determine if any injury has occurred during the course of the childbirth. Ideally this should be performed in the lithotomy position, particularly if there has been an instrumental delivery as cervical and upper vaginal tears under the pubic ramus and vault can be missed unless a careful inspection is made with a good light source and adequate exposure if necessary with the help of retractors and an assistant.

In closing vaginal lacerations, the apex should first be identified and the tear repaired from above downwards where possible. Any dead space should be obliterated to prevent paravaginal and pararectal hematomas. More details dealing with such tears are discussed in the chapter on postpartum hemorrhage. Repair of the perineum and the lower vagina requires infiltration with 10 ml of 1% lignocaine unless an epidural anesthetic is already in place. The perineal and pelvic floor musculature should be realigned to restore normal anatomy using either 2/O chromic catgut or dexon. Midline tears and episiotomies can be closed with continuous sutures, a deeper layer closing the musculature and interrupted sutures or a subcuticular layer approximating the skin edges.

More extensive lesions are better dealt with interrupted sutures in the perineal muscles and skin. Where there has been a third degree tear, it is essential to identify and close the tear in the rectal mucosa with interrupted catgut, and then to identify the divided portions of the external sphincter and approximate them with interrupted catgut sutures before closing the perineal musculature.

The volume of blood loss should be assessed although estimation of the blood loss in the third stage is grossly inaccurate when done by inspection alone. Although it is possible to collect some of the blood lost before and during the delivery of the patient, and to make allowances for contamination by amniotic fluid, faeces, urine, cleaning solutions and the soiling of bed linen, bleeding from the uterus occurring during the 24 hours after delivery is not usually measured accurately unless the loss is considerable and replacement is required. Nevertheless an effort should be made to calculate the blood loss during delivery and at least the first two hours after it to help with maternal management during the puerperium. An appreciable fall in the hemoglobin level may occur without a noticeable episode of hemorrhage especially when it is from lacerations. Exact measurement is not necessary but an approximation and the patient's blood pressure and pulse rate will indicate the likely loss and patient's reaction to it. If there is excessive bleeding and the patient shows evidence of shock, then an adequate amount of blood replacement is important. A more accurate method of determining the effects of blood loss and the amount to be replaced involves the measurement of the central venous pressure (O'Driscoll and McCarthy 1966) but is not necessary in cases with minor hemodynamic changes. More details of blood loss and replacement are discussed in the chapter dealing with postpartum hemorrhage.

Finally, the notes and the partogram should be completed and checked by a senior obstetrician to ensure that all the details of the labour have been entered fully for future reference.

Abnormalities of the third stage

Retained placenta   Physiologically, the placenta should be delivered within 30 minutes. Despite the routine use of oxytocics, the third stage of labour may be delayed. Possible explanations for this delay are inadequate uterine contraction and retraction and rarely, a morbidly adherent placenta.

The management of retained placenta has varied considerably from time to time but in modern practice, manual removal of the placenta is routinely employed if there is failure to deliver the placenta half an hour after delivery of the baby. The procedure may be performed earlier if the patient is bleeding and the placenta has failed to separate completely.

The patient with a retained placenta may be in shock, having had a postpartum hemorrhage. Adequate resuscitation is of prime importance before attempting manual removal. A repeat dose of oxytocic is administered, to encourage uterine contraction and placental separation and controlled cord traction applied. At times the placenta may have separated and be in the lower segment but further descent is prevented by a partially closed cervix. Following the cord digitally into the cervical canal whilst traction is applied on the cord will identify the placenta. Hooking a finger into the placental substance and traction along with cord traction may help to deliver the placenta. The finger may have to be hooked from the point of the cervical os to a higher level of the placenta in order to gradually deliver the placenta. Failure to deliver the placenta despite these measures indicates manual removal of the placenta in the theatre under general anesthesia. The patient is placed in the lithotomy position. One hand is placed abdominally on the uterine fundus to maintain its position in the abdomen and to allow counterpressure to be exerted. The vaginal hand is introduced through the cervical os and the retraction ring, if one is present, to the upper segment of the uterus, following the cord to its placental insertion. If it is difficult to introduce the hand through the cervical canal, gentle pressure must be continuously applied till the canal gradually opens. Tocolytics can be used as a bolus dose (Terbutaline 0.25 mg IV) which has to be reversed by propranolol (1 mg IV) or halothane can be administered by the anesthetist. The lower edge of the placenta is then located and with a sawing motion, the operator proceeds to detach the placenta from the uterus. When the placenta is totally separated and the cavity rechecked and found to be empty, it is removed. An intravenous oxytocic is administered to promote uterine contraction. A course of antibiotics is then given to prevent any infection following intrauterine manipulation.

There is no place for the use of vigorous fundal compression in the attempt to expel the placenta. This is dangerous and may cause complications, including inversion of the uterus, particularly if cord traction is applied at the same time.

If an active policy of management of the third stage is not practised, the indication to remove the placenta manually is bleeding from the uterine cavity with relaxation of the uterus. If there is no bleeding, it is a matter of convenience as to when the placenta should be removed but it should be done at the earliest to avoid sudden partial separation and hemorrhage. An intravenous injection of ergometrine may stimulate uterine contractions, and an attempt at placental delivery by cord traction may be made should sudden bleeding occur. If it is unsuccessful, it is usually advisable to prepare the patient for a general anesthetic. A placental cotyledon may occasionally be retained within the uterus. This may not give rise to immediate bleeding but during the puerperium there will be excessive blood loss with the likelihood of uterine infection. Often the placenta is reported as being complete in these patients at the time of delivery. Exploration and curettage are necessary if products are retained, although it is distressing and perhaps harmful to explore the uterus and to find no products (Beazley 1995). Malvern et al (1973) have shown that ultrasound can be helpful in detecting the presence of retained products but evacuation curettage must be undertaken with antibiotic cover when there is bleeding in order to arrest the hemorrhage of concern despite no definitive evidence of retained tissue.

Placenta accreta   When it is impossible to get a plane of cleavage to separate the placenta from the uterine wall, placenta accreta may be present. This arises because implantation of the ovum occurred in an area of the uterus in which the endometrium was deficient or damaged, possibly as a result of previous scarring or a congenital anomaly (Loring 1973). Placenta previa and previous caesarean section are two independent common predisposing causes (Fox 1972) and there is a strong association when placenta previa is on a previous caesarean section scar. Elderly multiparas are the most prone to this complication. The chorionic villi readily penetrate the endometrium and reach the myometrium.

Placenta increta refers to the penetration of the myometrium by the chorionic villi. When the villi reach the serosal aspect of the uterus, it is termed placenta percreta.

Placenta accreta is diagnosed when difficulty is encountered during delivery of the placenta and at manual removal. When the placenta is morbidly adherent and not removed, there are two possible outcomes. When there is no bleeding and the patient desires to preserve uterine function, it is possible to cut the cord high and to leave the placenta in situ and hope that autolysis will occur. This process can be enhanced by a short course of methotrexate (Arulkumaran et al, 1986). As the risk of uterine infection is considerable, antibiotic therapy will be required. The patient should be observed and warned of the possibility of secondary postpartum hemorrhage, which may occur 10–14 days after delivery or earlier.

If there is minimal bleeding and the patient is desirous of having more children, conservative treatment with oxytocics or prostaglandins can be tried first for a short period of 1–2 hours. No attempt at piecemeal removal of the placenta should be contemplated, because of the danger of severe hemorrhage. Internal iliac artery ligation or hysterectomy are the last resort. Hysterectomy is the safest and is the method of choice in a woman who has completed her family.

Perineal hematomas   The blood loss in this condition is into the tissues rather than external. It usually results from damage to a vessel wall without laceration of overlying tissues or if a bleeding vessel is not secured when a tear or episiotomy is sutured. This trauma may be the result of trauma during the normal course of labour, the application of forceps, or the result of the infiltration of a local anesthetic administered for paracervical or pudendal anesthesia.

The degree of discomfort to the patient is proportional to the size of the hematoma; if large, severe perirectal pain is experienced and shock may result.

The management of such a hematoma is immediate surgical drainage under anesthesia and establishment of hemostasis. Reflex retention of urine is common and a self-retaining catheter should be inserted for at least 24 hours. Blood transfusion and antibiotic therapy may be required.

Amniotic fluid embolism   Amniotic fluid embolism is rare (1:80,000 deliveries) and is associated with a mortality greater than 80 per cent (Morgan 1979; Mulder 1985). The underlying etiology is related to the passage of amniotic fluid and fetal squames into the maternal circulation causing an anaphylactic-like reaction. The onset is dramatic with the clinical manifestation of dyspnoea and cyanosis, together with pallor, chills, restlessness and perhaps convulsions. Shock usually follows rapidly and death may occur before any effective treatment can be initiated. In less severe forms, the patient survives, the thromboplastin contained in the amniotic fluid results in disseminated intravascular coagulation and a general bleeding tendency ensues.

High parity, maternal age of more than 35 years, over distension of the uterus, complete or partial uterine rupture, large babies and/or hypertonic labour, particularly that associated with the excessive use of oxytocic are features commonly found when amniotic fluid embolism occurs. However they are not specific and most women who have these features do not develop amniotic fluid embolism.

In the past, a definite diagnosis of amniotic fluid embolism was made by the pathologist at postmortem. More recently, examination of blood from the central circulation aspirated whilst using a pulmonary wedge catheter showing fetal squames has facilitated the diagnosis.

The treatment of amniotic fluid embolism is not specific but uses the general principles of treatment for shock. This includes oxygen administration and the maintenance of cardiac output. In the hypotensive patient, infusion of a dopamine drip 2–20 µg/kg/min may help. If necessary, administration of digoxin (0.5–1.0 mg in divided doses) may be beneficial. Treatment of the severe coagulopathy is accomplished by the use of fresh blood, fresh frozen plasma and cryoprecipitate.

Inversion of the uterus   This is an uncommon complication of the third stage of labour. The fundus of the uterus descends through the uterine body and cervix into the vagina and sometimes protrudes through the vulva. There are three degrees of inversion:

1. The inverted fundus reaches the internal os.
2. The whole body is inverted and emerging via the cervical os.
3. The uterus is completely inverted and is seen outside the introitus.

Acute inversion may be spontaneous or the result of mismanagement of the third stage of labour. Spontaneous inversion is often associated with a fundally located adherent placenta. Other associated factors are arcuate or unicornuate uterus (Das 1940).

Mismanagement and uterine inversion occurs when traction is attempted on the cord before uterine contraction and placental separation are established. Rarely it may follow a manual removal of the placenta when the abdominal hand is firmly pressed on the uterus and the vaginal hand is drawn too quickly. This results in the creation of a negative pressure and the uterus inverts.

The condition may be diagnosed in various ways. The most dramatic presentation is the complaint of severe lower abdominal pain and the feeling of prolapse followed by collapse and hemorrhage. In milder degrees of prolapse, the patient may complain of pain and hemorrhage. The shock produced by a uterine inversion is commonly neurogenic in origin as considerable traction is placed on the infundibulopelvic and round ligaments. The state of shock is often out of proportion to the amount of blood loss and in such cases inversion should always be suspected and a vaginal examination done.

If the condition is diagnosed at the time of delivery, replacement should be carried out instantly. At this time the pelvic soft tissues will be relaxed and there will be no spasm preventing replacement (Dewhurst and Bevis 1951). This should be followed by an intravenous dose of oxytocic to initiate uterine contractions. The patient should then be sent to the operating theatre for manual removal of the placenta. If the uterine inversion is only detected some time after the event, and the woman is in shock, it is best to resuscitate her with intravenous fluids and blood. Pain is alleviated by packing the vagina to relieve the tension on the infundibulopelvic ligaments. The patient should then be transferred to the operating theatre and a general anesthetic administered. Digital replacement under general anesthesia may be carried out but the hydrostatic method described by O'Sullivan (1945) may be more effective and safe. Warm sterile fluid (saline) is gradually instilled into the vagina by means of a douche can and tubing. Occlusion of the vagina should be achieved with the hands to prevent leak of water and as much as four or five litres may be required. The hydrostatic pressure reverses the inversion and results in the uterus being distended and returning to its normal intra-abdominal position. The fluid is then drained off and ergometrine is given, a hand remaining in the uterus until the fluid has escaped and the uterus is contracting satifactorily. If the placenta is still attached to the uterus, it should be removed manually and an oxytocic should be administered to ensure uterine contraction. Removal of the placenta before reduction will lead to uncontrollable hemorrhage. In order to relax the retraction ring whilst replacing the uterus, a bolus dose of terbutaline 0.25 mg in 5 cc of water over 5 minutes can be administered. Its action has to be reversed by propranolol 1 mg IV to avoid postpartum hemorrhage.

Obstetric shock

Shock may be defined as inadequacy of normal perfusion of the organs of the body. Shock in obstetrics may be cardiogenic, hypovolemic, neurogenic or septic.

The basic problem of shock is that there is not enough blood flow to carry oxygen and nutrients in the capillary vessels to supply vital organs. This has two major consequences:

1. Hypoxia of the tissues initially depresses their function and if unrelieved, eventually causes death.
2. Coagulation of the blood occurs in the smaller blood vessels from hypoxia and is hastened if thromboplastins are released at the same time. This disseminated intravascular coagulation adds to the hypoxia of the tissues.

Unless the shock is treated in time, it becomes irreversible and the patient will die.

Compensating mechanisms

1. *The sympathetic nervous system*   As the pressure falls in the large arteries and veins, there is an activation of the sympathetic nervous system. Blood is shunted away from the non-vital areas such as the skin (coldness and pallor), kidney (oliguria) and muscles, and the heart is stimulated (tachycardia).
2. *The fluid retaining mechanism*   The same stimuli described above activate two further mechanisms : antidiuretic hormone release from the posterior lobe of the pituitary and aldosterone release from the adrenal cortex, both of which help the kidney to conserve water.
3. *The fibrinolytic system*   This is activated in conditions of shock (plasminogen-plasmin) and is responsible for clearing the intravascular thrombosis which has formed.

Clinical features   These largely reflect the activity of the compensatory mechanisms as described above.

Tachycardia is usual in volume depletion shock and the pulse is weak and difficult to feel. The rate usually reflects the severity of shock. Bradycardia occurs in neurogenic shock. Skin pallor is usual, but normally there is much variation. A better sign is pallor of the conjunctiva and lips which, if noticeable, indicates significant anemia or blood loss. Skin temperature is usually low but may depend on room temperature. A fall in blood pressure is usual and is a reflection of the degree of shock. If the shock is mild the systolic pressure is usually 100 or more; if the shock is moderate it is 85–99; if marked, 70–84 and if critical below 70. Cyanosis is rare unless the lungs are affected (pulmonary embolism) or the heart is failing. Respiration may be initially faster and shallower, and deeper and irregular later.

Nausea and vomiting are relatively common as are periods of restlessness. The urine output is usually low (< 30ml/hr).

Treatment   The principles of management are discussed below. The treatment of individual conditions is discussed in Chapters 12 and 22 in the book.

General

1. All vital signs in the mother must be measured and recorded accurately including those in the conscious state.
2. The patient should be handled gently and offered reassurance. The situation should be explained so that she does not panic.
3. Laboratory tests : full blood count, blood for cross match, coagulation profile, serum urea electrolytes and creatinine, bacteriological and acid-base studies should be performed.

Replacement of circulating blood volume   Initial replacement is made with normal saline or Hartmann's solution. This will replace the lost blood volume without danger of transfusion reactions and will lower the blood viscosity. Colloid solutions like Haemaccel or Dextran may be given until proper grouped and cross-matched blood is available. In cases of disseminated intravascular coagulation, fresh blood, fresh frozen plasma and platelets may need to be added. (See Chapter 7 on Fluid Management in Labour.)

The amount of transfusion fluid required in a straightforward situation can be gauged by the recovery of vital signs to normal and urine flow. In complicated cases, central venous pressure (CVP) measurement is helpful to allow assessment of the correct volume of fluid replacement. In general a CVP value of 0–5 cm indicates hypovolemia; 6–10 cm indicates possible hypovolemia and a trial administration of fluid; 11 cm or more indicates normovolemia, hypervolemia or heart failure, and further fluid is not required.

Coagulation failure   If the blood does not clot normally, there is usually a deficiency of clotting factors. Fresh frozen plasma is usually given if the fibrinogen level is more than 1 g per litre. Cryoprecipitate which contains Factor VIII, Von Willie Brandt's and fibrinogen is given if the fibrinogen level is less than 1 g/L. Freeze dried fibrinogen should be available in the labour ward which can be reconstituted and given within a short period of time especially when fibrinogen is low (< 0.8g/L) and there is bleeding. Please see Chapter 22 on Management of Eclampsia for further details.

Oxygen   Oxygen should be administered by a mask and not intranasally, since the latter method is relatively ineffective. Giving oxygen by mask does not deliver uniform amounts and currently ventimasks are available. With minor adjustments to the valve and flow of oxygen, different concentrations of oxygen can be delivered uniformly.

Analgesia   Pethidine (IM or IV injection) or a similar narcotic is needed if the patient is in pain due to trauma or is anxious.

Vascular tone   Vasoconstrictor drugs such as dopamine (2–20 µg/kg/min), noradrenaline and angiotensin may be used to exaggerate nature's vasoconstrictive response. However it is less dangerous and more physiological to replace circulating blood volume. Vasodilator drugs such as isoprenaline and chlorpromazine are used to offset the vasoconstrictive response and lessen tissue hypoxia. If they are employed, early and adequate replacement of circulatory volume is also required.

Antibiotics These will be necessary in massive doses if the shock is due to sepsis. Cover must be provided against both aerobic and anerobic organisms. The exact choice of antibiotic will be determined by the severity of the infection, patient allergy, organism if known and urinary output.

Mannitol This is an osmotic diuretic and is useful in the early phase of oliguria and to combat the effect of stress. If there is a suggestion of oliguria due to reduced blood volume because of hemorrhage, which may lead to diuresis it should be corrected. Despite adequate blood volume correction (based on CVP), if oliguria persists, diuretics can be used.

Hydrocortisone Adrenal cortical hormones are used to assist the circulation and combat the effect of stress. Depending on the situation hydrocortisone 100 mg IV can be given, 4 to 6 hourly.

Other measures Assisted ventilation, therapy for cardiac arrest and digitalisation may be required for cardiac failure.

Active management of the third stage of labour with prophylactic oxytocics and controlled cord traction have gone a long way to make the third stage of labour less hazardous. Careful vigilance during the short interval between the delivery of the baby and the expulsion of the placenta and its membranes are of great help in the prevention of retained placenta, in uterine inversion and other associated complications.

References

Arulkumaran S, Ng CSA, Ingemarsson I and Ratnam SS 1986. Medical treatment of placenta accreta with methotrexate. *Acta Obstet Gynecol Scand* 65:285-286.

Benirschke K 1965. Birth Defects (original article series). The National Foundation, *March of Dimes*:53.

Beazley JM 1995. Complications of the third stage of labour. In: Whitfield CR, ed. Dewhurst's Textbook of Obstetrics and Gynecology. London. pp 368-376.

Botha MC 1968. *S Afr J Obstet Gynecol* 6:30.

Das P 1940 Inversion of the uterus. *J Obstet Gynecol Br Emp* 46:525-548.

Dewhurst CJ, Bevis DCA 1951. Acute puerperal inversion of the uterus. *Lancet* i:1394-1396.

Embrey MP 1961. Simultaneous intramuscular injection of oxytocin and ergometrine: a tocographic study. *BMJ* I:1737-1738.

Enkin M, Keirse MJNC, Chalmers I 1989. The third stage of labour. In: Enkin M, Keirse M, Chalmers I, eds. A Guide to Effective Care in Pregnancy and Childbirth. New York: pp 234-239.

Fliegner JR, Hibbard BM 1966. Active management of the third stage of labour. *BMJ* ii:622-623.

Fox H 1972. Placenta accreta 1945-1969. *Obstet Gynecol Surv* 27:475-490.

Loring TW 1973. Pregnancy and uterine malformations. *Am J Obstet Gynecol* 116:505-510.

Macpherson J, Wilson JK 1965. A radiological study of the placental stage of labour. *J Obstet Gynecol Br Cwlth* 63:321-330.

Morgan M 1979. Amniotic fluid embolism. *Anesthesia* 34:20-32.

Mulder JI 1985. Amniotic fluid embolism: An overview and case report. *Am J Obstet Gynecol* 152:430-435.

O'Driscoll K, McCarthy JR 1966. Abruptio placentae and central venous pressures. *J Obstet Gynaecol Br Cwlth* 73:923-929.

O'Sullivan JV 1945. Acute inversion of the uterus. *BMJ* ii:282.

Reports on Confidential Enquiries into Maternal Deaths in England and Wales 1967-69; 1973-75; 1982-84; 1988-90 (1972;1979;1989; 1994). London: HMSO.

Yao AC, Hirvensal M, Lind J 1968. Placental transfusion rate and uterine contraction. *Lancet* i:380-383.

Yao AC, Lind J 1969. Effect of gravity on placental transfusion. *Lancet* ii:505-508.

Yao AC, Moinian M, Lind J 1969. Distribution of blood between infant and placenta after birth. *Lancet* ii:871-873.

Yuen PO, Chan ST, Yim SO and Chang AMZ 1995. A randomised double blind comparison of syntometrine and syntocinon in the management of the third stage of labour. *Br J Obstet Gynecol* 102:377-380.

12

The Management of Postpartum Hemorrhage

S Arulkumaran
R Haththotuwa
S Chua

Over the years we have seen advances in the management of most obstetric conditions, but relatively less in postpartum hemorrhage (PPH). This is because more work has been done on the first and second stage of labour compared to the third stage (Gilbert et al 1987). PPH is a nightmare even to the present day obstetrician as it is sudden, frequently unpredicted and can be catastrophic. The clinical picture changes so rapidly that unless timely action is taken, maternal death could occur in a short period. About 500,000 mothers die in childbirth each year even in this decade (Royston and Armstrong 1989; Kwast 1991). The widespread introduction of blood transfusion services, the availability of antibiotics like penicillin and sulphonamides, changes in the socioeconomic status and the improvement of the nutritional and educational status of the mother have contributed to the marked decline of the mortality rate (Moir 1955). At the turn of the century PPH was the commonest cause of maternal death (Thilaganathan et al 1993). The introduction of oxytocic preparations for the management of PPH has contributed to a marked reduction in maternal mortality (Moir 1955). Although the introduction of oxytocics has reduced the maternal mortality due to PPH from one in 3,000 births in 1930 to one in 20,000 births in 1950 (Greenhill 1951), PPH still remains an important cause of maternal death (Gilliant 1949; DHSS 1982; Hall et al 1985; Embrey et al 1963). In the 1980s the maternal mortality due to PPH was around one in 60,000 births in the United Kingdom (DHSS 1986).

Maternal deaths and morbidity due to PPH is fifty times commoner in developing countries (Kwast et al 1986) than in England and Wales (DHSS 1989) and the difference is probably due to the prophylactic use of oxytocics in the management of the third stage of labour in the developed countries (WHO 1990).

Primary PPH is defined as the loss of 500 ml or more of blood per vaginum during the first 24 hours after the delivery of the baby. But the minimum quantity of blood loss taken to diagnose PPH by various authors has varied from 300 ml (Ratnam and Rauff 1989) to 600 ml (Lourdes St George and Grandon 1990) although 500 ml is the generally accepted quantity (Samil 1992). In most Asian countries the lower value is taken because Asian women are unable to cope with a larger amount of blood loss as they are smaller built and therefore have less blood volume, are less well nourished and tend to have a lower antenatal Hb value than their western counterparts (Ratnam and Rauff 1989). As the blood loss is usually estimated visually, the quantity is often underestimated (Gilbert et al 1987) and has a wide variation. The problem of estimating the amount of blood loss accounts for the wide range of incidence of PPH quoted in the literature, which varies from 2–11% (Gilbert et al 1987; Hall et al 1985; Brant 1967). When quantitative measurements of blood loss are taken, the incidence rises up to 20% (Brant 1967). An error of about 45% was found by Newton et al (1961) between the visual estimation and the quantitative measurement of blood loss. The clinical examination of the patient may indicate the blood loss in an indirect manner and is given in Table 1.

Table 1: Clinical symptoms and signs related to the amount of blood loss

Blood loss (% of blood volume)	Systolic blood pressure (mmHg)	Symptoms and signs
10–15	Normal	Postural hypotension Mild tachycardia
15–30	Slight fall	Tachycardia Thirst Weakness
30–40	60–80	Pallor Oliguria Confusion Restlessness
40+	40–60	Anuria Air hunger Coma Death

Source: Ratnam SS and Rauff M (1989)

Etiology

Knowledge about the etiology of PPH helps to take necessary steps to prevent it. Hemostasis is achieved after the third stage of labour by the mechanical constriction of blood vessels due to uterine muscle contraction and retraction, and by clots sealing off the raw surface in the placental bed. The causes of PPH can be broadly classified into:

1. uterine atony
2. traumatic injury to the genital tract
3. retained placenta
4. uterine inversion
5. coagulation disorders

1. *Uterine atony*

Uterine atony accounts for about 80% of the cases of PPH (Prendiville and Elbourne 1990; Weeks and O'Toole 1956; Hesler 1975; Hayashi 1990). Bleeding is the result of blood vessels not being obliterated by the contraction of uterine muscle. The bleeding could be brisk or slow and is usually intermittent, coinciding with uterine relaxation. There are several factors which may predispose to uterine atony and are given below.

a. *Overdistension of the uterus*   There is an increased risk of PPH due to overdistension of uterus in cases of multiple pregnancies, polyhydramnios and large babies (B.Wt > 4 kg) (Stones et al 1993). Uterine over-distension by a large baby causing PPH has been cited as early as 1904 (Ahlfield and Aschoff 1904). A large placental area (Samil 1992), possibly encroaching on the lower uterine segment, may contribute to PPH in cases of multiple pregnancy.

b. *Induction of labour*   Increased risk of PPH has been shown to occur with induced labour as opposed to spontaneous labour (Gilbert et al 1987; Lourdes St George and Grandon 1990; Brinsden and Clark 1978; Mackenzie 1979). The incidence in induced labour has been twice as high as that seen in spontaneous labour. Oxytocin and amniotomy for the induction of labour appears to carry a higher risk of PPH than the use of pro-staglandin pessaries (Lourdes St George and Grandon 1990; Mackenzie 1979). It is thought that intravenous oxytocin used to induce labour tends to reduce the myometrial efficiency following delivery, causing a poor response to the subsequent parenteral bolus of oxytocin (Mackenzie 1979; Leader 1974). Because of these findings, primary PPH is another compli-cation which must be considered when the induction of labour is being planned (Ratnam and Rauff 1989).

c. *Prolonged labour*   Prolonged labour has been found to be associated with an increased risk of PPH (Gilbert et al 1987; Lourdes St George and Grandon 1990). The duration of pushing in the second stage of labour does not show any relationship to the incidence of PPH but the total du-ration of the second stage has some correlation (Gilbert et al 1987). In the prevention of PPH, the length of the second stage of labour should be considered.

d. *Epidural analgesia*   There are conflicting reports about PPH and epidural analgesia. Lourdes St George and Grandon (1990) found an in-creased incidence of PPH in association with epidural analgesia while Studd et al (1980) did not find any definitive association. The prolonged second stage and increased incidence of instrumental deliveries associated with epidural analgesia (Studd et al 1980), may have an indirect relation-ship to PPH.

e. *Drugs.*   Halothane used in anesthesia and tocolytic drugs, especially beta mimetic drugs used to inhibit labour by uterine relaxation will cause PPH. If beta mimetics like ritordrine or terbutaline are administered and if delivery occurs in a short time, then the action of the beta mimetic drug should be counteracted using 1–2 mg propranalol given intravenously to prevent PPH (Anderson et al 1974).

f. *Antepartum hemorrhage*   Both placenta previa and abruptio placenta have been associated with an increased incidence of postpartum hemorrhage.

g. *Retained products of conception*   Placental cotyledons, membranes and succenturiate lobe of placenta can cause poor uterine contractions leading to PPH.
i. *Grandmultipara*   The age of the woman is significant.
j. *Sitting up position for delivery*   This position adopted in the second stage has been associated with PPH (Stewart et al 1983).
k. *Mismanagement of the third stage of labour*   Pulling on the cord with an uncontracted uterus may cause partial separation of the placenta and thus bleeding from the placental bed.

2. Injuries to the genital tract

When the uterus is well contracted, bleeding may occur from extraplacental sites, following injuries to the uterus, cervix, vagina, vestibule or perineum. This is more so with difficult vaginal and operative deliveries.

Primigravidas have been said to have higher blood loss compared with women who have their second or third deliveries (Gilbert et al 1987; Coon et al 1941; Newton et al 1961). But Bullough et al (1989) did not find an increase of PPH in primigravidas and they attributed this to the fact that none of the patients had episiotomies and that the incidence of perineal tears was low.

Prophylactic management

The primary aim of the obstetrician in the management of PPH should be its prevention. For this purpose women with a high risk of developing PPH (for example, grandmultiparas, women with multiple pregnancies, and prolonged labour) should be identified. These women should be managed more carefully as opposed to low risk patients.

High risk patients

During the antenatal period anemia should be identified, and the third stage should be managed by an experienced midwife or a medical officer.

On admission in labour, a full blood count should be done and blood cross matched. It is preferable to have an intravenous line with a wide bore cannula (16 or 18 G) prior to the second stage of labour. The third stage should be managed actively, administering 0.5 mg of ergometrine intravenously with the delivery of the anterior shoulder of the baby. In patients with hypertension and cardiac disease, ten units of intravenous syntocinon should be given instead of ergometrine.

Some women as well as some physicians have challenged active management of the third stage of labour (Chamberlain 1985; Milton 1985; Dunn 1985). The meta-analysis of controlled trials shows that the routine use of oxytocics in the third stage of labour reduces the risk of PPH by about 30–40% (Prendiville et al 1988).

Though there is widespread use of oxytocics in the prevention of PPH, the type of oxytocic used varies widely. Oxytocin is mainly used in much of North America and Canada, syntometrine in the United Kingdom and ergometrine is preferred in Denmark and most of Africa. Prendiville and Elbourne who analysed 17 trials, did not find that ergometrine had a definite advantage over syntocinon

(Prendiville and Elbourne 1990). Syntometrine has also not been found superior to oxytocin (McDonald et al 1993). But oxytocin has helped to reduce the incidence of nausea, vomiting and hypertension. Syntocinon, 10 units, has shown a better efficacy than 5 units, indicating a dose-dependent effect in preventing PPH (McDonald et al 1993).

Though prostaglandins are shown to rise in maternal blood within five minutes of delivery (Ilancheran and Ratnam 1990) and are used for the treatment of PPH, they are not widely used for its prevention. But it has been shown that an intra-muscular injection of 125 ug of 15(S) 15 methyl $PGF_{2\alpha}$ (Prostodin 15 m) can be used for the active management of the third stage of labour and that it prevents PPH (Anjaneyulu et al 1988). Gastrointestinal side effects like diarrhoea and vomiting have been very low.

Cord drainage of placental blood in the actively managed third stage of labour has been studied. This study showed no reduction in the incidence of retained placenta, in the length of the third stage of labour, in the amount of hemorrhage or transfusion rates (Thomas et al 1990).

Though oxytocics have been shown to reduce the incidence of PPH, unfortunately it is not available to about half the women in developing countries who deliver without the attendance of a trained midwife. The need to refrigerate oxytocics (Walker et al 1988) has also contributed to the difficulties in giving oxytocics routinely in developing countries. The oxytocin level is increased on preparation for breast feeding (McNeilly et al 1983) and again three minutes after commencement of suckling (Weitzman et al 1980). Based on this knowledge, early suckling has been advocated to prevent PPH, although some studies have failed to prove this effect (Bullough et al 1989).

Low risk patients

Syntometrine intramuscularly for normotensive patients and 10 units of syntocinon intravenously for hypertensive patients should be given with the delivery of the anterior shoulder of the baby. But controversy still exists as to whether active management of the third stage of labour reduces blood loss when compared with physiological management in women with low risk of developing PPH (Beard 1993).

Treatment of postpartum hemorrhage

Awareness that PPH is associated with a high maternal mortality rate is the first step towards its good management (Hayashi 1982). The condition should be identified early and action should be prompt. The obstetric team should be alerted, and medical methods should be instituted first in a stepwise manner before resorting to surgical methods. Another basic principle in the management of PPH is that if one method fails, the next step should be tried without losing time, adopting an expectant approach. This is because the longer the time taken to control bleeding, the higher the chances are of the patient needing a hysterectomy, developing coagulopathy or dying.

General management

The general condition of the patient, the amount of blood loss and the degree of hypovolemia should first be assessed quickly. At the same time blood should be sent for full blood count and cross matching with a request for four to six units of blood. Preferably two intravenous (IV) lines with a 16 or 18 gauge cannula should be set up. Crystalloids or colloids should be given, depending on the condition of the patient. When the patient has hypotension and is not shocked, two litres of crystalloids can be given in 1–2 hrs and if there is no response or if the condition deteriorates, colloids, plasma or blood should be given immediately. If the patient is in shock she should be resuscitated. The second IV line with a 16 gauge cannula should be set up if it was not started earlier and colloids, plasma or blood started immediately. As uterine atony is the cause of PPH in about 80% of instances, the uterus should be massaged continuously to induce contractions and to assess whether it is contracting. Massaging should be done properly so that the uterine muscle is massaged and not the abdominal wall, and it should not be so vigorous as to cause severe pain to the patient or a broad ligament hematoma. The vital parameters such as the level of consciousness, pulse rate, blood pressure, intake/output, level of the uterine fundus and the amount of blood loss should be monitored carefully.

Clinicians should remember that estimated blood loss is often very much less than measured blood loss, especially when there is postpartum hemorrhage. Care must be taken to assess the patient's condition, possibly with the help of ancillary investigations like hemoglobin estimation, instead of relying solely on the clinical estimation of blood loss. Clinical parameters in relation to blood loss are given in Table 1.

Use of the military anti shock trouser (MAST) suit

The use of an inflatable pneumatic suit to envelop the legs and abdomen of a patient in order to control hypotension in head and neck surgery was first reported in 1903. Subsequently, the MAST suit was developed based on the same principle and has proved valuable in patients with active uncontrollable bleeding and hypotension (Pearse et al 1984)). When used in this situation the MAST suit provides a rapid increase in blood pressure and slows down active bleeding, and as a result improves perfusion to the vital organs and probably decreases the incidence of the adult respiratory distress syndrome and acute tubular necrosis; it allows easier intravenous needle placement in the patient in hemorrhagic shock, and permits time for resuscitation and definitive procedures to control bleeding.

Specific management

Alongside initial management if the bleeding continues, the cause for the bleeding should be established. Checking the contractility of the uterus, rechecking the entirety of the placenta and membranes and looking for injuries to the genital tract will help to ascertain the cause.

If uterine atony is suspected, while continuing to massage the uterus, ergometrine 0.5 mg IV should be given. If there is no response within ten minutes it should be followed by an infusion of 100 units of syntocinon and 0.5 mg of ergometrine in 500 ml of N saline. An infusion rate of 90 drops a minute may be adequate. This will help to contract the uterus and expel any blood clots which might have accumulated during the phase of atony. A full blood count report should be traced and blood should be sent for a clotting screen. At least six units of blood should be cross matched and fresh frozen plasma kept in reserve.

If no response is forthcoming within ten minutes it will be prudent to increase the syntocinon dose to 300 units with 0.5 g of ergometrine in 500 ml of N saline given at a rate of 90 drops per minute.

Prostaglandins should be used if PPH continues despite the above measures for ten minutes. Analogues of PG have been shown to be more potent than parent compounds. Prostaglandins $PGF_{2\alpha}$, PGE_2 and the analogues 15 methyl $PGF_{2\alpha}$ (Carboprost), 16-phenoxy-W-17,18,19,20 tetranor PGE_2 methyl sulphonamide and 15-methyl $PGF_{2\alpha}$ tromethamine (Hembate sterile solution) have been used.

Prostaglandins have been used by various routes. PGE_2 used as vaginal pessaries (Hertz et al 1980) has been unsatisfactory and continued bleeding is likely to expel the drug. Continuous irrigation of the uterine cavity with a low concentration of PGE_2 has been shown to be effective in controlling severe PPH without side effects (Peyser et al 1990). Intramyometrial injection of $PGF_{2\alpha}$ has been shown to be effective by several authors (Jacobs and Arizas 1979; Toppozada 1986). Carboprost used intramuscularly (Toppozada 1986) has been shown to be more effective than that used intramyometrialy. Sulprostone has been used successfully intravenously and intramyometrialy.

Carboprost, 0.25 mg every 15–30 minutes, to a maximum of 2 mg should be given intramuscularly or sulprostone 1,000 ug in 500 ml of N saline should be given at 60–80 drops per minute. The vital parameters should be monitored carefully as occasionally cardiac complications could occur. If this fails, sulprostone can be used intramyometrialy; 500 ug is diluted in 10 ml of normal saline and injected into the four uterine quadrants transabdominally. The desired effect with these measures should be achieved in 10–15 mins.

If medical intervention does not bring about the desired effect the next step should be exploration under anesthesia and other surgical methods.

Surgical treatment

Under general anesthesia and good lighting, tears and lacerations should be excluded from the cervix downwards. Great care must be taken to look for lacerations in the endocervix. If the tear is seen extending into the uterus, laparotomy may be advisable.

The uterus should be explored with care to detect any retained placental tissue and to confirm that it is empty. A light curettage may be done using a large sharp curette, taking care not to perforate the soft uterus.

A hot douche could be considered if there is a general ooze despite the uterus being well contracted. Another procedure which was used historically (Stander 1945), but which fell out of favour from the 1960s to the 1980s was uterine packing. Though its use is controversial, its value in controlling PPH due to uterine atony, placenta accreta and placenta previa has been reported (Druzin 1989). Effort should be taken to pack the uterine cavity completely and uniformly. There has been no incidence of serious infections following this procedure (Druzin 1989; Lester et al 1965; Maier 1993). An oxytocin infusion must be continued to keep the uterus contracted over the pack, till the time of removal 12 – 24 hrs later. More, recently the successful use of a Sengstaken-Blakemore tube has been described to control massive PPH (Katesmark et al 1994). Balloon tamponade was achieved with a gastric balloon, and the aspiration channel provides a drain for any blood that collects above the balloon. Gradual reduction of the volume of the balloon by aspiration allows the uterus to contract over a period of hours. As with uterine packing, the myometrial tone is maintained with a syntocinon infusion. Prophylactic antibiotics are useful to prevent subsequent infection of the pelvic organs.

If the patient continues to bleed, bilateral ligation of the internal iliac arteries should be done. Although extensive collateral blood flow to the distal internal iliac artery persists, pulse pressure is reduced by 85% and the blood flow by about 48% in the distal vessel (Burchell 1968). Fertility does not seem to be impaired even when combined with ligation of infundibulopelvic vessels medial to the ovary (Likeman 1992). Bilateral internal iliac artery ligation is a safe, rapid and effective way of controlling bleeding from the uterus and the lower genital tract. Both the decision and performance of bilateral iliac artery ligation should be the responsibility of the obstetrician and should not be delegated to the vascular surgeon. The procedure should be taught to all the trainees (Maier 1993). The infundibulopelvic vessels and the uterine vessels also could be tied if necessary.

Other vascular methods which have been used are vasopressin infusion (Sacks et al 1982) or angiographic embolisation of the internal iliac arteries and its branches (Paris et al 1980; Minck et al 1984; Sproule et al 1994). In addition to achieving the hemostasis, the volume of tissue infarcted is kept to the minimum (Sproule et al 1994). Recently, super-selective catheterisation of the peripheral branches with a diameter of less than 2 mm, performed in order to occlude vessels both proximal and distal to the bleeding point has been reported to prevent the problem of continuing bleeding from the rich collaterals in the pelvis. This has been made possible with coaxial catheters through which embolic agents such as small absorbable gelatin sponges and microcoils can be injected.

The last resort in the management of PPH due to uterine causes is hysterectomy. It should be reserved for instances where all other measures have failed and should be performed only as a life saving procedure. In most instances subtotal hysterectomy which is much simpler, quicker, safer and associated with less blood loss, will be sufficient. But it may not be effective in instances where the source of bleeding is in the cervical branch of the uterine artery supplying the lower segment, as in placenta previa with accreta (Clark et al 1984) and tears in the lower segment. A statistically significant association has been seen with hysterectomy for atony and the following features: amnionitis, oxytocin augmentation of labour, caesarean section for labour arrest, preoperative $MgSO_4$ infusion and heavy fetal weight (Clark et al 1984).

Management of special circumstances

Injuries to the genital tract   The patient's condition can deteriorate rapidly if bleeding from the vaginal or cervical lacerations are not brought under control. It is important to have a good IV line, to give a rapid infusion and to get two to four units of blood cross matched. According to the condition of the patient the rate of infusion and quantum of cross matched blood will vary. Good light source, adequate exposure (may need optimal positioning, an extension of episiotomy, the use of Dewer's or special vaginal retractors), appropriate assistants and satisfactory analgesia or anesthesia are important. Whilst getting these organised, the amount of bleeding can be minimised using packs. Suturing may need long needle holders and it is essential that the uppermost point of bleeding should be arrested by suturing above the apex of the tear before gradually descending to suture the rest of the tear. The wound margins can be infiltrated with a vasopressor substance to reduce bleeding. Suturing should not be continuous as it may narrow the space available within the vagina. Individual sutures need not necessarily appose the two sides of the tear on the vaginal wall if such attempts leads to tearing of the vaginal wall. Each side of the tear can be sutured separately with individual sutures and the introital area apposed. The raw area left within the vagina re-epithelialises with no scarring.

Retained placenta　　Retained placenta is diagnosed if the placenta is not expelled within 15–30 mins of delivery of the baby. Different rates of success have been reported when 10 units of syntocinon has been milked up the umbilical vein to enhance expulsion of the placenta (Golan et al 1983). In the management of retained placenta a last attempt should be made to deliver the placenta by controlled cord traction prior to manual removal. If this fails, the placenta should be removed manually under general anesthesia. During this procedure the external hand should steady the uterus by pressing on the fundus to facilitate removal of the placenta and to reduce the risk of perforating the uterus. Once the procedure is over, it should be confirmed that the uterus is empty and the oxytocin/ergometrine infusion should be continued to enhance the uterine contractions.

Placenta accreta　　This is a condition where the placenta has penetrated up to the myometrium or the peritoneum of the uterus. A fourfold increase in the incidence of accreta has been reported with placenta previa over a previous caesarean scar (Read et al 1980). Repeated terminations of pregnancy, myomectomies and caesarean sections causing scarring have been postulated as causative factors (Weekstein et al 1986). Ultrasound has been claimed to be useful in the antenatal diagnosis of placenta increta (Pasto et al 1983).

　　Many complications including gangrene of the uterus, peritonitis, life threatening hemorrhage (Mahmood and Kok 1990) especially traumatic rupture during vigorous removal have been reported. In most instances the treatment is hysterectomy. If the bleeding is not of concern, conservation of the uterus is preferred. Provided adequate facilities for monitoring and management of the patient are available a conservative approach could be adopted. Here the placenta is left alone and no further treatment is given. Alternatively the patient could be treated with a cytotoxic agent like methotrexate. Ultrasound and serum ß-HCG levels have helped to follow up these patients (Arulkumaran et al 1986).

Acute inversion of the uterus　　About 50% of all uterine inversions are due to mismanagement of the third stage, either from excessive cord traction or fundal pressure (Watson et al 1980). They could also occur spontaneously in patients with an atonic uterus, when the abdominal pressure increases while coughing or sneezing. The shock is out of proportion to the blood loss, and the inversion is best corrected immediately.

If detected immediately, it can be corrected easily by manual replacement. If diagnosed later the patient should be resuscitated and the inversion corrected using the hydrostatic method or manually under general anesthesia with uterine relaxation. A bolus dose of terbutaline 0.25 mg in 5 ml saline has been found to relax the uterus to reduce the inversion. The relaxation effect has to be reversed by propranolol 1–2mg IV. If replacement from below is not possible due to constriction ring, laparotomy may become necessary. The inversion may be then reduced by upward traction on the fundus, but if it fails the constriction ring in the cervico-isthmic portion should be incised posteriorly and the uterus replaced (Lucas 1980).

If the placenta has not been delivered, it should be removed only after the correction of the inversion and oxytocics should be continued for some time till the uterus contracts well to prevent PPH and reinversion.

Disseminated intravascular coagulation   Disseminated intravascular coagulation (DIVC) can occur with abruption, sepsis, massive blood loss/transfusion, severe preeclampsia or amniotic fluid embolism which is rare. In cases of sepsis and abruption, emptying the uterus may prevent initiation or progression of disseminated intravascular coagulation. Better understanding of disseminated intravascular coagulation has helped the management of patients. Uncontrolled bleeding without clot formation may be due to elevated fibrinogen degradation products (FDP) which prevent clotting or the consumption of platelets, fibrinogen and clotting factors due to usage in the disseminated intravascular coagulation process or while trying to arrest bleeding before or after delivery of the placenta, thus depleting factors essential for clotting. Unless the FDP levels are extremely high the presence of minimum concentration of the factors needed for clotting should arrest bleeding. With commercially available latex, agglutination test kits using anti FDP, ranges of the FDP present can be assessed in 10 to 15 minutes. Currently components of fibrinogen, or fibrin degradation products (X, Y, D or E) can be measured. Fragment D or E can be individually measured. In disseminated intravascular coagulation there is a breakdown of both fibrin and fibrinogen. The D dimer component is specific for fibrin breakdown and is usually 200 ng/ml and reaches levels of > 2,000 mg/ml in disseminated intravascular coagulation. Table 2 shows the critical level of factors needed for clotting. Replacement of these factors by fresh blood and specific blood products can be rewarding in emergency situations. Standard blood products, their quantity and concentration in each pack is shown in Table 3. The hemotherapy profile of a patient showing the clotting factors at different times and the essential elements replaced to achieve hemostasis are discussed in the chapter on eclampsia. This illustrates judicious and rational management with required blood products instead of irrationally transfusing many units of stored blood. Careful monitoring with such a hemotherapy chart is useful in any disseminated intravascular coagulation state. Adequate blood banking facilities should be available to manage cases of PPH with coagulation problems, but a limited amount of blood or blood products can be utilised if facilities are available to measure fibrinogen and platelets. In the absence of such facilities the administration of fresh frozen plasma or two or three units of fresh blood units will save the trouble of transfusing large amounts of stored blood despite which the patient may continue to bleed.

Table 2: Critical level of clotting factors and FDP in DIVC

* Fibrinogen	< 0.8 g/L — critical
	> 1.0 g/L — safe

With < 0.6 g/L of fibrinogen, the thrombin time gets prolonged

* Platelets < 40,000 in addition to the clinical picture
* Fibrinogen/fibrin degradation products that may prevent clotting—100 mg/L

< 10 mg/L	—	normal
10–40 mg/L	—	post surgery or deep vein thrombosis
40–80 mg/L	—	on the way to DIVC
> 80 mg/L	—	situation of DIVC
Mode of action	—	1. interferes with polymerisation of fibrin
		2. antiplatelet function

* D-dimer > 200ug/L — presence of DIVC

Table 3: Blood products used in situations of clotting deficiency

*1 Pack cryoprecipitate	— from 1 donor and is approximately 200 ml in volume
	— Platelets nil
for useful therapy use 10–15 packs	— Fibrinogen approximately 0.2 g/pack
	— Factor VIII — average 80 units/pack
*1 Pack fresh frozen plasma	— from 1 donor and is approximately 200 ml in volume
	— Platelets nil
for useful therapy use 4–5 packs	— Fibrinogen approximately 0.4 g/pack
	— Factors — all (V, VIII etc)
Platelet concentrate	1. Each pack of 50–60 ml is from a single unit of whole blood and has a minimum of $5.5 \times 10^{10}/1$. For useful therapy use 6 packs or
	2. From platelet phoresis — pack of 200 ml containing at least $4 \times 10^{11}/1$.

The management of PPH starts prior to and during pregnancy and consists of the detection of anemia and correction. Healthy nutrition, and iron and folic acid supplements are essential. A woman who is not anemic will withstand a certain degree of hemorrhage. The next step would be to identify the high risk category: those with a previous history of PPH; a large uterus due to multiple pregnancy, polyhydramnios or a large baby; patients with a history of any APH. Prolonged labour and operative delivery fall into the high risk category. Prophylaxis by oxytocics in the third stage of labour is essential. Steps should be taken to provide this simple and cheap treatment to every labouring woman. In the event of PPH, quick remedial action should be taken; if one treatment strategy fails, the next step should be taken within minutes. The use of parenteral prostaglandin has reduced the number of cases that might have needed surgical intervention like hysterectomy. Every general practitioner should be armed with oxytocics which is a cheap but valuable life-saving drug. There is evidence that despite these drugs being stored at higher temperatures of 37° and 42°C they retain at least half their potency at the end of a year (Chua et al 1993). There is now new evidence that breastfeeding can promote more uterine contractions and may contribute to reduced blood loss (Chua et al 1994). A Sengstaken-Blakemore tube is easily stored in a general practice clinic and it provides a balloon tamponade to control massive PPH (Katesmark et al 1994). Colloid solutions like gelofusion or hemocel should be stored by family practitioners as they can be stored at room temperature and can be used as plasma expanders. When a rapid infusion of crystalloids does not raise the blood pressure or when the blood pressure is very low, colloids should be used after taking blood for group and crossmatch as the use of colloids may interfere with cross matching. In the absence of investigatory facilities for clotting profile and unavailability of specific blood products if DIVC is suspected, fresh blood should be transfused after emergency cross matching. Calling additional doctors and nurses before the patient is too ill and prompt action in a stepwise manner as described is essential in order to reduce this life threatening situation.

References

Ahlfield and Aschoff 1904. cited In: Helman LM, Pitcharrd JA, eds. 1971. Williams' Textbook of Obstetrics, 14th ed. New York: Appleton Century Croft, p 957.

Anderson KE, Ingemarsson I, Persson GGA 1974. Effects of terbutaline on human uterine motility at term. *Acta Obstet Gynecol Scand* 53 (S-1):1-8.

Anjaneyulu R, (Late) Devi PK, Jain S, Kanthamani CR, Vijaya R, Raghavan KS 1988. Prophylactic use of 15 (S) 15 methyl PGF$_{2\alpha}$ by intramuscular route. A controlled clinical trial. *Acta Obstet Gynecol Scand Suppl* 145: 9-11.

Arulkumaran S, Ng CSA, Ingemarsson I, Ratnam SS 1986. Medical treatment of placenta accreta with methotrexate. *Acta Obstet Gynecol Scand* 65: 285-286.

Beard R 1993. Management of the third stage of labour in women at low risk of postpartum hemorrhage. *Eur J Obstet Gynecol Reprod Biol* 48: 19-22.

Brant HA 1967. Precise estimation of postpartum hemorrhage: difficulties and importance. *Br Med J* i: 398-400.

Brinsden PRS and Clark AD 1978. Postpartum hemorrhage after induced and spontaneous labour. *Br Med J* 855-856.

Bullough CHW, Msukee RS, Karoade L 1989. Early suckling and postpartum hemorrhage: controlled trial in deliveries by traditional birth attendants. *Lancet* Sept 2: 522-525.

Burchell RC 1968. Physiology of internal iliac artery ligation. *J Obstet Gynecol Br Cwlth* 75: 642-51.

Chamberlain GVP 1985. Discussion. In: Chamberlain GVP, Or CJB, Sharp F, eds. Litigation and Obstetrics and Gynecology. London: RCOG, p 272.

Chua S, Arulkumaran S, Adaikan G and Ratnam SS 1993. The effect of oxytocins stored at high temperature on postpartum uterine activity. *Br J Obstet Gynecol* 100: 813-814.

Chua S, Arulkumaran S, Lim I and Ratnam SS 1994. Influence of breastfeeding and nipple stimulation on postpartum uterine activity. *Br J Obstet Gynecol* 101:804-5.

Clark SL, Yeh SY, Phelan J, Samuel B, Paul RH 1984. Emergency hysterectomy for obstetric hemorrhage. *Obstet Gynecol* 64: 3; 376-380.

Coon LC, Vant JR, Cantor MM 1941. A critical analysis of blood loss in 2,000 obstetric cases. *Am J Obstet Gynecol* 42: 768-85.

Department of Health and Social Security 1982. Report on confidential enquiries into maternal deaths 1976-1978, London: Her Majesty's Stationery Office.

Department of Health and Social Security, Welsh Office, Office of Population Censuses and Surveys 1989. Maternal Hospital. In patient enquiry, maternity tables 1977-1981, England and Wales, London: HMSO.

Department of Health and Social Security 1986. Report on confidential enquiries into maternal deaths 1979-1981. London: Her Majesty's Stationery Office.

DHSS 1989. Report on confidential enquiries into maternal deaths 1982-1984. London: Her Majesty's Stationary Office.

Druzin ML 1989. Packing of lower uterine segment for control of post-caesarean bleeding in instances of placenta previa. *Surg Gynecol Obstet* 169:543-5.

Dunn P M 1985. Management of childbirth in normal women: the third stage and fetal adaptation. In: Perinatal medicine; Report of the IX European Congress Perinatal Medicine, Dublin. Lancaster: MTP Press.

Embrey MP, Barber DTC, Scudmore JN 1963. Use of syntometrine in the prevention of postpartum hemorrhage. *Br Med J* i:1387-1388.

Gilbert L, Porter W, Brown VA 1987. Postpartum Hemorrhage - A continuing problem. *Br J Obstet Gynecol* 94: 67-71.

Gilliant WI 1949. Transactions of the 12th Congress of Obstetrics and Gynecology, Canada, p 271.

Golan A, Lider AB, David MP 1983. A new method for the management of the retained placenta. *Am J Obstet Gynecol* 46: 708-709.

Greenhill JP 1951. Year Book of Obstetrics and Gynecology. Chicago: Year Book Publishers, p 230.

Hall MH, Halliwell R, Carr-Hill R 1985. Concomitant and repeated happenings of complications of the third stage of labour. *Br J Obstet Gynecol* 92: 732-738.

Hayashi RH 1982. Heading off disaster in postpartum hemorrhage. *Contemp Obstet Gynecol* 20: 91-96.

Hayashi RH 1990. The role of prostaglandin in the treatment of postpartum hemorrhage. *J Obstet Gynecol* 10 (Suppl:2) 521-524.

Hertz RH, Sokal R, Dieker LJ 1980. Treatment of postpartum uterine atony with prostaglandin E$_2$ vaginal pessaries. *Obstet Gynecol* 56: 120-130.

Hesler JD 1975. Postpartum hemorrhage and devaluation of uterine bleeding. *Obstet Gynecol* 45: 501.

Ilancheran A, Ratnam SS 1990. Effect of oxytocics on prostaglandin levels in the third stage of labour. *Gynecol Obstet Invest* 29: 177-180.

Jacobs MM, Arizas F 1979. Intramyometrial prostaglandin F$_{2\alpha}$ in the treatment of severe postpartum hemorrhage. *Obstet Gynecol* 55: 665-666.

Katesmark M, Brown R, Raju KS 1994. Successful use of a Sengstaken - Blakemore tube to control massive postpartum hemorrhage. *Br J Obstet Gynecol* 101: 259-260.

Kwast BE, Rochat RW, Kidane-Mariano W 1986. Maternal Mortality in Addis Ababa, Ethiopia. *Stud Fam Plann* 17:288-30.

Kwast B 1991. Postpartum hemorrhage, its contribution to maternal mortality. *Midwifery* 7:64-7.

Leader 1974. A time to be born. *Lancet* 2: 1183-1184

Lester WM, Bartholomew RA, Colvin ED, Grimes WH, Fish JS, Galloway WH 1965. Reconsideration of the uterine pack in postpartum hemorrhage. *Am J Obstet Gynecol* 93: 321-6.

Likeman RK 1992 The boldest possible for checking the bleeding - A new look at an old operation, and a series of 13 cases from an Australian hospital. *Aust NZ J Obstet Gynecol* 32; 3: 256-261.

Lourdes St George, Alex J Grandon 1990. *Aust NZ J Obstet Gynecol* 30: 52-56.

Lucas William E 1980. Postpartum hemorrhage. *Clin Obstet Gynecol* 23: 2, 637-46.

Mackenzie IZ 1979. Induction of labour and postpartum hemorrhage, *Br Med J* 1:750.

Mahmood TA, Kok KP 1990. A review of placenta accreta at Aberdeen Maternity Hospital, Scotland. *Aust NZ J Obstet Gynecol* 30: 108-10.

Maier RC 1993. Control of postpartum hemorrhage with uterine packing. *Am J Obstet Gynecol* 169: 317-23.

McDonald S, Prendiviller J, Blair E 1993. Randomised controlled trial of oxytocin alone versus oxytocin and ergometrine in active management of third stage of labour. *Br Med J* 307: 1167-1171.

McNeilly AS, Robinson I CAF, Houston MJ, Howie PW 1983. Release of oxytocin and prolactin in response to suckling. *Br Med J* 286: 257-59.

Milton PJD 1985. Natural childbirth and home deliveries - Clinical aspects. In: Chamberlain GVP, ed. Litigation and Obstetrics and Gynecology. London: Royal College of Obstetricians and Gynecologists, pp 279-299.

Minck RN, Palestrant A, Cherny WB 1984. Successful management of postpartum vaginal hemorrhage by angiographic embolization. *Ariz Med* 41: 537-8.

Moir JC 1955. The history of present day use of ergot. *Can Med Assoc J* 72: 727-34.

Newton M, Mosey LM, Egli GE, Gifford WB and Hulls CT 1961. Blood loss during and immediately after delivery. *Obstet Gynecol* 17: 9-18.

Paris SO, Glickman M, Schwartz P, Pingoud E, Berkowitz R 1980. Embolization of pelvic arteries for control of postpartum hemorrhage. *Obstet Gynecol* 55: 754-58.

Pasto ME, Kurtz AB, Rifkin MD, Cole-Beuqlete, Wagner RJ, Goldberg BB 1983. Ultrasonographic findings in placenta increta. *J Ultrasound Med* 2: 155-159.

Pearse CS, Magrina JF, Finley BE 1984. Use of MAST suit in obstetrics and gynecology. *Obstet Gynecol* 39:416-22.

Peyser M, Reuben, Kupferomine MJ 1990. Management of severe postpartum hemorrhage by intrauterine irrigation with prostaglandin E_2. *Am J Obstet Gynecol* 162: 694-696.

Prendiville W, Elbarne D, Chalmers I 1988. The effects of routine oxytocic administration in the management of the third stage of labour; an overview of the evidence from controlled trials. *Br J Obstet Gynecol* 95: 3-16.

Prendiville W and Elbourne D 1990. Care during the third stage of labour in effective care. In: I Chalmers, M Enkin, MJNC Keirse, eds. Pregnancy and Childbirth Vol 2. Oxford: Oxford University Press, pp 1145-1169.

Ratnam SS, Rauff M 1989. In: Sir Alec Turnbull, Chamberlain G eds. Postpartum hemorrhage and abnormalities of the third stage of labour. London: Churchill Livingstone, pp 867-875.

Read J, Cotton D, Millar F 1980. Placenta Accreta: Changing clinical aspect and outcome. *Obstet Gynecol* 56: 31-34.

Royston E, Armstrong S 1989. Preventing maternal deaths. Geneva: World Health Organization, pp 30-42.

Sacks B, Palestrant AM, Cohen W 1982. Internal iliac artery vasopressin infusion for postpartum hemorrhage. *Am J Obstet Gynecol* 143: 601-3.

Sproule MW, Bendomir AM, Grant KA, Reid AW 1994. Embolization of massive bleeding following hysterectomy, despite internal iliac artery ligation. *Br J Obstet Gynecol* 101:908-909.

Stander HJ 1945. ed. Textbook of Obstetrics. 3rd edn, New York: Appleton-Century-Crofts, pp 1125-27.

Stewart P, Hillan E, Calder A 1983. A randomized trial to evaluate the use of a birth chair for delivery *Lancet* i, 1296-1298.

Stones WR, Catherine M, Paterson and Nigel J St, Saunders G 1993. Risk factors for major obstetric hemorrhage. *Eur J Obstet Gynecol Reprod Biol* 48: 15-18.

Studd J, Crawford J, Duignan N, Rowbotham CJP and Huges AO 1980. The effect of lumbar epidural analgesia on the rate of cervical dilatation and the outcome of labour of spontaneous onset. *Br J Obstet Gynecol* 87: 1015-1021.

Samil Suprapti R 1992. Postpartum Hemorrhage In: Ratnam SS, Bhasker Rao K, Arulkumaran S, eds. Obstetrics and Gynecology for Postgraduates, Vol 1. Madras (India): Orient Longman Ltd, pp 143-150.

Thilaganathan B, Canter A, Latimer J and Beard R 1993. Management of the third stage of labour in women at low risk of postpartum hemorrhage. *Eur J Obstet Gynecol Reprod Biol.* 48: 19-22.

Thomas IL, Jefferes TM, Brazler JM, Burst CL and Barr KE 1990. Does cord drainage of placental blood facilitate delivery of the placenta? *Aust NZ J Obstet Gynecol* 30; 4: 314-318.

Toppozada MK. 1986. Postpartum hemorrhage, In: M Bygdeman, Berger GS, Keith LG, eds. Prostaglandins and Their Inhibitors in Clinical Obstetrics and Gynecology. Lancaster: MTP Press, pp 233-251.

Walker GJA, Hogerzeil HV, Hillgren U 1988. Potency of ergometrine in tropical countries. *Lancet.* i: 3-16.

Watson P, Besch N, Bowes WA 1980. Management of acute and subacute puerperal inversion of the uterus. *Obstet Gynecol* 55: 12-16.

Weeks LR, O'Toole DM 1956. Postpartum hemorrhage. A five year study of Queen of Angels Hospital. *Am J Obstet Gynecol* 71: 45.

Weekstein LN, Masserman JSH, Garitie TS 1986. Placenta accreta: A problem of increasing clinical significance. *Obstet Gynecol* 69: 480-482.

Weitzman RE, Leake RD, Rubin RT, Fisher DA 1980. The effect of nursing on neurohypophyseal hormones and prolactin in human subjects. *J Clin Endocrinol Metab* 51: 836-39.

WHO Report of Technical Working Group 1990. The prevention management of postpartum hemorrhage. Geneva: World Health Organization (WHO/MCH/90.7).

13

Prostaglandins in Labour

K S Raghavan

Prostaglandins, first described and named by von Euler (1935), remained dormant for more than 20 years before being taken up for investigation. With the elucidation of the structure of primary prostaglandins, PGE_2 and $PGF_{2\alpha}$ by Bergstrom and his team (Bergstrom et al 1962) the subsequent total synthesis by E.J. Corey at Harvard (Corey et al 1969) and at the Upjohn Company, the interest in this group of compounds became universal.

Chemistry

Prostaglandins are 20 carbon atom fatty acids with a 5-membered (cyclopentane) ring and two side chains (Fig 13.1).

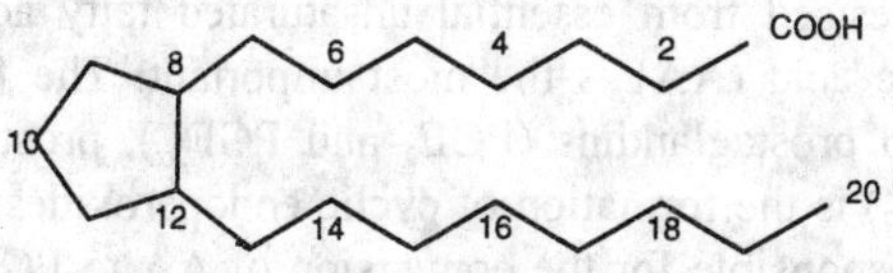

Fig 13.1 Structure of prostanoic acid

Prostaglandins are named A to I depending upon the structure of the carbon ring (Fig. 13.2).

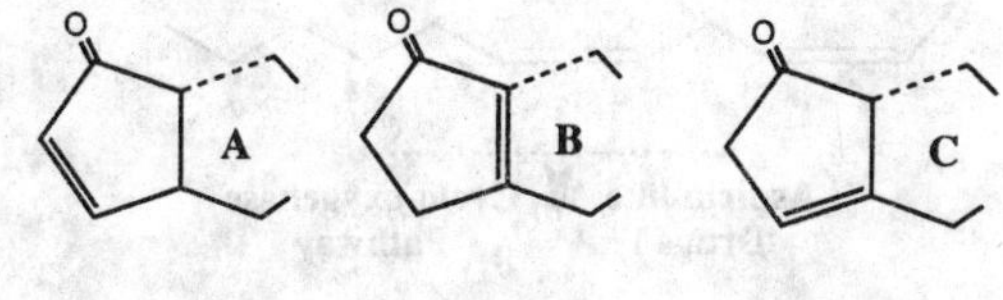

Fig 13.2 Prostaglandins A to I

The side chains of prostaglandins have one or more double bonds. The number of double bonds are indicated by the numerical subscript, e.g. PGE_1, PGE_2, and PGE_3 (Fig. 13.3).

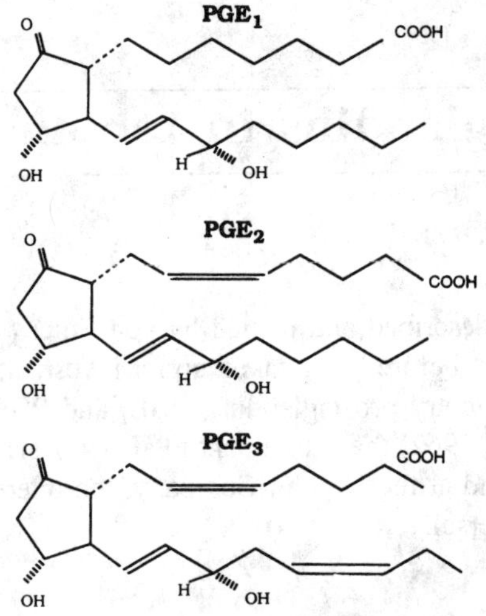

Fig 13.3   The structure of prostaglandins E_1, E_2 and E_3

Biosynthesis

Prostaglandins are synthesised from essential unsaturated fatty acids (Fig 13.4). Among them arachidonic acid (AA) is the most important. The first step in the bio-conversion of AA to prostaglandins (PGE_2 and $PGF_{2\alpha}$), prostacyclins (PGI_2) and thromboxanes (TXA_2) is the formation of cyclic endoperoxides: prostaglandins G and H. The enzyme responsible for the conversion of AA to PGH_2 is known as

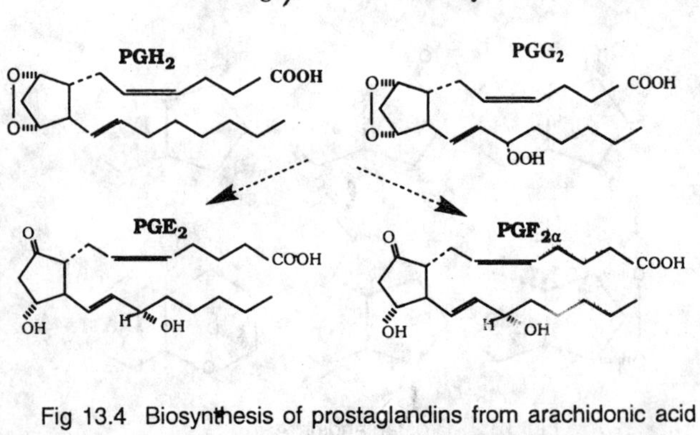

Fig 13.4   Biosynthesis of prostaglandins from arachidonic acid

'fatty acid cyclo-oxygenase' or 'prostaglandin endoperoxide synthetase' or 'PGH synthase'.

Non-steroidal anti-inflammatory drugs (NSAIDs) like aspirin and indomethacin can inhibit the action of cyclo-oxygenase and thereby the formation of prostaglandins (Fig 13.4). Depending on the tissue, the endoperoxides (PGG_2 and PGH_2) are further converted non-enzymatically into PGE_2, $PGF_{2\alpha}$, PGI_2 and TXA_2 (Samuelsson et al 1975; Samuelsson et al 1978). These conversions are extremely rapid and occur in all mammalian tissues. Once the biosynthesis is initiated, it is completed within a few minutes in the in vitro systems (Hamberg, Svensson and Samuelsson 1975; Christensen and Green 1983).

Metabolism

Natural prostaglandins are metabolised rapidly. The main route of metabolic degradation is by oxidation at the site of carbon 15 that gives rise to 15 keto prostaglandins, which are biologically inactive. A further reduction of the double bond at carbon 13 leads to the formation of 15 keto 13,14 dihydroprostaglandins (Fig 13.5). The enzymes involved in the initial conversion are found in the lungs, liver and kidney (Anggard, Larsson and Samuelsson 1971). 15 keto 13,14 dihydro prostaglandins are formed rapidly following the intravenous injection of primary prostaglandins in humans (Samuelsson et al 1975). Within 90 seconds of an intravenous injection of tritium labelled PGE_2, less than 5% remains as PGE_2 and 50%

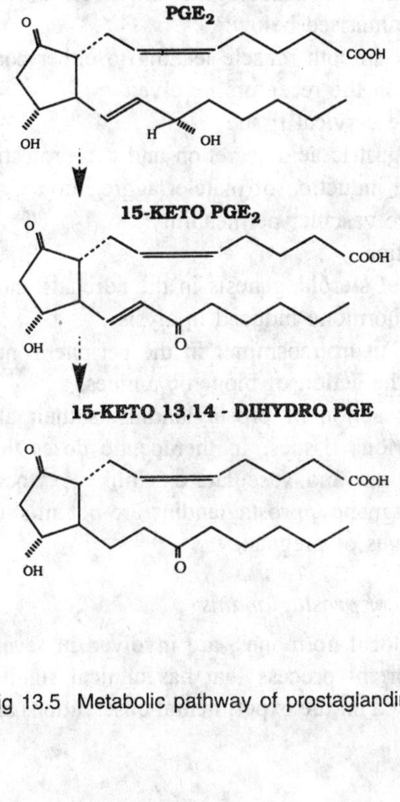

Fig 13.5 Metabolic pathway of prostaglandins

as 15 keto 13,14 dihydro prostaglandin in the peripheral circulation (Hamberg and Samuelsson 1971). The estimated half life of PGE_2 is about 15 seconds and that of the metabolite eight minutes.

Prostaglandin analogues

The rapid inactivation of natural prostaglandins necessitates continuous administration of the drug to obtain the desired pharmacological actions. The understanding of the metabolism has lead to the development of analogues that are resistant to inactivation, while retaining their biological activity. 15 methyl $PGF_{2\alpha}$ (Carboprost) was one of the first analogues to be developed for human use. It has a half life of 8 minutes, about 10 times more potent than $PGF_{2\alpha}$ (Green, Christensen and Bygdeman 1981) and suitable for other routes of administration. The following analogues were produced and tested in humans for their action on the uterus.

    1. 15(S)-15-methyl-$PGF_{2\alpha}$ (Carboprost)
    2. 16-phenoxy-ω-tetranor-PGE_2 sulfonylamide (Sulprostone)
    3. 16,16-dimethyl-trans-Δ^2-PGE_1 (Gemeprost)
    4. 9-deoxo-16,16-dimethyl-9 methylene-PGE_2 (Meteneprost)

Prostaglandin analogues provide an opportunity to formulate vehicles for different routes of administration. Thus they can be administered by both intramuscular and vaginal routes compared to primary prostaglandins, which have to be administered by the intravenous route.

Pharmacological actions

Prostaglandins exert their pharmacological action on almost all tissues. The best known actions are summarised below:

    1. stimulation of smooth muscle leading to either contraction or relaxation, depending upon the receptors involved
    2. changes in the cervical tissue
    3. inhibition of gastric acid secretion and cytoprotection
    4. inhibition and induction of platelet aggregation
    5. increase in the vascular permeability
    6. thermoregulation
    7. modification of steroidogenesis in the adrenals and gonads
    8. inhibition of hormone induced lipolysis
    9. the release of neurotransmitter in the peripheral nervous system and potentiation of the action of biogenic amines.

The most potent action of prostaglandins is their ability to stimulate the smooth muscle of various tissues. In therapeutic doses they act on the smooth muscle of the uterus, gut and vasculature. Unlike oxytocin, which is relatively ineffective in early pregnancy, prostaglandins are potent stimulators of the uterine myometrium at all stages of pregnancy.

The physiological role of prostaglandins

Prostaglandins, being local hormones, are involved in several physiological processes. The most important process that has clinical significance is their role in human parturition. Based on the experimental observations and clinical effects, they are now established firmly in obstetric practice. Prostaglandins are implicated in (a) the initiation of labour, (b) cervical ripening and (c) postpartum hemostasis.

1. *Initiation of labour*   In humans prostaglandins can induce uterine contractions at any time of gestation. Prostaglandin synthesis inhibitors are known to inhibit uterine contractions; thus prostaglandins may have a key role in the initiation of labour (Lewis and Schulman 1973; Thiery and Amy 1975; Collins and Turner 1975; Wiqvist 1979). The control of the biosynthesis of uterine prostaglandins and therefore labour seems to be under the influence of hormones. Steroid hormones were reported to modulate the prostaglandin production. Progesterone inhibits the prostaglandin synthesis in vivo and phospholipase A_2 activity in vitro (Wilson et al 1986), whereas oestrogen has the opposite effect (Skinner et al 1984). No changes in the concentration of progesterone and oestrogen were detected in humans at term either in the plasma or the myometrial nuclear receptor occupancy. Moreover, antiprogestational compounds like RU 486 (Mifepristone) when administered at term did not always result in labour. Only a third of the treated women went into labour within four days and there was no marked response in the cervix of women who failed to respond (Frydman et al 1992). Further Bokstrom, Norstrom and Wiqvist (1995) have shown that the administration of Mifepristone did not increase the cervical PGE_2 and $PGF_{2\alpha}$ and concluded that Mifepristone induced cervical changes are not mediated through alteration in the prostaglandin synthesis.

Prostaglandins probably represent the final link between the endocrine control and translation of these messages into the process of labour. The evidence in favour of the participation of prostaglandins in human labour comes from the measurement of prostaglandins and their metabolites in maternal and fetal circulation, the amniotic fluid and the fetal membranes. The presence of PGE_2 and $PGF_{2\alpha}$ in the amniotic fluid and their increase in women in labour was first reported by Karim and Devlin (1967). They reported that the amniotic fluid PGE concentration increases during late pregnancy and labour, while $PGF_{2\alpha}$ levels rose only during labour. Nieder and Augstin (1983) showed that the amniotic fluid PGE and F remain unchanged till about 34 weeks of gestation and then increase exponentially. They also noted that in the last 6 weeks of pregnancy, the PGF levels increase thirteen-fold following cervical dilation while the PGE equivalent remains static. Recently Romero et al (1994) estimated PGE_2, $PGF_{2\alpha}$, PGFM ($PGF_{2\alpha}$ metabolite), TXB_2 and 6 keto $PGF_{1\alpha}$ (PGI_2 metabolite) in the upper amniotic fluid compartment of women during the course of spontaneous labour. They found that the amniotic fluid prostanoid concentration in women in early labour (cervical dilatation of ≤ 3 cm) was significantly higher than those who were not in labour. Women with a cervical dilatation of 4 to 7 cm did not have higher amniotic fluid prostanoids than those in early labour. However, the amniotic fluid concentration of PGE_2, $PGF_{2\alpha}$ and PGFM were higher in women with a cervical dilatation of 8 to 10 cm as compared to early labour. MacDonald and Casey (1993) argue that the accumulation of prostaglandins in the amniotic fluid is an after effect of labour and not indicative of their role in human parturition. They estimated the PGE_2, $PGF_{2\alpha}$, PGFM concentrations in the forebag and the upper compartment of the amniotic sac during labour. They found a marked increase only in the forebag, which they attributed to the production and entry of prostaglandins into the amniotic fluid during and not before the onset of labour, from the lining of the forebag (decidua parietalis, the principle site of formation of prostaglandins). Sahmay et al (1988) suggest that though there is an increase in the prostaglandin level in maternal and fetal plasma and amniotic fluid, the ratio of $PGE_2/PGF_{2\alpha}$ is an important factor for the initiation of labour. A decrease in the ratio from 1.5 at the third trimester to 0.88 during labour was reported by Sharma et al (1982).

Norman and Reddi (1990) reported that in women with dysfunctional labour there is a decrease in amniotic fluid $PGF_{2\alpha}$ levels compared to women in labour or prelabour. They propose that PGE_2 is the dominant prostaglandin for the onset of labour while the progress of labour requires an adequate concentration of $PGF_{2\alpha}$. The increase in the $PGF_{2\alpha}$ seems to dominate during the progress of labour, while the increase in PGE_2 levels precedes labour. There appear to be two different switches for the control of synthesis and release of PGE_2 and $PGF_{2\alpha}$. If dysfunctional labour is due to the inhibition of prostaglandin production, this may be at the level of prostaglandin synthetase or further down the pathway.

The evidence for the participation of prostaglandins in the initiation of labour is shown at the molecular level by Bennett et al (1992). They have studied the expression of gene coding for cyclo-oxygenase, and the central enzyme in prostaglandin synthesis during pregnancy, before and after the onset of labour in the human placenta and fetal membranes. They found that after spontaneous onset of labour, there was a significant 2.5 and 3.5-fold increase in the gene expression in the trophoblast and amnion respectively. They concluded that the increase of prostaglandin synthesis is a result of both increase in the substrate (namely, arachidonic acid) and the gene expression.

There are still gaps in the knowledge of the events that lead to the initiation of labour and the influence of prostaglandins on these events. Though the signals initiating parturition are obscure, they may depend upon the mature fetus.

2. *Cervical ripening*   The human cervix is an organ of diverse properties. During pregnancy it is rigid and preserves the growing fetus in the uterus. At term it gradually becomes soft, effaced and dilated. The main body of the cervix consists of stroma made primarily of connective tissue containing bundles of collagen embedded in ground substance made of large proteoglycan molecules that incorporate a number of glycosaminoglycans. In addition, elastin is also found in human cervical connective tissue along with collagen and proteoglycans. It has characteristic elastic fibres that can be stretched to several times their length and that rapidly return to their original shape and size. Danforth et al (1960), using microscopy, reported that prior to labour, the collagen fibres appear to be swollen and enlarged. Several studies have shown that the hydroxyproline (a measure of collagen content) is significantly less in the cervix during labour and immediately after delivery compared to the cervix of nonpregnant women (Uldbjerg et al 1983; Kleissl et al 1978; Yamamoto et al 1981 and Yoshida et al 1993).

Ripening of the cervix takes place during the prelabour phase resulting in increased softening, effacement, distensibility and early dilatation. Two important components constitute this change: (1) softening and increased compliance (2) a change in the shape of the cervix as a whole (Calder 1994). These changes are achieved through a series of alterations in the bio-mechanical properties of the cervical tissue. These are (a) reduction in collagen concentration, (b) increase in water content and (c) change in glycosaminoglycans.

Prostaglandins, particularly PGE_2, have a role in the physiological process of cervical ripening. This is substantiated by the clinical efficacy of PGE_2 for this purpose. Though it is not clear whether the PGE_2 induced reduction in the collagen content of the cervix is the direct result of collagen breakdown, increased collagenase activity following PGE_2 was reported by Szalay et al (1989). Rath et al (1987) found no such changes in women treated with sulprostone, and their findings were supported by the absence of collagen degradation products in the cervical tissue electrophoresis. The other possible mechanism is that PGE_2 brings about the changes through the alteration of the composition of proteoglycan complexes that would modify the tissue hydration and collagen binding. Johnston et al (1993) have shown that the administration of PGE_2 in late pregnancy provokes a rise in circulating levels of chondroitin similar to those observed in spontaneous labour, thereby supporting the concept that PGE_2 may induce a breakdown of the proteoglycans complex.

Whichever physiological mechanism operates the process of cervical ripening, clinically it is proved beyond any doubt that local administration of PGE_2 results in the ripening of the cervix similar to spontaneous labour.

3. *Postpartum hemostasis*   In the third stage of labour, the uterus continues to contract and retract rhythmically. The measurement of oxytocin levels in maternal circulation show that they reach the peak during the second stage and subsequently fall to below the first stage levels during the third stage of labour (Dawood et al 1978; Mapa 1981), thereby suggesting that the uterine activity during the third stage is maintained by substances other than oxytocin.

Postpartum hemostasis is probably achieved by a combination of myometrial contraction and retraction, vasoconstriction and thrombosis. The postpartum uterus continues to contract, though at reduced frequency. At the same time there is an increase in the intensity of contractions which exceeds the intensity of the first stage of labour and is almost always associated with an elevation of basal tone. This pressure is adequate to stop the myometrial blood flow by mechanical compression of the vessels.

During the periods of myometrial relaxation between the contractions, mechanisms other than compression must play a part in hemostasis. The short phase of high amplitude contractions in the postpartum period may be sufficient to maintain a decreased uterine size and assist in achieving clinical hemostasis. Infusion of $PGF_{2\alpha}$ during the postpartum period produces hypertonus with superimposed irregular contractions with gradually increasing amplitude. This was different from those observed with oxytocin infusion, suggesting a different mechanism of action (Forman et al 1983).

Among the prostaglandins that are synthesised by the pregnant uterus, PGI_2, PGD_2 and to a lesser extent PGE_2 are vasodilators and potent inhibitors of platelet aggregation, while TXA_2 is a powerful vasoconstrictor and promotes platelet aggregation. It induces rapid and irreversible platelet aggregation in humans. On the other hand $PGF_{2\alpha}$ has little or no effect on platelet aggregation (Toppozada 1979).

Concentration of PGI_2 and its metabolite in the plasma of pregnant women increases towards term, rises significantly during labour and reaches below prelabour levels within two hours after delivery (Ylikorkala et al 1981; Kimball 1983; Seed et al 1983). The significance of this finding could be related to the properties of PGI_2. It is a potent inhibitor of platelet aggregation and a vasodilator. During labour, it is produced in the uterus to ensure adequate blood supply to the placenta and the fetus during uterine contractions by keeping the blood vessels dilated to maintain the blood flow. Once the fetus is delivered it has no further role to play and therefore its production is 'switched off', which is reflected in the decreased blood levels during the third stage of labour. The two prostaglandins that may be participating in the postpartum hemostasis are $PGF_{2\alpha}$ and TXA_2. $PGF_{2\alpha}$ acts through its ablity to produce uterine contraction thereby squeezing the vasculature, while TXA_2 facilitates the platelet adhesion, promotes clotting and eventually plugs the open sinuses following placental separation. The release of prostaglandins during the third stage of labour could be due to increased uterine contractions produced by circulating oxytocin, whose levels reach a peak during the second stage of labour. Increased levels of prostaglandins during the third stage of labour were reported by Zuckerman et al (1978), Sellers et al (1982), and Ilancheran and Ratnam (1990).

A sensitive system probably controls the hemostatic balance through an interaction between platelets and the vascular endothelium mediated through PGE_2, $PGF_{2\alpha}$ and TXA_2. Local release of prostaglandins after delivery are therefore important for hemostasis. It is possible that during the third stage of labour, prostaglandins and not oxytocin have a major role in hemostasis. Any disruption in such a mechanism can lead to atony and postpartum hemorrhage.

The clinical uses of prostaglandins

The ability of prostaglandins to produce uterine contraction at any stage of pregnancy was fully exploited for use in obstetric practice. One of the earliest clinical uses of prostaglandins was for induction of labour. In Sweden, Bygdeman et al (1968) used PGE_2 infusion in escalated doses in seven women, while in Uganda Karim and his colleagues (Karim et al 1969) used intravenous $PGF_{2\alpha}$ at the rate of 3 µg/min to induce labour in 35 women.

The three main areas in which prostaglandins find use during labour are cervical ripening, labour induction and the third stage and its complications.

1. *Cervical ripening*   Prostaglandins, particularly PGE_2 is found to be effective to ripen the cervix and is used extensively for this indication. In patients in whom labour is indicated either for maternal (PIH, diabetes, PROM etc) or fetal reasons (Rh-isoimmunisation, IUGR, post date etc) PGE_2 is effective in ripening the cervix. It is effective by different routes of administration like extra-amniotic, vaginal and intracervical. Though extra-amniotic route requires smaller dose, it was soon given up for less invasive procedures like vaginal or intra cervical routes.

Several studies were published on the use of PGE_2 using different dosage forms and schedules (2–5 mg pessaries: Varma and Norman 1984; 1–3 mg gel: Graves et al 1985; 3 mg suppository: Gransrom et al 1987, and repeated 3 mg pessaries: El-Leil et al 1993).The pessary or gel is placed in the posterior fornix and the patient is advised to remain in the supine position for at least 30 minutes after placing the drug. Intracervical route requires a single application of 0.5 mg PGE_2 (Ulmsten et al 1982; Floberg et al 1983; Bernstein et al 1987 and Trofatter 1993) The drug is commercially supplied in ready to use sterile syringe with a catheter (3 g of gel containing 0.5 mg of PGE_2 is the usual preparation). The gel is placed in the cervical canal after centralising it with the help of two specula and visualising the external os. The catheter is inserted till it reaches the internal os and then slowly withdrawn while pushing the plunger to expel the gel into the cervical canal. The procedure is repeated till all the gel in the syringe is expelled. Part of the gel may leak into the vagina, which is of no consequence. However entry of the gel into the extra-amniotic space may result in stimulation of uterine contractions or hypertonus. Care should be taken to avoid extra-amniotic spillage of the drug.

Some of the studies compared prostaglandins with placebo or no treatment. Several studies were published from India in the last few years comparing 0.5 mg intracervical PGE_2 with placebo or oxytocin or 'no treatment' (Baveja et al 1988; Bhide and Daftary 1993; Patki et al 1993).

Prostaglandin E_2 gel is also used for cervical ripening in patients with premature rupture of the membranes (Gonen et al 1994), previous caesarean section (Stone et al 1994) and breeech presentation (O'Herlihy 1981), though these were considered as contraindications.

Though analogues of prostaglandin E (for example, sulprostone, gemeprost, meteneprost) are available for clinical use, none of them have been used at term. These are used either for first or second trimester termination. Prostaglandin E_2, when used for cervical ripening, does not act exclusively on the cervix. It tends to increase the myometrial activity. Cervical ripening is the first step for labour induction and therefore should not be used unless there is a valid reason for inducing labour. In such patients prostaglandins can be beneficial for ripening the cervix.

2. *Labour induction*   Labour Induction was one of the first indications for the use of prostaglandins in obstetrics. Initially PGE_2 and $PGF_{2\alpha}$ were used by the intravenous route for inductions. Subsequently other formulations were available for the induction of labour. Two routes are in vogue to administer PGE_2 for the induction of labour, oral and vaginal.

(a) Oral PGE_2   Prostaglandin E_2 tablets are available in a strength of 0.5 mg. The usual dose is one tablet hourly which can be escalated in case of inadequate uterine contractions to three tablets. The lowest possible dose that produces adequate uterine activity is maintained till delivery. The side effects include GI effects like nausea, vomiting, diarrhoea and fever. These side effects are transient and self limiting. The Table 1 summarises the published data.

Oral PGE_2 can also be used for the augmentation of labour in the absence of inadequate uterine activity. High success rates (100% in multipara and 50% in primipara) were reported with oral PGE_2 for the augmentation of labour (Gordon-Wright, Dutt and Elder 1979).

Table 1: The effectiveness and side effects of oral PGE$_2$ in
induction of labour according to various workers

Authors	No of Cases	Dosage Regimen	Success Rate (%)	Uterine Hyper-tonus	Vomiting	Diarrhoea
Freidman and Sachtleben 1974	45	0.5–1.5 mg/hr	86.7	3	12	7
Elder and Stone 1974	70	0.5 mg/hr	85.7	–	17	–
Basu and Rajan 1975	100	0.5–1.0 mg/hr	96.0	–	7	–
Gabert and Herbertson 1976	60	0.5–1.0 mg/hr	91.6	–	8	–
Wesel and Massart 1978	41	0.5–1.5 mg/hr	75.6	–	–	–
Ang et al 1978	153	0.5–1.0 mg/hr	91.3	0	7	3
Lange et al 1981	99	0.5–1.5 mg/hr	97.0	–	8	3
Hingorani et al 1988	459	0.5–1.5 mg/hr	74.5	16	33	–
Krishna et al 1990	15	0.5–1.5 mg/hr	100.0	2	2	–
El-Qarmalawi et al 1990	50	0.5 mg/hr	96.0	1	1	–
Roztocil et al 1990	141	0.5–1.5 mg/hr	96.5	–	15	–
Agarwal et al 1993	100	0.5 mg/hr	67.0	2	8	3

(b) Vaginal PGE$_2$ PGE$_2$ is also used by vaginal route for labour induction
and cervical ripening. It is available for vaginal use in three different forms: 1. Pessary, 2. Tablets, 3. Gel.

Pessaries or suppositories were first developed for the management of second
trimester terminations which were later found useful by obstetricians for cervical
ripening and labour induction. They are used as single dose by cutting a 20 mg
suppository (Buchanan et al 1984) or using 2 doses of 3 mg suppositories (Kurup
et al 1991; El-Leil et al 1993; Andersson et al 1985). Vaginal tablets are also
available for induction of labour (Kennedy et al 1982; Lo et al 1994). Gel preparations were used by vaginal route for cervical ripening and labour induction. They

were either home-made containing 2.5 or 5 mg PGE_2 (Prins et al 1983), 2 mg (Chatterjee et al 1990), 4 mg in cellulose base (Johnson et al 1985) and commercially available triacetin based gel containing 1–3 mg (Graves et al 1985).

Pessaries/tablets/gel are placed in the posterior fornix and the patient should be asked to lie in supine position for at least one hour. The action of the vaginal prostaglandins can be seen within 5–7 hours and most patients go into spontaneous labour. However in some, labour has to be induced with oxytocin or prostaglandins can be used. In patients with premature rupture of membranes, vaginal prostaglandins can be used.

Vaginal administration of PGE_2 requires higher dose than intracervical route, however it has the dual advantage of cervical ripening and labour induction. Hypertonia is one of the side effects to reckon with.

Prostaglandin analogues like sulprostone or carboprost should not be used for induction of labour. Due to their longer half life and higher potency than the natural prostaglandins, they can cause hypertonus and uterine rupture (Prasad and Ratnam, 1992).

3. *The third stage and its complications*   Management of the complications of the third stage of labour will depend upon the cause. They are summarised in Table 2.

Table 2: Causes of the complications of the
third stage of labour and their management

Cause	Management
Injury to genital tract	Repair the cervix or uterus
Retained placenta or placental fragments	Manual removal of placenta or fragments under anesthesia and observe for further bleeding
Retained blood clots	Remove the clots by curettage
Coagulation defects	Carry out lab investigations, replace blood and blood products to promote the clotting.
Chrioamnionitis	Usually unresponsive to oxytocics including prostaglandins, alert operation theatre for a hysterectomy.

Prostaglandins seem to have a role to play in the third stage of labour. $PGF_{2\alpha}$ and its analogue 15 methyl $PGF_{2\alpha}$ (Carboprost) are potent uterine stimulants. Carboprost is the drug of choice for the management of PPH due to uterine atony. There are several reports on the use of prostaglandins for the treatment of PPH (Corson and Bolognese 1977; Toppozada et al 1981; Hayashi et al 1981; Jain et al 1984; Ananthasubramaniam et al 1988; Dasgupta et al 1988; Oleen and Mariano 1990) and is now used universally.

More than 80% of the women with PPH will respond to a single injection of 250 μg carboprost. If the response is inadequate or the bleeding is not arrested the same dose can be repeated at an interval of 30 to 90 minutes. If the bleeding is not arrested in spite of the uterus contracting, the patient should be reexamined for possible injury to genital tract. In patients who do not respond to even eight doses of carboprost hysterectomy or internal iliac ligation should be considered. The uterine atony in patients with chorioamnionitis usually does not respond to oxytocics including carboprost; in such patients early surgical intervention could be life saving (Ananthasubramaniam et al 1988).

Carboprost has the advantage that it can be given by the intramuscular route and the action lasts for several hours (Green et al 1981). Granstrom et al (1989) have used an intravenous infusion of carboprost very effectively to control PPH. Few investigators have reported the efficacy of prostaglandins by a direct intramyometrial injection (Takagi et al 1976; Bigrigg et al 1991; Bruce et al 1982).

Intravenous PGE_2 (Sarkar and Mamo 1990), intramuscular sulprostone (Laajoki and Kivikoski 1986; Phuapradit et al 1993) and intrauterine gemeprost (Barrington and Roberts 1993) were also used to control PPH due to uterine atony.

Based on the properties of carboprost, its usefulness for the management of third stage of labour was reported by several researchers. Compared to methyl ergometrine or no treatment, carboprost in a dose of 125 µg – 250 µg seems to reduce both the duration of the third stage and blood loss (Devi et al 1988; Anjaneyulu et al 1988; Bhattacharya et al 1988; Abdel-Aleem et al 1993; Patki et al 1993; Singh and Megh 1995). However recent studies (Chou and MacKenzie 1994) in a double blind randomised trial using 125 µg of carboprost by the intramyometrial route showed that it was no better than 20 units of i.m. oxytocin. Double blind randomised trials on the efficacy of these drugs by the same route of administration are required to confirm their finding.

Uterine inversion

Acute puerperal uterine inversion can be a life threatening complication. After repositioning, if the tone is not established with conventional measures like oxytocin infusion or fundal massage, carboprost should be used (Heyl et al 1984; Catanzarite et al 1986).

Prostaglandins, being local hormones, have a physiological role in the process of labour. The available experimental evidence indicates their involvement in human parturition. This is further substantiated by the clinical efficacy of prostaglandins in cervical ripening, induction of labour, the management of the third stage and control of postpartum hemorrhage.

References

Abdel-Aleem H, Abol-Oyoun E M, Moustafa SAM et al 1993. Carboprost trometamol in the management of the third stage of labor. *Int J Gynecol Obstet* 42: 247-250.

Agarwal S, Gupta B, Kulashreshtha S 1993. Comparaive evaluation of prostaglandin E_2 and oxytocin for induction of labour at term pregnancy. *J Obstet Gynecol India* 43:923-927.

Ananthasubramaniam L, Kuntal Rao, Sivaraman R et al 1988. Management of intractable postpartum hemorrhage secondary to uterine atony with intramuscular 15(S)15 methyl $PGF_{2\alpha}$ *Acta Obstet Gynecol Scand Suppl.* 145: 17-19.

Ananthasubramaniam L, Sivaraman R, Premalatha 1988. Clinical trial of injection 15

(S) 15 methyl PGF$_{2\alpha}$ in severe postpartum hemorrhage. *J Obstet Gynecol India* 39:208-211.

Andersson B, Bock JE, Larsen J 1985. Induction of labour : A double blind randomized controlled study of prostaglandin E$_2$ vaginal suppository with intranasal oxytocin and with sequential treatment. *Acta Obstet Gynecol Scand* 64: 157-161.

Ang LT, Ng KH, Sivanesaratnam V et al 1978. Inducing labor with oral prostaglandin E$_2$ tablets. *Int J Gynecol Obstet* 15: 415-418.

Anggard E, Larsson C, Samuelsson B 1971. The distribution of 15-hydroxy-prostaglandin-dehydrogenase and prostaglandin -13- reductase in different tissues of the swine. *Acta Phys Scand* 81: 396-404.

Anjaneyulu R, Devi PK, Jain S et al 1988. Prophylactic use of 15(S)15-methyl-PGF$_{2\alpha}$ by intramuscular route - A controlled clinical trial. *Acta Obstet Gynecol Scand Suppl* 145: 9-11.

Barrington JW, Roberts A 1993. The use of gemeprost pessaries to arrest postpartum hemorrhage. *Br J Obstet Gynecol* 100: 691-692.

Basu HK, Rajan KTJ 1975. Induction of labour with prostaglandin E2 tablets. *J Int Med Res* 3: 73-76.

Baveja R, Bhattacharya SK, Coyaji CJ et al 1988. Prostaglandin E$_2$ gel and placebo for cervical ripening. *J Obstet Gynecol India* 38: 289-292.

Bennett PR, Henderson DJ, Moore GE 1992. Changes in expression of cyclooxygenase gene in human fetal membrane and placenta with labor. *Am J Obstet Gynecol* 167: 212-216.

Bergstrom S, Ryhage R, Samuelsson B et al 1962. The structure of prostaglandin E$_1$, F$_1$ and F$_2$. *Acta Chem Scand* 16: 501-502.

Bernstein P, Leyland N, Gurland P, et al 1987. Cervical ripening and labor induction with prostaglandin E$_2$ gel: A placebo controlled study. *Am J Obstet Gynecol* 156: 336-339.

Bhattacharya P, Devi PK, Jain S et al 1988. Prophylactic use of 15(S) 15 methyl PGF$_{2\alpha}$ by intramuscular route for control of postpartum bleeding - A comparative trial with methylergometrine. *Acta Obstet Gynecol Scand Suppl* 145: 13-15.

Bhide A, Daftary SN 1993. Preinduction cervical softening with endocervical PGE$_2$ gel. *J Obstet Gynecol India* 43: 729-733.

Bigrigg A, Chui D, Chissell S et al 1991. Use of intramyometrial 15 methyl prostaglandin F$_{2\alpha}$ to control atonic postpartum haemorrhage following vaginal delivery and failure of conventional therapy. *Br J Obstet Gynecol* 98: 734-736.

Bokstrom H, Norstrom A, Wiqvist N 1995. Cervical mucus concentration of prostaglandin E$_2$ and F$_{2\alpha}$ after pretreatment with mifepristone in the first trimester of pregnancy. *Prostaglandins* 49: 41-48.

Bruce SL, Paul RH, Van Dorsten JP 1982. Control of postpartum uterine atony by intramyometrial prostaglandin. *Obstet Gynecol* 59: 47S-50S.

Buchanan D, Macer J, Yonekura ML 1984. Cervical ripening with prostaglandin E$_2$ vaginal suppositories. *Obstet Gynecol* 63: 659-663.

Bygdeman M, Kwon SU, Mukherjee T et al 1968. Effect of intravenous infusion of prostaglandin E$_1$ and E$_2$ on motility of the pregnant human uterus. *Am J Obstet Gynecol* 102: 317-326.

Calder AA 1994. Prostaglandins and Biological Control of Cervical Function. *Aust NZ J Obstet Gynecol* 34: 347-351.

Catanzarite VA, Moffitt KD, Baker ML et al 1986. New approaches to the management of acute puerperal uterine inversion. *Obstet Gynecol* 68: 7S-10S.

Chatterjee MS, Ramachandran K, Ferlita J et al 1990. Prostaglandin E$_2$ (PGE$_2$) vaginal gel for cervical ripening. *Eur J Obstet Gynecol Reprod Biol* 38: 197-202.

Chou MM, MacKenzie IZ 1994. A prospective double blind randomised comparison of prophylactic intramyometrial 15 methyl prostaglandin F$_{2\alpha}$ 125 micrograms, and intravenous oxytocin 20 units for the control of blood loss at elective caesarean section. *Am J Obstet Gynecol* 171: 1356-1360.

Christensen NJ, Green K 1983. Bioconversion of arachidonic acid in human pregnant reproductive tissues. *Biochem Med* 30: 162-180.

Collins E, Turner G 1975. Menstrual effects of regular salicylate ingestion in pregnancy. *Lancet* 2: 335-337.

Corey EJ, Weinshenker NM, Schaaf TK et al 1969. Total synthesis of prostaglandins. *J Am Chem Soc* 91: 567.

Corson SL, Bolognese RJ 1977. Postpartum uterine atony treated with prostaglandins. *Am J Obstet Gynecol* 129: 918-919.

Danforth DN, Buckingham JC, Roddick JW 1960. Connective tissue changes incident to cervical effacement. *Am J Obstet Gynecol* 80: 939-945.

Dasgupta S, Chatterji M, Heera P et al 1988. Prostaglandins in the management of postpartum hemorrhage. *J Obstet Gynecol India* 38: 572-574.

Dawood MY, Raghavan KS, Pociask C et al 1978. Oxytocin in human pregnancy and parturition. *Obstet Gynecol* 51: 138-143.

Devi PK, Sutaria UD, Raghavan KS 1988. Prophylactic use of 15(S) 15 methyl PGF$_{2\alpha}$ for control of postpartum bleeding. *Acta Obstet Gynecol Scand Suppl* 145: 7-8.

Elder MG, Stone M 1974. Induction of labour by low amniotomy and oral administration of a solution compared with a tablet of prostaglandin E$_2$. *Prostaglandins*. 6: 427-432.

El-Leil Abou LAA, Nasrat AA, Fayed HM 1993. Prostaglandin E$_2$ vaginal pessaries in the grand multipara with an unripe cervix, a comparison of different parity groups. *Int J Gynecol Obstet* 40: 119-122.

El-Qarmalawi AM, Elmardi AA, Saddik M et al 1990. A comparative randomised study of oral prostaglandin E$_2$ (PGE$_2$) tablets and intravenous oxytocin in induction of labor in patients with premature rupture of membranes before 37 weeks of pregnancy. *Int J Gynecol Obstet* 33: 113-119.

Floberg J, Allen J, Belfrage P et al 1983. Experience with industrially manufactured gel PGE₂ for cervical priming. *Arch Gynecol* 233: 225-228.

Forman A, Gandrup P, Andersson KE et al 1983. Effect of nifedipine on oxytocin and prostaglandin F₂α induced uterine activity in postpartum uterus. *Am J Obstet Gynecol* 144: 665.

Freidman EA, Sachtleben MR 1974. Oral Prostaglandin E₂ for induction of labour at term. *Obstet Gynecol* 43: 178-185

Frydman R, Lelaidier C, Baton-Saint-Mleux C et al 1992. Labor induction in women at term with mifepristone (RU-486): A double blind randomised placebo controlled study. *Obstet Gynecol* 80: 972-975.

Gabert HA, Herbertson RM 1976. The use of oral prostaglandin E₂ to induce labor at term. *J Reprod Med* 16: 276-280.

Gonen R, Samberg I, Degani S 1994. Intracervical prostaglandin E₂ for induction of labor in patients with premature rupture of membranes and an unripe cervix. *Am J Perinatol* 11: 436-438.

Gordon-Wright AP, Dutt TP, Elder MG 1979. The routine use of oral prostaglandin E₂ tablets for induction or augmentation of labour. *Acta Obstet Gynecol Scand* 58: 23-26.

Granstrom L, Ekman G, Ulmsten U 1987. Cervical priming and labor induction with vaginal application of 3 mg PGE₂ suppositories in term pregnant women with premature rupture of amniotic membranes and unfavorable cervix. *Acta Obstet Gynecol Scand* 66: 429-431.

Granstrom L, Ekman G, Ulmsten U 1989. Intracervical infusion of 15 methyl prostaglandin F₂α (PROSTINFENEM) in women with heavy postpartum hemorrhage. *Acta Obstet Gynecol Scand* 68: 365-367.

Graves GR, Baskett TF, Gray JH et al 1985. The effect of vaginal administration of various doses of prostaglandin E₂ gel on cervical ripening and induction of labor. *Am J Obstet Gynecol* 151: 178-181.

Green K, Christensen N, Bygdeman M 1981. The chemistry and pharmacology of prostaglandins with reference to human reproduction. *J Reprod Fertil* 62: 269-281.

Hamberg M, Samuelsson B 1971. On metabolism of prostaglandins E₁ and E₂ in man. *J Biol Chem* 246: 6713-6721.

Hamberg M, Svensson J, Samuelsson B 1974. Prostaglandins endoperoxides. A new concept concerning the mode of action and release of prostaglandins. *Proc Nat Acad Sci* 71: 3824-3828.

Hayashi RH, Castillo MS, Noah ML 1981. Management of severe postpartum hemorrhage due to uterine atony using an analogue of prostaglandin F₂α. *Obstet Gynecol* 58: 426-429.

Heyl PS, Stubblefield PG, Phillippe M 1984. Recurrent inversion of puerperal uterus

managed with 15 (S) 15-methyl PGF₂α. *Obstet Gynecol* 63: 263.

Hingorani V, Nair S, Patel D et al 1988. Randomised clinical trial with oral PGE₂ tablets and intravenous oxytocin for induction of labour. *J Obstet Gynecol India* 38: 658-662.

Ilancheran A, Ratnam SS 1990. Effect of oxytocics on prostaglandin levels in the third stage of labour. *Gynecol Obstet Invest* 29: 177-180.

Jain S, Bharati P, Gupta A et al 1984. The effect of intramuscular 15 (S)-15 methyl prostaglandin F₂α in refractory postpartum hemorrhage. *J Obset Gynecol India* 34: 228-231.

Johnson IR, Macpherson MBA, Welch CC et al 1985. A comparison of lamicel and prostaglandin E₂ gel for cervical ripening before induction of labour. *Am J Obstet Gynecol* 151: 604-607.

Johnston TA, Hodson S, Greer IA et al 1993. Plasma glycosaminoglycans and prostaglandin concentrations before and after the onset of spontaneous labour. *Proceedings of 3rd European Congress on Prostaglandin in Reproduction,* Edinburgh.

Karim SMM, Devlin J 1967. Prostaglandin content of amniotic fluid during pregnancy and labour. *J Obstet Gynecol Br Cwlth* 74: 230-234.

Karim SMM, Trussell RR, Hillier K et al 1969. Induction of labour with prostaglandin F₂α. *J Obstet Gynecol Br Cwlth* 76: 769-782.

Kennedy JH, Stewart P, Barlow DH et al 1982. Induction of labour: A comparison of a single prostaglandin E₂ vaginal tablet with amniotomy and intravenous oxytocin. Br J Obstet Gynecol 89: 704-707.

Kimball FA 1983. Role of prostacyclin and other prostaglandins in pregnancy. In: Lewis PJ, Moncada S., O'Grady J, eds. Prostacyclin and Pregnancy. New York: Raven Press, pp 1-13.

Kleissl HP, Van der Rest M, Naftolin F et al 1978. Collagen changes in the human uterine cervix at parturition. *Am J Obstet Gynecol* 130: 748-753.

Krishna UR, Mandlekar A, Vaze M et al 1990. Oral prostaglandins in induction of labour. *J Obstet Gynecol India* 40: 370-373.

Kurup A, Chua S, Arulkumaran S et al 1991. Induction of labour in nulliparas with poor cervical score: Oxytocin or prostaglandin vaginal pessaries? *Aust NZ J Obstet Gynecol* 31: 223-226.

Laajoki VI, Kivikoski AI 1986. Sulprostone in the control of postpartum hemorrhage. *Acta Chirurgica Hungarica* 27: 165-168.

Lange AP, Secher NJ, Nielsen FH et al 1981. Stimulation of labor in cases of premature rupture of the membranes at or near term. A consecutive randomised study of prostaglandin E₂ tablets and intravenous oxytocin. *Acta Obstet Gynecol Scand* 60: 207-210.

Lewis RB, Schulman JD 1973. Influence of acetylsalicylic acid, an inhibitor of prostaglandin synthesis, on the duration of gestation and labor. *Lancet* 2: 1159-1161.

Lo L, Ho MW, Leung P 1994. Comparison of prostaglandin E_2 vaginal tablet with amniotomy and intravenous oxytocin for induction of labour, *Aust NZ J Obstet Gynecol* 34: 149-153.

MacDonald PC, Casey ML 1993. The accumulation of prostaglandins (PG) in amniotic fluid is an after effect of labour and indicative of a role for PGE_2 or $PGF_{2\alpha}$ in the initiation of human parturition. *J Clin Endocrinol Metab* 76:1332-1339.

Mapa MK 1981. Role of oxytocin in initiation of labour and control of myometrial activity. Ph.D. Thesis: Postgraduate Institute of Medical Education and Research, Chandigarh.

Nieder J, Augustin W 1983. Increase of Prostaglandin E and F equivalence in amniotic fluid during late pregnancy and rapid PGF elevation after cervical dilatation. *Prostaglandins Leukotrines and Medicine.* 12:289-297.

Norman RJ, Reddi K 1990. Prostaglandins in dysfunctional labour: Evidence of altered production of prostaglandin $F_{2\alpha}$. *Reprod Fertil Dev* 2: 563-574.

O'Herlihy C 1981. Vaginal prostaglandin E_2 gel and breech presentation. *Eur J Obstet Gynecol Reprod Biol* 11: 299-303.

Oleen MA, Mariano JP 1990. Controlling refractory atonic postpartum hemorrhage with hemabate sterile solution. *Am J Obstet Gynecol* 162: 205-208.

Patki A, Mane S, Desai S et al 1993. Active management of third stage of labour with Carboprost ($PGF_{2\alpha}$). *J. Obstet Gynecol India* 43: 734-737.

Patki A, Mane S, Lenka S et al 1993. Use of prostaglandin E_2 for cervical ripening and induction of labour, *J Obstet Gynecol India* 43: 928-932.

Phuapradit W, Saropala N, Rangsipragarn R 1993. Treatment of atonic postpartum hemorrhage with a prostaglandin E2 analogue. *J Med Assoc Thai* 76: 304-307.

Prins RP, Bolton RN, Mark III C et al 1983. Cervical ripening with intravaginal prostaglandin E_2 gel. *Obstet Gynecol* 61: 459-462.

Rath W, Adelmann-Grill BC, Pieper U et al 1987. The role of collagenases and proteases in prostaglandin induced cervical ripening. *Prostaglandins.* 34: 119-127.

Romero R, Baumann P, Gonzalaz R et al 1994. Amniotic fluid prostonoid concentrations increase early during course of spontaneous labour at term. *Am J Obstet Gynecol* 171: 1613-1620.

Roztocil A, Paral V, Jelinek J 1990. Our experience with induction of labour with oral prostaglandin E_2. *Scripta medica.* 63: 23-28.

Sahmay S, Coke A, Hekim N et al 1988. Maternal, umbilical, uterine and amniotic prostaglandin E and $F_{2\alpha}$ levels in labour. *J Int Med Res* 16: 280-285.

Samuelsson B, Boldyne M, Granstrom E et al 1978. Prostaglandins and Thromboxanes. *Ann Rev Biochem* 47: 997-1029

Samuelsson B, Granstrom E, Green K et al 1975. Prostaglandins. *Ann Rev Biochem* 44: 669-695.

Sarkar PK, Mamo J 1990. Successful control of atonic primary postpartum hemorrhage and prevention of hysterectomy using IV prostaglandin E2. *BJCP.* 44: 756-757.

Seed MP, Williams KI, Bamford DS 1983. Influence of gestation on prostacyclin synthesis by human pregnant myometrium. In: Lewis PJ, Moncada S, O'Grady J, eds. Prostacyclin and Pregnancy. New York: Raven Press, pp 141-146.

Sellers SM, Hodgson HT, Mitchell MD et al 1982. Raised prostaglandin levels in the third stage of labor. *Am J Obstet Gynecol* 144: 209-212.

Sharma SC, Walzman M, Molloy A et al 1982. Relationship of total ascorbic acid to prostaglandin F_2 and E_2 levels in the blood of women during third trimester of normal pregnancy. *Int J Vitan Nutr Res* 52: 312-319.

Singh PD, Megh MG 1995. Carboprost traomethamine in the active management of third stage of labour. *Ind Pract* 43: 103-105.

Skinner SJM, Liggins GC, Wilson T et al 1984. Synthesis of prostaglandin F by cultured human endometrial cells. *Prostaglandins* 27: 821-828.

Stone JL, Lockwood CJ, Berkowitz G et al 1994. Use of cervical prostaglandin E_2 gel in patients with previous cesarean section. *Am J Perinatol* 11: 309-311.

Szalay S, Husslein P, Grunberger W 1989. Local application of prostaglandin E_2 and its influence on collagenolytic activity of cervical tissue. *Sing J Obstet Gynecol* 12: 15.

Takagi S, Yoshida T, Togo Y et al 1976. The effects of intramyometrial injection of prostaglandin $F_{2\alpha}$ on severe postpartum hemorrhage. *Prostaglandins* 12: 565-579.

Thiery M, Amy JJ 1975. Induction of Labour with Prostaglandins. In: SMM Karim, ed. Advances in Prostaglandin Research. Prostaglandins and Reproduction. Baltimore: University Park Press, p.149.

Toppozada MK 1979. Prostaglandins and their synthesis inhibitors in dysfunctional uterine bleeding. In: Karim SMM, ed. Practical Applications of Prostaglandins and their Synthesis Inhibitors. Lancaster: MTP Press, pp 237-266,

Toppozada M, El-Bossaty M, El-Rahman HA et al 1981. Control of intractable atonic postpartum hemorrhage by 15 methyl prostaglandin $F_{2\alpha}$. *Obstet Gynecol* 58: 327-330.

Trofatter Jr KF 1993. Effect of preinduction cervical softening with dinoprostone gel on outcome of oxytocin induced labor. *Clin Therap* 15: 838-844.

Uldbjerg N, Ekman G, Malmstrom A et al 1983. Ripening of human uterine cervix related to changes in collagen, glycosaminoglycans and collagenolytic activity. *Am J Obstet Gynecol* 167: 662-666.

Ulmsten U, Wingerup L, Belfrage P et al 1982. Intracervical application of prostaglandin gel for induction of term labor. *Obstet Gynecol* 59: 336-339.

Varma TR, Norman J 1984. A comparison of three dosages of prostaglandin E₂ pessaries for ripening of unfavourable cervix prior to induction of labour. *Acta Obstet Gynecol Scand* 63: 17-21.

von Euler US 1935. Uber die spezifische blutdrucksenkende substanz des menschlichen Prostata - und samenblasensekretes. *Klin Wochschr* 14: 1182-1183

Wesel S, Massart JC 1978. Labour induction with prostaglandin E₂ tablets followed by amniotomy. *Acta Therapeutica* 4: 153-159.

Wilson T, Liggins GC, Aimer GP et al 1986. The effect of progesterone on the release of arachidonic acid in human endometrial cells stimulated by histamine. *Prostaglandins.* 31: 343-360.

Wiqvist N 1979. The use of inhibitors of prostaglandin synthesis in Obstetrics. In: Keirse MJNC, Anderson ABM, Gravenhorst JB, eds.

Human Parturition. Netherlands: Leiden University Press, p.189.

Yamamoto S, Hirayama H, Seida A et al 1981. Studies on prolyl hydroxylase activity, hydroxyproline content and solubility of collagen in the human uterus during pregnancy, delivery and postpartum involution. *Acta Obstet Gynecol Jpn* 33: 1703-1710.

Ylikorkala O, Makarainen L, Viinikka L 1981. Prostacyclin production increase during human parturition. *Br J Obstet Gynecol* 88: 513-516.

Yoshida K, Tahara R, Nakayama T et al 1993. Effect of dehydroepiandrosterone sulphate, estrogens and prostaglandins on collagen metabolism in human cervical tissue in relation to cervical ripening. *J Int Med Res* 21: 26-35.

Zuckerman H, Reiss U, Atad J et al 1978. Prostaglandin F in human blood during labor. *Obstet Gynecol* 51: 311-314.

14

Induction of Labour

A Biswas
S Arulkumaran

Induction of labour is the non-spontaneous initiation of uterine contractions that result in progressive cervical effacement and dilatation with descent of the presenting part. The aim of successful induction is to achieve vaginal delivery when continuation of pregnancy presents a threat to the life or wellbeing of the mother or her unborn child. The infant should be delivered in good condition within an acceptable time-frame and with a minimum of maternal discomfort or side effects. In current obstetric practice induction is usually performed for medical indications and is rarely done for a patient's or care-provider's convenience. Induction of labour for the latter indications, often termed as social induction, comprises a small proportion of the total inductions especially in teaching institutions. Induction rates vary greatly between different countries, population groups and hospitals. In a recent survey from Finland, Jarvelin et al (1993) showed that the practice of induction of labour is not consistent in different hospitals within the same country. The opinions of individual practitioners and staff routines influence the induction policy nearly as much as medical reasons do. Despite the safety of induction, a liberal induction policy leads to an increase in operative deliveries creating potential risks for the mother and child and greater expense. Nevertheless, the 1980's saw the incidence of induction varying from 4% (Pearson and Andrews 1980) to 40% (McNaughton 1980) in teaching institutions of the UK and figures as high as 55% in nonteaching institutions (Tipton and Lewis 1975).

Indications for induction

The obstetrician who is considering induction of labour must take into consideration one issue above all others : a detailed risk-benefit analysis must indicate that the woman and her fetus are more likely to benefit from than be harmed by, the artificial initiation of labour. While in a few circumstances the advantages of elective delivery by induction are clear, for example, to prevent maternal morbidity in fulminating preecalmpsia, the advantages are less clear when it is done for so called possible fetal compromise. Maternal indications for induction are few as the pregnant mother is directly accessible for examination and investigation. The majority of inductions are done for fetal indications and are mainly based on epidemiological evidence (Butler and Bonham 1963; Chamberlain et al 1975) derived from studies that were carried out two decades ago when tests for fetal wellbeing were less advanced than at the present time. The wide variation in induction rate between different countries and institutions partly reflects the differences in opinion about the indications of induction of labour in the presence of markers of increased fetal risk and also the differences in the assessments of risks associated with elective delivery (Keirse and Chalmers 1989).

Induction rates have also been influenced by several reports (Baird et al 1954; McNay et al 1977; Howie 1977; McNaughton 1980) which claimed that an active induction policy led to substantial reduction in perinatal mortality, especially from unexplained stillbirths after 37 weeks. The existence of such a cause-effect relationship has been questioned and the reduction in perinatal mortality has been attributed to other factors like improved socio-economic standards, good intrapartum care and improvement in neonatal intensive care services (Chalmers et al 1976 a and b; Pearson and Andrews 1980). In a recent review of perinatal mortality at the National University Hospital, Singapore, it was shown that between 1982 and 1992, the marked reduction in perinatal mortality was actually accompanied by a reduction in induction rates (Biswas et al 1995).

Finally, attention should be paid to women's views on induction, especially when the indications for induction are not well founded. Many women believe that induced labour, not being natural, is more painful than spontaneous labour and that in induced labour they are not in control of what is happening to them during childbirth. Such negative attitudes may partly reflect inadequate provision of information regarding induction.

Factors influencing the outcome of induced labour

The aim of induction of labour is to achieve a safe vaginal delivery for the fetus without causing any harm to the mother. Failed induction may be associated with a poor neonatal outcome and/or long labour with physical and emotional disturbances for the mother. Failed induction was defined by Duff et al (1984) as the failure to enter the active phase of labour after 12 hours of regular uterine contractions. Failed induction is diagnosed when a patient who was induced did not deliver vaginally in the absence of fetal distress, with acute events like abruption or cord prolapse and a failure to progress due to cephalopelvic disproportion or malposition, and if the patient has not entered the active phase of labour despite adequate management for 12 hours (Arulkumaran et al 1985a).

The success of any method of induction depends largely on the parity and the state of the cervix at the beginning of induction. The process of prelabour cervical softening, shortening and eventual dilatation (cervical ripening) is a part of a continuum which culminates in spontaneous labour. The success of any method of induction in a particular circumstance depends largely on the point in this continuum at which the efforts of induction start. In most centres Bishop's score (1964) or a modified version of it is used to assess the favourability of the cervix. The characteristics of the cervix and the station of the head are considered. A modified scoring system with a maximum of 10 points is given below.

The influence of parity and the cervical score on the success of the time honoured methods of induction with amniotomy and oxytocin was well demonstrated in a study carried out in Singapore during 1982/1983 (Arulkumaran et al 1985a).

Cervical score

Score	0	1	2
Position of cervix	Posterior	Axial	Anterior
Length of cervix	2 cm	1 cm	< 0.5 cm
Dilatation of cervix	0 cm	1 cm	> 2 cm
Consistency of cervix	Firm	Soft	Soft and stretchable
Station of presenting part	−2	−1	0

Table 1 summarises the typical risks of caesarean section for failed induction of labour, classified by parity and the cervical score, derived from that study. The rate of caesarean section in multiparas and nulliparas with a good cervical score was not high. However nulliparas with a cervical score of 3 or less had a CS rate of 65% for all indications and 45% for failed induction. Those who had CS for failed induction of labour did not have a maximum cervical dilatation of more than 4 cm and thus did not enter the active phase of labour despite an intravenous infusion of oxytocin for a period of 10–12 hr. Nulliparas with a score of 3 or less had a one in two chance of CS for failed induction and this was 1 in 10 if the cervical score was 4 to 6.

Table 1: Caesarean section rate for failed induction of labour according to parity and cervical score

	Para 0		Para 1 or more	
Cervical score	n	%	n	%
0 – 3	27/59	45.8	2/26	7.7
4 – 6	30/292	10.3	10/257	3.9
7 – 10	3/208	1.4	2/215	0.9

The parity and cervical score not only influenced the caesarean section rate but also influenced the other characteristics of labour and their outcome. Women with poor cervical score had longer labours, required higher doses of oxytocin and had a poorer neonatal outcome (Arulkumaran et al 1985a). Cervical priming methods to improve the cervical score in this group of women improves the chance of successful induction.

Methods of cervical priming

During the last 15 years the use of different methods to render the cervix more favourable for induction or cervical priming before the formal induction, have become popular. However it must be realised that the distinction between cervical priming and induction of labour is artificial, as it attempts to compartmentalise the latent prelabour phase from the active 'acceleratory' labour. The process of functional transformation of the cervix from a sphincteric organ acting to preserve and contain the growing fetus within the uterus to a canal which softens, shortens and dilates to facilitate the passage of the fetus, starts well before the actual labour itself. Depending on the time of initiation during this transformation process, a method used for cervical priming might act as a method to induce labour. The same dose of prostaglandin E_2 used to prime a cervix with a poor score, may induce labour in a woman with a more favourable cervix. Depending on the primary intention for use and based on parity and the cervical score, the same agent or method may act as a method of cervical priming or a method of induction.

During the process of cervical ripening, important structural and biochemical changes take place and create a cervix that requires less uterine work to achieve cervical dilatation (Arulkumaran et al 1985b). Histochemical studies have shown that cervical ripening is associated with gradual dissociation and scattering of previously densely packed collagen bundles, along with changes in both the type and content of the proteoglycans in the ground substance. Both mechanical and pharmacological methods have been used to hasten the process of cervical ripening.

1.   Pharmacological methods of cervical ripening

Prostaglandins   Both prostaglandin PGE_2 and $PGF_{2\alpha}$ have been used for this purpose, although PGE_2 seems to be more effective than $PGF_{2\alpha}$ (MacKenzie and Embrey 1979). Synthetic prostaglandin analogues have generally been avoided for priming or induction at term with a live fetus, mainly because of uncertainities over their effects on the fetus-neonate. In addition to ripening of the cervix, prostaglandins lead to an increase in myometrial activity which includes an enhanced uterine responsiveness to oxytocin. There may also be an improvement in the quality of uterine contractions by enhanced formation of gap junctions between the myometrial muscle fibres. PGE_2 has been used through various routes : orally, extra-amniotically, intracervically and vaginally. Oral PGE_2 is associated with significant systemic side effects and uterine contractions, while extraamniotic administration appears to be too invasive with a possible risk of infection and membrane rupture. Both vaginal and intracervical methods are currently popular methods of administration of PGE_2. Published reports suggest that a single application of PGE_2 2–5 mg as biodegradable vaginal pessaries and gel or 5–10 mg as non-biodegradable formulations introduced to the posterior fornix as appropriate. The lower dose is probably as effective as the higher dose. Intracervical instillation is usually done as PGE_2 0.5–1G in viscous cellulose gel.   It must be noted that significant difference in absorption rates necessitates a vast difference in dosage in these two different routes of application. Recent double-blind studies have shown both routes to be safe, but the vaginal route is probably better because of its greater ease of administration and slightly higher efficacy (Hales et al 1994). A second dose of PGE_2 after 6–8 hours may be tried in cases with poor response, but repeated doses are usually unhelpful and cause delay in delivery. The use of controlled release hydrogel pessaries may reduce the incidence of hyperstimulation and fetal distress associated with topical prostaglandins (MacKenzie 1993). A couple of recent studies from the University Hospital of Jamaica have evaluated the use of vaginal misoprostol (PGE$_1$ methyl analogue) 0.1 mg for cervical ripening and have found it to be a safe, equally effective and cheaper alternative to PGE$_2$ (Fletcher et al 1993; Fletcher et al 1994). Further studies on this are eagerly awaited.

Oxytocin   Regular uterine contractions achieved with intravenous infusions of oxytocin or buccal oxytocin or demoxytocin would result in cervical ripening in many cases. Before the introduction of prostaglandins this was the usual method for women with a poor cervical score. However it is a laborious approach necessitating constant monitoring and may require several 8–15 hours sessions spaced over a number of days. Controlled studies have shown it to be a less satisfactory method than local prostaglandin application (Roberts et al 1986).

Other topical pharmacological agents   Oestradiol (150–300 mg) in tylose gel has been used extra-amniotically, intracervically or vaginally for effecting pre-induction cervical ripening (Craft and Yovich 1978; Tromans et al 1981). The improvement in the cervical score appears to be equivalent to that of a local PGE$_2$ application with minimal uterine activity. However the labour outcome following formal induction 24 hours later was not significantly different. Purified porcine ovarian relaxin (1–4 mg) in a gel, applied vaginally or intracervically has also been found to be effective (MacLennan et al 1980). Recombinant human relaxin (1.5 mg) in methylcellulose gel, studied in a small randomised placebo controlled trial, was not found to be effective at this dosage (Bell et al 1993). Recently, RU-486 (mifepristone), an anti-progestin, has been used in France for preinduction cervical ripening at term. The dosage used was 200 mg orally for 2 days, 48 hours before the formal induction, and the initial results were very encouraging (Frydman et al 1991; Lelaidier et al 1994).

2. *Mechanical methods of cervical ripening*

Introduction of hygroscopic tents, such as natural laminaria tents or synthetic sponges impregnated with magnesium sulfate (Lamicel) into the cervical os, 12 hours prior to induction of labour, has been shown to improve the cervical score (MacPherson 1984). Similar results have been noted with the use of a Foley's catheter in the cervix with the balloon inflated with 30 ml of saline (Lewis 1983). Although they can effectively ripen the cervix, maternal and neonatal infections remain a risk with the use of these mechanical methods, especially if the attempt at induction is prolonged. Since it appears that mechanical agents bring about cervical ripening through a local release of tissue prostaglandins in the cervix or the lower uterine segment, there seems little rationale for their use where topical prostaglandins are available.

Methods of induction of labour

Historically, a wide variety of mechanical and chemical methods, some of them even bizarre, have been used for labour induction. Modern obstetric practice however uses only two broad approaches to induction of labour, namely, amniotomy and the use of oxytocic agents (oxytocin or one of the prostaglandins, used systemically or vaginally). A third method, which is widely used, but rarely as a formal method of induction, is sweeping or stripping of the membranes.

1. Sweeping of membranes

Sweeping or stripping of membranes from the lower segment, which was apparently introduced by Hamilton in 1810, has been widely used to induce labour. Although it is rarely considered as a formal method of induction of labour, it is still frequently employed at term, especially when the indications for induction are not strong enough. Uterine contractions are frequently established following the procedure, resulting from the release of endogenous prostaglandins. Despite its long history and wide use, very few controlled studies have been made to assess the efficacy and safety of the procedure. Swann (1958) reported that when the cervix was favourable, 69% of women would go into labour if the procedure was repeated daily for three days. A more recent randomised controlled study of the procedure in pregnancies longer than 40 weeks, found it to be safe and useful in reducing the incidence of post-term pregnancies (Allott and Palmer 1993). It may be a simple and useful attempt for women with a very good cervical score. If the procedure fails to induce labour within a few hours or a day, forewater amniotomy can be performed (MacKenzie 1994).

2. Amniotomy

Amniotomy or artificial rupture of the membranes, since its introduction by Thomas Denman more than 200 years ago, has had marked ups and downs in popularity. This is not surprising, since the procedure represents one of the most irrevocable interventions in pregnancy and more than any other procedure, calls for a firm commitment to delivery.

Amniotomy alone would result in vaginal delivery in most women with a good cervical score, the main disadvantage being the occassional unpredictably long interval between the procedure and the onset of regular uterine activity of labour. Patterson (1971) found that 15% of primigravidas and 22% of multigravidas were not in established labour more than 24 hours after amniotomy. In current practice, amniotomy is usually combined, immediately or after a variable interval, with intravenous oxytocin, in order to reduce the induction-delivery interval.

Hind-water or high amniotomy with a Drew-Smythe catheter is hardly used in modern obstetrics, except for cases of polyhydramnios with a firm indication for induction. The claimed advantages of reduced risk of infection and cord prolapse, and controlled release of amniotic fluid has never been assessed in randomised trials. The procedure can cause damage to the fetus, placenta or maternal genital tract (Parker 1957) and hence should be undertaken by a senior clinician.

3. Oxytocin

Since the introduction of oxytocin as an intravenous infusion in the 1940s, it has come to be the most widely used method of labour induction. The principles of current clinical usage of intravenous oxytocin are based on the classic studies of Turnbull and Anderson (1968) who recognised the wide differences in the responsiveness of the pregnant uteri to oxytocin. These studies led to the concept of 'titration' of oxytocin dosage in response to uterine contractions.

Customarily oxytocin dosage titration is based on the clinical feedback of labour ward staff on the characteristics of uterine contractions: their intensity, duration and frequency. There is still wide variation in the use of oxytocin, especially with regard to the initial starting dose, dose increments, rate of escalation and use of delivery systems. Infusion solutions vary from oxytocin 2.5–10 units/500 ml of saline, N/5% dextrose-saline or 5% dextrose solution. The starting dose is usually 1 to 4 mu/min and the dosage is subsequently increased till effective contractions are established. Two approaches to dose escalation have been tried, the arithmetic escalation (Kurup et al 1991) or geometric escalation (Turnbull 1976). The arithmetic approach uses a starting dose of 2 or 2.5 milliunits/minute (mu/min) and then the dose is increased by 2 or 2.5 mu/min at intervals of 30 min. In the geometric method, a far more rapid dose escalation is used, doubling the dose every 20–30 min. The geometric method is more often associated with hyperstimulation and fetal hypoxia and is less preferred. The time interval between the dosage increments has been the subject of much debate. In a randomised controlled study involving 224 patients, Chua et al (1991) found no difference between a 15 min and a 30 min interval increment protocol, in terms of hyperstimulation and fetal distress. On the other hand, Orhue (1993) showed that increments at 30 min intervals were superior to 15 min incremental protocol in reducing the incidence of hyperstimulation. Satin et al (1994) also found that a 20 min interval is associated with more hyperstimulation, but fewer caesarean sections for dystocia when compared to a 40 min interval protocol. Based on most studies an escalation interval of every 30 min appears to be adequate and gives a similar outcome of labour as shorter increment intervals. Monitoring and management of patients is also easier with half hourly increment intervals. Hyperstimulation and fetal heart rate changes are real possibilities even with such a regime necessitating fetal heart rate and uterine contraction monitoring whenever oxytocin is used.

The dose schedule in induction should aim to initiate effective contractions and subsequently maintain them. There is evidence from the clinical studies of Beazley et al (1975) and Steer et al (1975) that the amount of oxytocin required to maintain labour is substantially less than that required to initiate it. However most dosage schedules retain the original approach of escalating the dose until effective contractions are established and subsequently maintaining the rate till delivery. The maximum dosage of oxytocin required is also highly variable. O'Driscoll et al (1973) used a standard concentratiom of 10 units/litre of infusion fluid, a maximum rate of 40 mu/min and an arbitrary limit of 1 litre of fluid to be infused. A number of studies have shown that in the majority the desired frequency of uterine contractions can be achieved with doses less than 11 mu/min (Steer et al 1985; Arulkumaran et al 1985c). Based on these observations it appears safe to titrate oxytocin starting from 2 to 2.5 mu/min up to 14 to 15mu/min till a contraction frequency of 4 to 5 in 10 min is reached with each contraction lasting for > 40 sec. If an adequate response is not observed after reaching 14 to 15 mu/min it is reasonable to increase the oxytocin dose in increments of 4 to 5 mu/min every 30 min (up to a maximum of 30 to 40 mu/min) till the desired contraction frequency is achieved.

The question of what the desired contraction frequency or uterine activity should be which will maximise the chances of vaginal delivery and minimise the length of labour and the risk of fetal hypoxia, has proved to be rather difficult to answer. Traditionally oxytocin titration is based on the assessment of the frequency of uterine contractions either by palpation or by external or internal tocography. With the use of internal tocometry, total uterine activity can be continuously computed from the area under the contraction curve above the baseline (Steer 1977). However neither intrauterine pressure measurements by internal tocography (Chia et al 1993), nor attempts to acheive preset uterine activity (Arulkumaran et al 1987) have been found to confer any benefit over external tocography in the monitoring of uterine contractions in induced labour. Since the amount of uterine work required to achieve vaginal delivery can vary greatly between individual cases, preset targets of uterine workload are not satisfactory. It can be concluded from these randomised controlled studies that external tocography or the traditional method of clinical palpation are dependable and satisfactory methods of monitoring uterine activity in induced labour.

Various delivery systems have been used for the titration of oxytocin during induced or augmented labour. Either a gravity-fed system with a manual compression switch or peristaltic pumps controlled mechanically or electronically, are used. The precision of dosage delivery is important for oxytocin infusions mainly because of the risk of hyperstimulation and consequent fetal hypoxia or uterine rupture with an inadvertent high dosage. Peristaltic infusion pumps or drip counters are preferred as they can control the delivery of precise doses of oxytocin, while gravity-fed systems are not dependable. Automatic infusion systems governed by feedback from intrauterine contraction pressure have also been tried. At first, an open-loop system was devised. The Cardiff automatic infusion system (Francis et al 1970) was of the open-loop type in not being directly dependent on the input from contraction assessment. It automatically doubled the oxytocin dosage every 12.5 min but the operator had to select the appropriate maximum dose based on contractions assessed manually or by external or internal tocography. Carter and Steer (1980) devised a closed loop automatic infusion system programmed to control the infusion based on preset active contraction areas derived from intrauterine pressure measured by a Sonicaid FM3 R fetal monitor with a special uterine activity integral (UAI) module. While Steer et al (1985) demonstrated a marked reduction of the total and mean maximum dose of oxytocin used, Gibb et al (1985) failed to find any advantage with the use of the system over the conventional peristaltic pump infusion. Maeda and Suzumara (1984) developed a closed-looped system based on the feedback from external tocography. This system was evaluated by Arulkumaran et al (1986), who found no particular advantage of the system over manual titration. In general, automated infusion systems have not found wide acceptance, because primarily of the high cost of the equipment and lack of confidence over the safety of these systems. In addition, automated systems are not popular with the patients themselves, as it denies them the personal care and attention provided during the manual titration method.

Amniotomy is usually combined with oxytocin infusion during induction. However there is some variation in the timing of amniotomy between different centres. Most obstetricians start with an amniotomy followed, immediately or within an hour, by oxytocin infusion. In cases with a high presenting part, it may be prudent to start the oxytocin infusion first and delay the amniotomy till effective contractions are established. Amniotomy can be performed when the head descends and fits the brim of the pelvis.

4. *Prostaglandins for induction of labour*

Both prostaglandins $PGF_{2\alpha}$ and PGE_2 have been used for cervical priming as well as for labour induction. Depending on the cervical score and the dosage, prostaglandins cause cervical priming or result in induction of labour. Initially, the intravenous route was used and Karim et al (1968) were the first to use intravenous $PGF_{2\alpha}$ for induction of labour. Infusions usually start with $PGF_{2\alpha}$ 2.5–5 ug/min, which is then titrated like oxytocin to a maximum dose of 18–40 μg/min. Since PGE_2 is almost 10 times as potent as $PGF_{2\alpha}$ in its uterotonic action, it is started at an initial infusion dose of 0.1–0.5 μg/min and increased to a maximum dose of 2 – 4 μg/min. However, intravenous prostaglandins have not found wide clinical acceptance because of the associated gastrointestinal side effects and local phlebitis. From the point of efficacy, they are only as effective as intravenous oxytocin (Lange 1986).

In 1971, Karim and Sharma reported on the use of oral prostaglandins for the induction of labour. Prostaglandin $PGF_{2\alpha}$ is not used orally as it is less effective and gives rise to more gastrointestinal side effects compared to oral PGE_2. In a typical regime, oral PGE_2 is started at a dose of 0.5 mg/ hour. The dose is increased by 0.5 mg every 4 hours up to a maximum dose of 1.5–2.0 mg/hour (Tsakok et al 1975). The treatment is continued till labour is established. Amniotomy is performed at the onset if the cervical score is favourable or when labour is established. In a randomised controlled study of over 200 patients, Ratnam et al (1974) found oral PGE_2 to be as effective as intravenous oxytocin.

From 1973 onwards, various local forms of PGE_2 (as gels, pessaries or films) have been used for application to the vagina or the cervix (Calder and Embrey 1974; Arulkumaran et al 1989). Extra-amniotic infusions have also been used with no demonstrable advantage. The most widely adopted mode of administration of PGE_2 has become the vaginal route. When the cervical score is good, a single vaginal application of PGE_2, 2–5 mg, has been reported to induce labour and avoid the necessity for formal oxytocin-amniotomy induction in 65.9% of nulliparas and 87.5% of multiparas with a concomitant reduction in CS rates (MacKenzie and Embrey 1978). However for women with a good cervical score, failed induction is usually not a problem (Arulkumaran et al 1985a). For this group of patients, amniotomy and oxytocin infusion should be the preferred method as it is less expensive and allows better control over uterine contractions than vaginal prostaglandins. A number of studies have shown that, compared to oxytocin infusion, hyperstimulation does not occur more often with prostaglandins. When it occurs, reversal could be achieved by using tocolytics like 0.25 mg terbutaline in 5 ml of saline given intravenously over 5 minutes. In the case of hyperstimulation with oxytocin infusion, the drip can be stopped, and if necessary a tocolytic can be used. For nulliparous women with a poor cervical score (score < 6), vaginal prostaglandins are preferable as demonstrated by the study of Kurup et al (1991). With the use of two PGE_2 3 mg pessaries inserted 4 hours apart followed by amniotomy and oxytocin infusion if required, 24 hours later, 52% started labour within 24 hours of the first pessary insertion. The caesarean section rate was reduced from 43.5% in the oxytocin-amniotomy group to 23.7% in the prostaglandin group.

Prostaglandin analogues have not been commonly used for induction of labour in term pregnancy because of the lack of data on their fetal and neonatal effects. Recently, in a randomised trial comparing intravaginal misoprostol and intravenous oxytocin infusion for labour induction, Sanchez-Ramos et al (1993) found vaginal misoprostol to be an effective agent for labour induction but it was associated with an unacceptably high rate of uterine hyperstimulation.

Induction of labour in special circumstances

Intrauterine fetal death   Induction of labour is often the kindest procedure following the unfortunate occurrence of intrauterine fetal death. However induction of labour in the presence of a dead fetus differs from normal term pregnancy in a number of ways. Firstly, the uterine sensitivity to oxytocic agents appear to be less; and secondly, the cervix is often unfavourable. Certain methods of induction of labour like amniotomy and the intra-amniotic instillation of prostaglandins may be effective but not suitable, because of the possible risk of sepsis, especially if the induction-delivery interval becomes unduly prolonged.

Prior to the introduction of prostaglandins, high doses of oxytocin infusion were commonly used in this situation. However uterine responsiveness to oxytocin varies enormously and it is desirable to start with a low dose of oxytocin. Subsequently dose escalation can be done in a geometric manner till effective contractions are established. Unfortunately, oxytocin alone is not always effective and very high doses of dilute oxytocin can lead to water intoxication and electrolyte disturbances through its antidiuretic properties.

Prostaglandins PGE_2 and $PGF_{2\alpha}$ and their various analogues have been used via different routes for induction of labour in the presence of intrauterine death. Intraamniotic instillation is best avoided because of the risk of sepsis and erratic absorption through devitalised membranes. Prostaglandin analogues, like sulprostone or gemeprost, appear to be more effective and have fewer side effects compared to the parent prostaglandins. Intramuscular injection of 16,16 dimethyl PGE_2 p-benzaldehyde semicarbazone ester 150 µg every 6 hr till delivery is achieved has been shown to be effective (Prasad and Ratnam 1987). Sulprostone (Nalador) can be used intravenously 500 µg in 500 ml saline, titrated with incremental doses escalated every half an hour till the desired frequency of contractions is achieved. Sulprostone has also been used in doses of 200 µg intramuscularly every 2 hr upto a maximum of 1,000 µg per day and the drug repeated the next day in the same manner in those who did not deliver (Grunberger 1987). The results were good but the intramuscular use of this drug has been withdrawn recently by the manufacturers because of the reported rare occurrences of anaphylactic reaction. Gemeprost (Cervagem) 1 mg pessaries can be used vaginally at 3 hourly intervals for a maximum of 5 doses and the course may be repeated after an interval of 24 hours in cases of failure. PGE$_2$ pessaries may be used for either cervical ripening or for induction in cases of intrauterine death, much in the same way as it is used for the induction of labour in the presence of a live fetus. Thus, there is a wide choice of different prostaglandins and analogues used through different routes, all of which are of similar efficacy. The method a particular obstetric unit chooses should depend on the local experience and the availability of the drug.

Previous caesarean section, breech presentation and multiple pregnancy   Although previous low transverse caesarean delivery, multiple pregnancy and breech presentation are traditionally considered as relative contraindications for induction of labour, under compelling circumstances labour can be induced in most such cases after careful selection. For women with a previous lower segment caesarean scar, induction of labour with rupture of the membranes and oxytocin infusion can be carried out with fair safety, when the cervix is favourable and the pelvis appears clinically adequate. In presence of a poor cervical score, PGE$_2$ vaginal pessaries may be used for labour induction. In a large series of 439 cases with previous caersarean section undergoing induction of labour with PGE$_2$ vaginal pessaries, MacKenzie (1990) found a scar damage in 1%, which is not significantly different from that reported following oxytocin-induced labour and spontaneous labour (Arulkumaran et al 1992).

Although very little has been written about induction of labour in twin pregnancies and even less about the use of prostaglandins in these situations, induction may often become necessary because of the high incidence of maternal and fetal complications. When the first twin is in cephalic presentation and cervical score is favourable, induction of labour by amniotomy and oxytocin infusion is usually effective. A PGE$_2$ pessary and gel can be used for cervical priming in the presence of an unfavourable cervix. However with twin pregnancies, an unfavourable cervical score is rare at term.

Although breech presentation is considered as a relative contraindication to induction of labour, in well selected cases where the chances of achieving vaginal delivery are reasonable, labour may be induced by amniotomy and oxytocin infusion. Since prolapse of the cord is a significant risk with incomplete breech presentations, induction should only be attempted in cases of extended breech with the presenting part well settled in the pelvis. Vaginal PGE$_2$ has also been used for induction of labour in cases of breech presentation where the cervix is unfavourable (Shepherd et al 1981). With prostaglandin induction, forewater amniotomy can be delayed till the breech is well descended in the pelvis, thereby reducing the risk of cord prolapse.

In these special circumstnces, the rate of progress of labour in the active phase should be monitored closely and early recourse to caesarean section should be taken when the progress is slow.

Stabilising induction   In patients with a transverse or oblique lie with no apparent cause, especially in multiparae, stabilising induction at 38 – 40 weeks may be a valid option of management (Edwards and Nicholson 1969). In this, external cephalic version is performed first, converting the fetal lie to longitudinal. A titrated intravenous infusion of oxytocin is commenced to stimulate uterine contractions. Once the uterine contractions are established and the fetal head is firmly sitting on the pelvic brim, a low amniotomy is performed. Amniotomy may also be performed prior to oxytocin stimulation in cases where the fetal head can be made to enter the pelvic brim after the external cephalic version. During the procedure of stabilising induction, the obstetrician should be in constant attendance till labour is well established, as cord prolapse is a real possibility. When performed with adequate precautions and where it is successful, the procedure will allow the prevention of an operative abdominal delivery.

Risks and complications of induction of labour

Induction of labour is a potentially hazardous obstetric intervention. There are three broad groups of risks associated with induction of labour. Firstly, the risks associated with terminating the pregnancy artificially before the spontaneous onset of labour; secondly, those that are associated with the artificial stimulation of uterine contraction; and finally, those attributable to the specific method of labour induction.

Any attempt at initiation of labour is associated with a chance of failure. Failed induction equates to caesarean section. Therefore if the induction of labour itself was unnecessary, the consequent failed induction would also result in an unnecessary operative delivery. The risks of failed induction have been discussed earlier. Inadvertent preterm delivery is a risk with any induction. An accurate determination of the gestational age is therefore a necessary prerequisite. Any pharmacologic agent used to stimulate uterine contractions could lead to uterine hyperstimulation, which in turn could lead to fetal hypoxia and fetal death. Occasionally, especially in the higher order multipara and in patients with a previous caesarean section, uterine hyperstimulation could lead to uterine rupture. Atonic postpartum hemorrhage occurs more commonly following induced labour than with spontaneous labour and may be related to the length of labour, which is usually longer with induction (Brinsden and Clark 1978). It probably occurs less commonly following prostaglandin induction compared to oxytocin induction.

There are certain specific hazards associated with individual techniques and pharmaceutical agents. Low amniotomy, especially with a high presenting part or a flexed breech presentation, could result in prolapse of the cord. This does not always occur at the time of amniotomy, but may become evident when labour eventually starts. Another potential risk associated with amniotomy is the introduction of pathogenic organisms. The risk of a clinically significant infection is largely dependent on the aseptic procedure practised at the time of amniotomy and the interval between amniotomy and delivery.

Use of oxytocin in labour has been associated with an increased incidence of neonatal jaundice (Ghosh and Hudson 1972). This could be due to the direct toxic effect of the drug on red cell membranes or due to the relative immaturity of the fetus. Prolonged infusion of relatively high doses of oxytocin in dilute solutions can lead to maternal water intoxication, hyponatremia, coma and even death. Similar disturbances in neonatal biochemistry, leading to seizures, could also occur in severe cases.

The specific hazards associated with prostaglandins relate mainly to their effect on the gastrointestinal tract. These effects are greater with $PGF_{2\alpha}$ compared to

PGE$_2$ and occur less commonly with endocervical and extraamniotic administration compared to oral, intravenous or vaginal use (Keirse and Chalmers 1989). Prostaglandins, particularly PGE$_2$, may also cause pyrexia due to their direct effect on thermoregulatory centres in the brain. Pyrexia, together with a rise in leucocyte count, which can also be stimulated by prostaglandins, may lead to an erroneous diagnosis of intrauterine infection. More worrying than these specific risks associated with their use is the concern that the simplicity of their administration may encourage their use for trivial indications and that inadequate attention may be paid to proper monitoring of uterine contractions and fetal wellbeing.

'The spontaneous onset of labour is a robust and effective mechanism .... and should be given to operate on its own. We should only induce labour when we are sure that we can do better.'

Turnbull (1976)

The most important decision to be made when considering induction of labour is whether or not the induction is justified. How it is to be achieved is a secondary decision. Whatever method is chosen to implement a justified decision to induce labour, uterine contractility and maternal and fetal wellbeing should be monitored closely. Induction of labour is one of the common interventions in obstetrics and is not without risk. In many circumstances, induction of labour may either result in an increase or a decrease in maternal or perinatal morbidity. These uncertainities are reflected in the wide differences in induction policies between different obstetric units and will not be resolved till substantial evidence is accumulated from properly controlled, large, randomised trials regarding the indications and methods of induction of labour.

References

Allott HA, Palmer CR 1993. Sweeping the membranes: a valid procedure in stimulating the onset of labour? *Br J Obstet Gynecol* 100: 898-903.

Arulkumaran S, Gibb DMF, TambyRaja RL, Heng SH, Ratnam SS 1985a. Failed induction of labour. *Austr NZ J of Obstet Gynecol* 25: 190-193.

Arulkumaran S, Gibb DMF, Heng SH, Lun KC, Ratnam SS 1985b. Total uterine activity in induced labour - an index of cervical and pelvic tissue resistance. *Br J Obstet Gynecol* 92:693-697.

Arulkumaran S, Gibb DMF, TambyRaja RL, Heng Sh, Ratnam SS 1985c Rising caesarean section rates in Singapore. *Sing J Obstet Gynecol* 16:6-15.

Arulkumaran S, Gibb DMF, Heng SH, Ratnam SS 1985d. Perinatal outcome of induced labour. *Asia Oceania J Obstet Gynecol* 11:33-37.

Arulkumaran S, Ingemarsson I, Ratnam SS 1986. Closed loop automatic infusion system for induction of labour based on external

tocography. *Asia Oceania J Obstet Gynecol* 12:221-226.

Arulkumaran S, Ingemarsson I, Ratnam SS 1987. Oxytocin titration to achieve preset active contraction area values does not improve the outcome of induced labour. *Br J Obstet Gynecol* 94: 242-248.

Arulkumaran S, Adaikan G, Anandakumar C, Viegas OAC, Piara Singh S, Ratnam SS 1989. Comparative study of a two dose schedule of PGE 3 mg pessary and 1700 ug film for induction of labour in nulliparae with poor cervical score. *Prostaglandins, leukotrienes and essential fatty acids* 38:37-41.

Arulkumaran S, Chua S, Ratnam SS 1992. Symptoms and signs of with scar rupture: value of uterine activity measurements. *Aust NZ J Obstet Gynecol* 32: 208-212.

Baird D, Walker J, Thompson AM 1954. The causes and preventions of stillbirths and first week deaths. *J Obstet Gynecol Br Cwlth.* 61:498-501.

Beazley JH, Banovic I, Feld MS 1975. Maintenance of labour. *BMJ* ii:248-250.

Bell RJ, Permezel M, MacLennan A, Hughes C, Healy D, Brennecke S 1993. A randomised, double-blind, placebo-controlled trial of the safety of vaginal recombinant human relaxin for cervical ripening. *Obstet Gynecol* 82: 328-33.

Bishop EH 1964. Pelvic scoring for elective induction. *Obstet Gynecol* 2: 266-268.

Biswas A, Chew S, Joseph R, Arulkumaran S, Anandakumar C, Ratnam SS 1995. Towards improved perinatal care - Perinatal audit. *Ann Acad Med Singapore* 24: 211-217.

Brinsden PRS, Clark AD 1978. Postpartum hemorrhage after induced and spontaneous labour. *BMJ* 2: 855-856.

Butler NR, Bonham DG 1963. Perinatal Mortality. Edinburgh: Churchill Livingstone.

Calder AA, Embrey MP 1974. Prostaglandins and the unfavourable cervix. *Lancet* ii: 1322-1323.

Carter MC, Steer PJ 1980. An automatic infusion system for the measurement and control of uterine activity. *Med Instrum.* 14:169-173.

Chalmers I, Lawson JG, Turnbull AC 1976 a. Evaluation of different approaches to obstetric care. Parts I and II. *Br J Obstet Gynecol* 83:921-933.

Chalmers I, Zlosnik JE, Johns KA, Campbell H 1976 b. Obstetric practice and outcome of pregnancy in Cardiff residents 1965-1973. *BMJ.* 1: 735-738.

Chamberlain R, Chamberlain G, Howlett B, Claireaux A 1975. *The First Week of Life.* In: Chamberlain G, ed. British births 1970, Vol 1. London: William Heinemann.

Chia YT, Arulkumaran S, Soon SB, Norshida S, Ratnam SS 1993. Induction of labour: Does internal tocography result in better obstetric outcome than external tocography. *Austr NZ J Obstet Gynecol* 33:159-161.

Chua S, Arulkumaran S, Kurup A, Tay D, Ratnam SS 1991. Oxytocin titration for induction of labour. A prospective randomised study of 15 versus 30 minute dose increment schedules. *Austr NZ J Obstet Gynecol* 31:134-137.

Craft I, Yovich J 1978. Oestradiol and induction of labour. *Lancet* ii: 208.

Duff P, Huff RW, Gibbs RS 1984. Management of premature rupture of membranes and unfavourable cervix in term pregnancy. *Obstet Gynecol* 63:697-702.

Edwards RL, Nicholson HO 1969. The management of unstable lie in late pregnancy. *J Obstet Gynecol Br Cwlth* 76:713-718.

Francis JG, Turnbull AC, Thomas FF 1970. Automatic oxytocin infusion equipment for induction of labour. *J Obstet Gynecol Br Cwlth* 77:594-602.

Fletcher HM, Mitchell S, Simeon D, Frederick J, Brown D 1993. Intravaginal misoprostol as a cervical ripening agent. *Br J Obstet Gynecol* 100: 641-4

Fletcher H, Mitchell S, Frederick J, Simeon D, Brown D 1994. Intravaginal misoprostol versus dinoprostone as cervical ripening and labour-inducing agents. *Obstet Gynecol* 83: 244-7.

Frydman R, Baton C, Lelaidier C, Vial M, Bourget P, Fernandez H 1991. Mifepristone for induction of labour. *Lancet* 337: 488-489.

Gibb DMF, Arulkumaran S, Heng SH, Ratnam SS 1985. Characteristics of induced labour. *Asia Oceania J Obstet Gynecol* 11: 3

Gibb DMF, Arulkumaran S, Ratnam SS 1985. A comparative study of methods of oxytocin administration for induction of labour. *Br J Obstet Gynecol* 92:688-692.

Ghosh A, Hudson FP 1972. Oxytocin and neonatal hyperbilirubinaemia. *Lancet* 2: 823.

Grunberger W. 1987 International colloquy on the management of intruterine fetal death. *Int J Obstet Gynecol* 25:185-197.

Hales KA, Rayburn WF, Turnbull GL, Christensen HD, Patatanian E 1994. Double-blind comparison of intracervical and intravaginal prostaglandin E_2 for cervical ripening and induction of labour. *Am J Obstet Gynecol* 171: 1087-91

Howie P 1977. Induction of labour, In: Chard T, Richards M, eds. Benefits and Hazards of the New Obstetrics. London: SIMP, pp 83-87.

Jarvelin MR, Hartikainen-Sorri AL, Rantakallio P 1993. Labour induction policy in hospitals of different levels of specialisation. *Br J Obstet Gynecol* 100: 310-5.

Karim SMM, Trussel RR, Patel RC, Hillier K 1968. Response of pregnant human uterus to $PGF_{2\alpha}$ -induction of labour. *BMJ* 4: 621-623.

Karim SMM, Sharma SD. 1971. Oral administration of prostaglandins for induction of labour. *BMJ* 1: 260-262.

Keirse MJNC, Chalmers I 1989. Methods for inducing labour. In: Enkin M, Keirse MJNC, Chalmers I, eds. Effective Care in Pregnancy and Childbirth. Oxford: Oxford University Press, pp 1057-1079.

Kurup A, Chua S, Arulkumaran S, Tham KF, Tay D, Ratnam SS, 1991. Induction of labour in nulliparas with poor score: Oxytocin or prostaglandin vaginal pessaries? *Austr NZ J Obstet Gynecol* 31: 223-226.

Lange AP 1986. Induction of labour. In: Bygdeman M, Berger CS, Keith LG, eds. Prostaglandins and their Inhibitors in Clinical Obstetrics and Gynecology. Lancaster: MTP Press. pp. 165-202.

Lelaidier C, Baton C, Benifla JL, Fernandez H, Bourget P, Frydman R 1994. Mifepristone for labour induction after previous caesarean section. *Br J Obstet Gynecol.* 101: 501-503.

Lewis GJ 1983. Cervical ripening before induction of labour with prostaglandin E2 pessaries or a Foley's catheter. *J Obstet Gynecol* 3: 173-176.

MacKenzie IZ, Embrey MP 1978. The influence of pre-induction vaginal prostaglandin E_2 gel upon subsequent labour. *Br J Obstet Gynecol* 86:657-671.

MacKenzie IZ, Embrey MP. 1979. A comparison of PGE$_2$ and PGF$_{2\alpha}$ vaginal gel for ripening the cervix before induction of labour. *Br J Obstet Gynecol* 85: 657-661.

MacKenzie IZ 1990. The therapeutic roles of prostaglandins in Obstetrics. In: Studd JW, ed. Progress in Obstetrics and Gynecology, Vol 8. Oxford: Churchill Livingstone, pp 149-173.

MacKenzie IZ 1993. The unripe cervix and its management for labour induction. *Ann Acad Med Singapore* 22: 151-7

MacKenzie IZ 1994. Labour induction including termination for fetal anomaly. In: James DK, Steer PJ, Weiner CP, Gonik B, eds. High Risk Pregnancy - Management Options. London: WB Saunders, pp. 1041-1060.

MacLennan AH, Green RC, Bryant-Greenwood GD, Greenwood FC, Seamark RF 1980. Ripening of the human cervix and induction of labour with purified porcine relaxin. *Lancet* i: 220-223.

MacPherson M 1984. Comparison of Lamicel with prostaglandin E$_2$ gel as a cervical ripening agent before the induction of labour. *J Obstet Gynecol* 4: 205-206.

Maeda K, Suzumara M 1984. Uterine contraction induction control system. Model DR 300-operation manual. Tokyo (Japan): Toitu Co Ltd.

McNaughton MC 1980. Induction of labour. The case for a high rate. In: Beard RW, Paintin DB, eds. Outcome of Obstetric Intervention in Britain. London: RCOG publication, pp 131-136.

McNay MB, McIlwaine GM, Howie PW, Mc Naughton MC. 1977. Perinatal deaths; analysis by clinical causes to asess values of induction. *BMJ* 1:347 - 350.

O'Driscoll K, Stronqe JM, Minoque M 1973. Active management of labour. *BMJ* 3:135-137.

Orhue AA 1993. A randomised trial of 45 minutes and 15 minutes incremental oxytocin infusion regimes for the induction of labour in women of high parity. *Br J Obstet Gynecol* 100: 126-9.

Parker RB 1957. The results of surgical induction of labour. *J Obstet Gynecol Br Cwlth* 64: 94-112.

Patterson WM 1971. Amniotomy with and without simultaneous oxytocin infusion. *J Obstet Gynecol Br Cwlth* 78:310-316.

Pearson JF, Andrews J 1980, Induction of labour. The case for a low rate. In: Beard RW, Paintin DB, eds. Outcome of Obstetric Intervention in Britain. London: RCOG publication. pp 137-149.

Prasad RNV, Ratnam SS 1987. International colloquy on the management of intrauterine fetal death. *Int J Obstet Gynecol* 25:185-197.

Ratnam SS, Khew KS, Chen C, Lim TC 1974. Oral prostaglandin E$_2$ in induction of labour. *Aust NZ J Obstet Gynecol* 14: 26-30.

Roberts WE, North DH, Speed JE, Martin JN, Palmer SM, Morrison JC 1986. Comparative study of prostaglandin, laminaria and minidose oxytocin for ripening of the unfavourable cervix prior to induction of labour. *J Perinatol* 6: 16-19.

Sanchez-Ramos L, Kaunitz AM, Del-Valle GO, Delke I, Schroeder PA, Briones DK 1993. Labour induction with the prostaglandin E$_1$ methyl analogue misoprostol versus oxytocin: a randomised trial. *Obstet Gynecol* 81: 332-6.

Satin AJ, Leveno KJ, Sherman ML, McIntire D 1994. High-dose oxytocin: 20- versus 40-minute dosage interval. *Obstet Gynecol* 83: 234-8.

Shepherd JH, Bennet MJ, Laurence D, Moore E, Sims CD 1981. Prostaglandin vaginal suppositories: a simple and safe approach to induction of labour. *Obstet Gynecol* 55:596-600.

Steer PJ, Little DJ, Lewis NL, Kelly McM, Beard RW 1975. Uterine activity in induced labour. *Br J Obstet Gynecol* 82: 433-441.

Steer PJ 1977. The measurement and control of uterine contractions. In: Beard RW, Campbell S, eds. The Current Status of Fetal Heart Rate Monitoring and Ultrasound in Obstetrics. London: RCOG, pp 46-48.

Steer PJ, Carter MC, Choong K, Hanson M, Gordon AJ, Pradhan P 1985. A multicentre prospective randomised controlled trial of induction of labour with an automatic closed loop feed back controlled oxytocin infusion system. *Br J Obstet Gynecol* 92:1127-1133.

Swann RO 1958. Induction of labour by stripping membranes. *Obstet Gynecol* 11: 74-78.

Tipton RH, Lewis BV. 1975. Induction of labour and perinatal mortality. *BMJ* 1: 391-393.

Tromans PM, Beazley JM, Shenouda PI 1981. Comparative study of oestradiol and prostaglandin E$_2$ vaginal gel for ripening the unfavourable cervix before induction of labour. *BMJ* 282: 679-681.

Tsakok FHM, Grudzinskas JG, Karim SMM, Ratnam SS 1975. The routine use of oral prostaglandin E$_2$ in induction of labour. *Br J Obstet Gynecol* 82: 894-898.

Turnbull AC, Anderson ABM 1968. Induction of labour. Part II. *J Obstet Gynecol Br Cwlth* 75: 24-31,

Turnbull AC 1976. Cited in Nowlan D. (1976) Obstetricians welcome reversal of trend in cases of induced labour. *Irish Times.* 30 June. p 3.

15

Prelabour Rupture of Membranes

S Chua
S Arulkumaran

Prelabour rupture of membranes (PROM) is associated with significant maternal and neonatal morbidity and/or mortality. It presents the obstetrician with a management dilemma. Despite the amount of research done in this area, there is still no universally accepted policy for management. The exact etiology of PROM is not known, so it cannot be predicted or prevented. It involves poorly understood infective, biochemical and mechanical pathways. Controversies surround the use of steroids, tocolytic drugs and prophylactic antibiotics in the preterm period.

Prelabour rupture of the membranes is the spontaneous breach of the chorioamnion with the release of amniotic fluid, with a latent period before the onset of labour. If the membranes rupture before 37 completed weeks of gestation, it is called preterm prelabour rupture of the membranes (PPROM). The latent period is the time interval between the rupture of the membranes to the onset of labour. The latent period varies on a host of factors like the presence or absence of infection, multiple pregnancy polyhydramnios and, to some degree, the gestational age.

The maternal problem associated with PROM in term pregnancies are risks of cord prolapse, infection and an unfavourable cervix for induction. The latter is associated with a high incidence of dysfunctional labour, chorioamnionitis, an increased rate of caesarean section, postpartum hemorrhage and endomyometritis, while the problems for the new born are those of infection.

In the preterm period, maturity in terms of gestation poses the greatest threat. Gestation of less than 34 weeks poses problems of bronchopulmonory dysplasia (if less than 26 weeks), hyaline membrane disease (leading to respiratory distress syndrome), intraventicular hemorrhage, necrotising enterocolitis, sepsis, other problems associated with prematurity, prolapse of the cord and postural deformities if the PROM to delivery interval is many weeks.

Fetal wastage and neonatal mortality and morbidity is high when PROM occurs in pregnancies of less than 32 weeks. The decision for appropriate management depends upon the assessment of gestational age, the likelihood of infection and the availability of neonatal intensive care facilities.

Incidence

The average incidence is 10%, but it varies from 2–18% (Gunn et al 1970). This wide range is due to a number of variables like the definition of the latent period and the methods used for the diagnosis of PROM. Approximately 60–80% of cases of PROM occur in term pregnancies (Allen 1991).

Although most cases of PROM occur at term, the main cause of concern arises predominantly from the 20 – 40% of cases of preterm PROM that occur before 37 weeks gestation (PPROM). PPROM is the commonest precipitating cause of preterm labour, and contributes disproportionately to the problem of prematurity and low birthweight.

Etiology

PROM usually occurs suddenly and unpredictably. The exact causative factor for PROM is not known. It is the result of a variety of biochemical and mechanical pathways (Polzin and Brady 1991) which cause weakness in the chorioamnion and allow rupture. Membranes from pregnancies associated with PROM are less elastic than normal chorioamniotic membranes (Lonky and Hayashi 1988). It is thought that PROM occurs when the intrauterine pressure is excessive or when intact membranes are weakened by exogenous factors that destroy the connective tissue framework which imparts tensile strength to membranes. Such factors constitute a system of collagenases, proteases and protease inhibiting factors.

Some of the risk factors associated with PROM include infection, polyhydramnios, trauma and an incompetent cervix, but are not present in the majority of cases.

1. *Maternal genital tract infection*

There is a strong association between infection and PROM. Studies have shown an increase in chorioamnionitis in populations with PROM compared to a normal population (Morales et al 1989; Beyduin and Yasin 1986). Additionally, bacteria have been demonstrated in the amniotic fluid before ROM in patients with preterm labour (Gravett et al 1986). The incidence of inflammation in fetal membranes in parturients with PROM is higher when compared with those with spontaneous ROM in labour (Naeye and Peters 1980).

Bacteria (whether an overgrowth of commensal bacteria or infection by pathogenic bacteria) have been shown to cause weakening of the amnion directly by induction of proteases, collagenases and elastases and also indirectly by the activation of the prostaglandin cascade. Neutorophils and other products of the inflammatory response mounted against the bacterial overgrowth also enhance this destruction of the amnion. Thus, chorioamnionitis may be both a cause as well as a sequelae of PROM. A large number of microorganisms including Group B streptococcus, Neisseria gonorrhoea, chlamydia, Trichomonas vaginalis, E coli, bacteriodes, fusobacteria, mycoplasma and ureaplasma have been associated with PROM.

2. *Incompetent cervix*

Mechanical decreased resistance of the cervix and opening of os can lead to less mechanical support of the membranes and chorioamnionitis followed by PROM.

3. *Increased intrauterine pressure*

Increased intrauterine pressure associated with polyhydramnios or multiple pregnancy can result in PROM.

4. *Prenatal diagnostic procedures*

Invasive procedures like amniocentesis or cordocentesis are associated with PROM.

5. *Cervical cerclage*

Placing emergency cervical cerclage in the presence of bulging membranes can puncture the membranes leading to PROM.

6. *Diet and habits*

Deficiency of ascorbic acid, zinc or copper has been incriminated as a cause of PROM. Cigarette smoking is also considered to be a risk factor.

7. *Coitus*

Sexual activity, especially when chorioamnionitis is present, can be a causative factor with spermatozoa helping in the ascending of bacteria. Seminal enzymes or prostaglandins can participate in the process of weakening the membranes and initiating uterine contractions.

8. *Placental pathology*

Placenta previa of a minor degree, abruption or marginal insertion of the cord has been linked to PROM although there is no strong association.

9. *Génetic disorders*

Ehlers-Danlos syndrome is an inherited connective tissue disorder which can cause weakening of the membranes.

10. *Unknown factors*

Most cases fall into this category: A prior history of PROM or preterm delivery could be associated with a possible recurrence.

Diagnosis

Diagnosis of PROM may be difficult either due to the presence of other fluids in the vagina or because there is no fluid. No test is available which can confirm the diagnosis in every case. It may require an integration of the history, physical examination and investigation involving cytological or biochemical methods. Prompt diagnosis is essential for proper management.

1. *History*

A history of sudden gush of fluid from the vagina followed by persistent leakage or constant wetting of the underclothing is suggestive of PROM. The diagnosis is made obvious when there is passage of meconium and/or vernix. Detailed history regarding the time of rupture, the colour of the fluid and associated symptoms like uterine contractions should be noted.

2. Physical examination

Sterile speculum examination usually confirms the diagnosis. Wetting of the vulva and vagina, the presence of an amniotic fluid pool in the posterior fornix and fluid emerging through the cervix provides the most reliable diagnosis. If the fluid cannot be seen, the patient can be asked to cough or strain (Vulsalva manoeuvre) which will help to provide the diagnosis. If in spite of all these methods fluid is still not seen, the woman is asked to constantly wear a pad. When soaked, the pad can be examined clinically and chemically by using colour change to a nitrazine stick to confirm the leak of amniotic fluid.

Opinion is divided as to whether vaginal examination introduces infection or intrauterine infection. A careful, sterile speculum examination should be carried out in all women with prelabour rupture of membranes to confirm the rupture of membranes, and fetal presentation, to exclude cord prolapse, and to assess cervical dilatation and effacement. Such examination also permits a cervical swab to be taken for bacteriological studies and the collection of the amniotic fluid for culture and for determination of the lecithin-sphingomyelin ratio or similar tests. Some advocate that all vaginal examinations, whether by gloved fingers or by speculum, should be avoided unless women are in active labour. A digital examination is best avoided if the decision has been to manage the pregnancy conservatively. There is insufficient data from controlled trials to identify the consequences of the alternative policies.

3. Investigations

Amniotic fluid must be differentiated from urine and cervical/vaginal secretions. There are a variety of tests which have been developed specifically for this purpose.

a. Nitrazine paper / Litmus paper test   Amniotic fluid is alkaline with a pH of 7.0 – 7.5. Nitrazine paper which is orange in colour turns blue when it comes in contact with alkaline fluid. Similarly, red litmus paper turns blue when in contact with amniotic fluid. False positive reactions may occur due to alkalinisation of the vagina by blood, semen, soap, antiseptic, infected urine and infection with Trichomonas or bacterial vaginosis.

b. Arborisation test   When the fluid from the vagina is dried on the slide and examined under the microscope, the formation of a fern pattern confirms the presence of amniotic fluid. Many studies have shown that the test has a sensitivity of 96 – 99%, a specificity of 96 – 98% and a negative predictive value of 90 – 99% (Davidson 1991).

c. Microscopy of fluid   The gross presence of specks of vernix caseosa and the microscopic detection of lanugo hair in the fluid from the vagina will confirm the presence of amniotic fluid.

d. Cytological methods for the detection of fetal cells in amniotic fluid   S o m e of these tests employ cytological methods for the detection of fetal cells (flourescence microscopy, Papanicolaou smear, staining for lipids in cells: Sudan III, Nile blue sulphate) in amniotic fluid. When the amniotic fluid is treated with Nile blue sulphate, fetal cells with a higher fat content take an orange colour stain against a blue background. But this test may not be reliable in cases of very preterm PROM as the percentage of the fetal cells with fat increase in the fluid only with an increase in gestational age.

e. Ultrasound   Ultrasound where available can play an important role in suggesting the diagnosis and management of PROM. It helps in the detection of oligohydramnios associated with PROM. Its further role is in the detection of gestational age, the weight of the baby and any congenital abnormality. The presentation and lie of the fetus can be confirmed and fetal health assessed by the biophysical profile. However ultrasound estimation of amniotic fluid volume in utero does not correlate with the presence or absence of PROM (Robson et al 1990).

f. Dye tests   The administration of certain dyes like indigo carmine, Evan's blue and sodium fluorescent into the amniotic sac causes staining of the pad with dye, which confirms the diagnosis. This test is usually not needed and the procedure is invasive with the associated risks of introducing infection and inducing preterm labour.

Methods to quantify alphafetoprotein, uric acid, protein and creatinine, which are present in amniotic fluid in higher concentrations than in urine, vaginal or seminal fluid, have all been used with varying degrees of accuracy to distinguish between intact and ruptured membranes.

Management

Management of prelabour rupture of the membranes is mainly based upon the presence or absence of intrauterine infection and the gestation at which PROM occurs. Evidence of infection at any gestation warrants early delivery of the fetus with appropriate antibiotic cover for the mother and the newborn. Cord prolapse will also warrant delivery by the appropriate route based on gestational maturity and cervical dilatation; usually being caesarean section in a viable fetus.

Once infection and cord prolapse are excluded in a case with a live fetus with no known fetal abnormalities, the gestation has to be confirmed. If preterm, attempts can be made to determine lung maturity. The patient should be observed for development of chorioamnionitis and signs of fetal distress. Determination of lie and presentation are of importance for the decision on the mode of delivery should labour start or should infection set in.

Estimation of gestational age

Gestational age should be calculated from the last menstrual period. If the dates are not certain then uterine size, a pregnancy test and ultrasound performed in early pregnancy should help to arrive at the dates. An ultrasound examination done on admission should determine the amount of liquor, the number of fetuses, any congenital abnormality, and the presentation and lie of the fetus. Estimated fetal weight by clinical and/or ultrasound fetal parameters will give some idea of the 'fetal maturity' which will help in planning the management.

Estimation of fetal lung maturity

Fetal lung maturity is determined by taking the amniotic fluid from the vaginal pool and determining the lecithin sphingomyelin ratio. A ratio of 2:1 or more confirms the lung maturity. The determination of L/S ratio from the vaginal pool is not entirely reliable and estimation of phosphatidyl glycerol may be more confirmatory.

Monitoring for chorioamnionitis

Chorioamnionitis refers to the microbial invasion of the fetal membranes which may lead to their being infected and subsequently the amniotic cavity as well. This is associated with maternal and neonatal sepsis and can become a life threatening condition. Once the chorioamnionitis is confirmed, prompt termination of pregnancy is required, irrespective of gestational age. Clinical manifestation includes maternal fever, fetal and/or maternal tachycardia, uterine tenderness, foul smelling vaginal discharge and maternal leucocytosis. Preclinical occult infection may be detected by abdominal amniocentesis. The amniotic fluid is obtained and examined microscopically for the presence of bacteria by doing Gram's staining. The fluid can also be sent for cultures and an antibiotic sensitivity test. Amniocentesis is not popular because it is an invasive procedure and in addition there may be failure of collection of fluid in cases with oligohydramnios. Rise in the leucocyte count and the level of C reactive protein in the maternal blood can predict infection as it precedes the onset of symptoms but in clinical practice it has not been found to be consistently useful.

The biophysical profile is of interest in the detection of fetal infection. Intra-amniotic infection affects fetal behaviour which leads to decreased body and breathing movements and an increased fetal heart rate. This reduces the biophysical profile score. Clinical observation of reduced fetal movements and fetal tachycardia should be a warning for the possibility of infection.

Monitoring for fetal distress

Signs of fetal distress like meconium stained amniotic fluid, an abnormal fetal heart rate pattern either on auscultation or on electronic fetal monitoring (tachycardia and cord compression variable decelerations) or abnormal biophysical profile should cause concern and expedite prompt termination of pregnancy if the fetus is viable. If there is suspicion of infection termination must be carried out irrespective of gestational age.

Determination of lie and presentation

Confirmation of lie and presentation will effect the mode of delivery. The aim should be to achieve vaginal delivery wherever possible. Abnormal lie and presentation may necessitate a caesarean section if there is an indication for delivery like the onset of labour, infection, cord prolapse or fetal distress.

Management of PROM at term

Prelabour rupture of the membranes at term is defined as spontaneous rupture of the membranes after 37 weeks of gestation and before the onset of regular painful contractions. It occurs in 3 – 10% of term deliveries (Grant and Keirse 1989).

Management of term PROM varies in different institutions. About 80% of women at term with PROM go into spontaneous labour within 24 – 48 hrs and only a minority of patients (10–25%) have a latent period from PROM to the onset of labour of more than 24 hr (Duff et al 1984; Gunn et al 1970; Kappy et al 1979). If the latent period is prolonged beyond 24 hr, the chance of infection increases. In the early sixties several investigators reported a significant increase in perinatal loss (Johnson et al 1981; Shubeck et al 1966), maternal morbidity (Lanier et al 1965; Russel and Anderson 1962) and even maternal deaths associated with PROM in term pregnancy (Johnson et al 1981; Webb 1967). These studies prompted a policy of immediate stimulation of labour after PROM at term, and whenever possible, delivery within 24 hr (Lanier et al 1965; Russel et al 1962). Such a policy, carried out usually by the administration of intravenous oxytocin in order to stimulate labour, has since been widely adopted in term pregnancies.

Controversies in the management of PROM at term

The case for expectant management

Much of the fear previously experienced with regard to infectious morbidity in term PROM has been overplayed in today's context. Many of the studies documenting an increase in infection rates for the mother and the fetus were retrospective studies, and lacked bacteriological confirmation of infection. The high rates of infectious morbidity and mortality in the early 1960s could have been due to factors other than the prolonged latent period, for example, host factors, repeated vaginal examination prior to the onset of labour and general patient activity. But a more important reason was that clinical chorioamnionitis was not diagnosed at an early stage of its development and once it was made, effective treatment as we know it today was often not instituted (broad spectrum antibiotics and termination of pregnancy within a reasonable period of time). The changing prognosis of PROM at term in the 1990s is readily apparent. The incidence of severe complications for both mother and baby has decreased markedly in recent years even after chorioamnionitis has set in (Koh et al 1979; Garite and Freeman 1982; Yoder et al 1983). In more recently conducted studies of PROM at term, maternal mortality is almost unknown, and even perinatal death from infection is rare (Yoder et al 1983).

Most women with PROM at term will go into labour soon after the membranes rupture; 69% will deliver within 24 hours and 86% will do so within 48 hours; 2–5% of women will remain undelivered after 72 hours and the same proportion will remain undelivered after seven days. The latter group probably represent a high risk group, with possible underlying dystocia (Grant et al 1989), and cervical dilatation is slow with conventional means of induction with oxytocin infusion.

Evidence has been presented that a conservative approach without stimulation, especially in patients with an unfavourable cervix might be justified (Duff et al 1984; Kappy et al 1979; Kappy et al 1982; Van der Walt and Venter 1989; Duncan and Beckley 1992; Grant et al 1992). The meta-analysis of the clinical trials published in the Oxford perinatal database (Grant et al 1989) suggests that active management by stimulation of labour with oxytocin leads to an increase in caesarean section and a longer and presumably less comfortable labour in the induced group. The overall rate of serious maternal and neonatal infection in the trials was very low (< 1%), but the meta-analysis suggests that there is a slightly increased risk of maternal infection with a routine policy of induction of labour. However there was no effect on neonatal infection with either form of treatment. Similarly, a recent review of the results of 12 trials of active management of PROM at 37+ weeks (Hannah 1993) indicates that active management at 37+ weeks is associated with a higher caesarean section rate, a lower risk of endomyometritis and a lower risk of neonatal infection than a policy of expectant management. These studies, which compared outcomes following expectant and immediate stimulation policies, excluded patients who had any medical or obstetric complications of pregnancy that warranted immediate intervention. Labour was stimulated promptly if evidence of maternal infection occurred, and efforts were made to minimise the number of vaginal examinations in early labour.

The case for immediate stimulation of labour

Recently conducted clinical trials have shown an increased need for caesarean section when labour was stimulated in term PROM, especially in the group of nulliparae with unfavourable cervices (Duff et al 1984; Morales et al 1986; Van der Walt and Venter 1989; Grant and Keirse 1989). However most centres still advocate stimulation of labour in term PROM because of reports of the association of delay between membrane rupture and delivery with an increased risk of sepsis and perinatal morbidity. In addition, immediate stimulation gives the patient a definite time frame for management and makes it unnecessary for her to go through the anxiety of uncertainty while waiting for events to occur.

In contrast to the studies which show a better outcome with expectant management, Rydhstrom et al (1991) found no benefit from conservative management for up to three days in women with PROM at term, compared with immediate stimulation of labour. There was a tendency to an increased rate of obstetric intervention in labour in the group treated conservatively. The neonatal infectious morbidity was slightly higher in the cases managed conservatively. These findings are in line with those of other studies (Wagner et al 1989) of delayed stimulation of labour in PROM at term. Comparative studies have shown no benefit from an overnight conservative policy and stimulation of labour next morning compared with immediate stimulation of labour (Arulkumaran et al 1988).

If an aggressive approach to PROM at term is practised, it appears that stimulation is more likely to be more successful if the cervix is favourable. A prospective study of 303 women from two different parts of the world showed that in nulliparae with an unfavourable cervix, the immediate use of oxytocics was associated with a higher rate of instrumental and caesarean delivery particularly for failed stimulation of labour (Rydhstrom et al 1986). A higher rate of ominous fetal heart rate changes in labour was also found in the group, compared with nulliparae with a favourable cervix, or in multiparae. When categorised by parity and a cervical score, nulliparae with a poor cervical score do poorly compared with multiparae and nulliparae with good scores, whether these women have been stimulated immediately, or managed by a policy of overnight conservatism (Arulkumaran et al 1988). Based on the studies available an immediate stimulation policy with oxytocin infusion appears to be a reasonable approach in multiparae and nulliparae with a good score. This will minimise the risk of infection or occasional cord complication without an increase in the caesarean section rate.

The use of prostaglandin in cases of PROM

Many trials have compared the obstetric outcome that follows stimulation of labour with prostaglandin as opposed to oxytocin in PROM at term, especially in nulliparae. In three of the older studies (Hauth et al 1977; Lange et al 1981; Westergaard et al 1983) oral PGE$_2$ tablets were compared with oxytocin for stimulation of labour. All three studies found that oral PGE$_2$ was a safe method for stimulation of labour, although gastrointestinal side effects were present in this group. Lange et al (1981) and Westergaard et al (1983) concluded that intravenous oxytocin was the drug of choice for stimulation of labour when compared with oral PGE$_2$ or oral oxytocin.

In subsequent trials, PGE$_2$ administered vaginally either as a pessary (Magos et al 1983; Van der Walt and Venter 1989; Chua et al 1991; Granstrom et al 1987; Ray and Garite 1992; Chua et al 1995) or as a gel (Eckman-Ordeberg et al 1985; Mahmood et al 1992; Chung et al 1992) was compared with intravenous oxytocin for stimulation of labour after PROM at term. Based on these trials, there appears to be no consensus as to whether the use of vaginal prostaglandin conferred any benefit over the use of intravenous oxytocin in terms of obstetric or neonatal outcome when both agents were used a few hours after PROM. Meta-analysis of recent trials shows a tendency (which is not statistically significant) for a reduced caesarean section rate with the use of vaginal prostaglandins compared with intravenous oxytocin at 37+ weeks (Hannah 1993).There was no difference in the incidence of infectious morbidity in the mother and baby when stimulation of labour was carried out with vaginal prostaglandins compared with oxytocin infusion. When meta-analysis included trials where prostaglandins were compared with oxytocin for PROM at 34+ weeks (Hannah 1993), results showed that active management with prostaglandins (with or without oxytocin) for PROM resulted in a lower caesarean section rate compared to when oxytocin was used. The use of prostaglandins did not appear to be associated with a higher or lower risk of other adverse maternal or fetal outcomes compared with the use of oxytocin (Hannah 1993).

Nulliparae with an unfavourable cervix

The subgroup of patients with PROM at term who are nulliparae and have an unfavourable cervix have a high caesarean delivery rate when labour is stimulated with oxytocin infusion on admission (Rydhstrom et al 1986; Van der Walt and Venter 1989; Duff et al 1984). When managed conservatively, those who become established in spontaneous labour fare well, although a significant proportion of those who require stimulation of labour after overnight conservative management require caesarean section for dystocia (Conway et al 1984). Conservative management as opposed to immediate stimulation with oxytocin has been reported to reduce the caesarean rate and infectious morbidity (Kappy et al 1979; Van der Walt et al 1989). However teaching and reports from large retrospective series suggest increased maternal and neonatal infectious morbidity with unlimited conservative management in term pregnancies (Johnson et al 1981).

Prostaglandins are claimed to give a better obstetric outcome. Eckman-Ordeberg et al (1985) studied 20 nulliparous women with a poor cervical score in their randomised trial and concluded that the use of 4 mg PGE$_2$ gel gave better results than oxytocin, both agents being used a few hours after admission. Van der Walt et al (1989) randomised 60 patients at term who had PROM and an unfavourable cervix to receive three treatment modalities. They compared expectant management, oxytocin stimulation by infusion and use of PGE$_2$ vaginal tablets for cervical ripening/stimulation of labour, and concluded that prostaglandin induced cervical ripening is the method of choice in handling term patients with PROM and an unfavourable cervix. In a more recent study (Chua et al 1991), 94 nulliparous women with a poor cervical score who had PROM at term were randomised either for immediate stimulation of labour with oxytocin infusion or for two PGE$_2$ 3 mg pessaries 4 hours apart, followed by oxytoicn infusion 4 hours later if regular painful contractions and progressive cervical changes were not observed. The results showed that the interval between the initiation of therapy to the onset of labour was significantly longer in the PG group, although the length of labour was similar in both groups. The caesarean delivery rate was not significantly different in the two groups. The incidence of maternal and neonatal infectious morbidity was small and not significantly different in the two groups.

In similar studies conducted by Mahmood et al (1992) the caesarean section rate with the use of PGE$_2$ was 12%, which is half the caesarean section rate observed in the study by Chua et al(1991). Other authors have also reported less than 10% caesarean section rate in the groups treated with PGE$_2$ (Granstrom et al 1987; Van der Walt and Venter 1989). The reason for such a reduction may have been due to the fact that PGE$_2$ gels were left to act for 18 – 24 hours compared with only 8 hours given in the trial by Chua et al (1991). In a subsequent double blind randomised trial of prostaglandin versus placebo study in the same centre, 155 women with PROM after 36 weeks and an unfavourable cervical score were randomised to receive either a PGE$_2$ 3 mg vaginal pessary or an identical placebo pessary. If labour did not start after 12 hours, it was stimulated with oxytocin. In this study, when labour was not stimulated until 12 hours after admission to the study, the caesarean section rate was not statistically significantly less in the PG group (13.9%) compared with the group of women who received a placebo (15.8%) (Chua et al 1995). However the caesarean section rates were lower than that in a similar population in the previous study when labour was stimulated immediately on admission (14.9% in the group stimulated immediately with oxytocin and 19.1% in the group who had 2 PGE$_2$ pessaries inserted 4 hours apart followed by oxytocin infusion 4 hours later).

Role of prophylactic amnioinfusion

Intrapartum prophylactic amnioinfusion refers to infusing normal saline at an appropriate rate into the amniotic cavity to augment amniotic fluid volume. The idea is to prevent cord compression due to oligohydramnios and hence to decrease the incidence of variable decelerations of the fetal heart rate pattern and thus the operative delivery rate. This method is still experimental and should not be encouraged till further evidence accumulates regarding its beneficial and harmful effects.

Role of prophylactic antibiotics

Older trials (Lebherz et al 1963; Brelje et al 1966) in the 1960s failed to show any reduction in the incidence of fetal and neonatal infection after the use of prophylactic antibiotics for the mother. Brelje et al, using nitrofurazone pessaries in the antenatal period, did not show any decreased risk of amnionitis in the treated group when compared with the untreated group. However Leberz et al have showed a decrease in postpartum infection in the mother when dimethylchlorotetracycline was used prophylactically in the antenatal, intrapartum and postnatal periods. In these trials, antibiotics were utilised which would be contraindicated today. Unfortunately there have been no large properly controlled trials recently to show that women and babies without overt signs of infection after PROM at term benefit by antibiotic prophylaxis.

The main cause of intrauterine infection with PROM is ascending infection from the vagina into the uterine cavity. Information on the presence of bacteria which cause fetal and neonatal infections would be useful in the treatment of these patients. However the demonstration of vaginal colonisation with bacteria does not mean that intrauterine or fetal infection will follow, and the necessity and efficacy of treating all patients prophylactically is debatable. In a retrospective study of 117 patients with PROM at term, 4 infants developed septicaemia, and all the four mothers, though asymptomatic, grew Group B beta streptococcus in the high vaginal swabs taken on admission with PROM (Chua et al 1995). Screening for Group B beta streptococcus (GBS) colonisation would be helpful if intrapartum antibiotics prevent the transmission of infection from mother to baby. Data from a meta-analysis of five randomised controlled trials have demonstrated a major reduction in GBS colonisation in infants born to mothers treated with intrapartum antibiotics compared with infants of mothers in the control group. The incidence of sepsis in infants with GBS was reduced in the treated groups in the three trials that reported sepsis rates (Wang and Smaill 1989). The available data also show a reduction in neonatal deaths from infection. As intrapartum prophylaxis of colonised pregnant women offers the possibility of reducing the incidence of infant sepsis, rapid methods for identifying GBS in women with PROM would be useful.

A protocol for management of PROM at term

The treatment for term PROM can be immediate stimulation of labour or expectant management depending upon the parity, the favourability of the cervical score and the presence or absence of chorioamnionitis. Cord prolapse or fetal distress warrants immediate delivery. The following protocol of management may be observed when women come with PROM at term.

  a. Speculum examination to confirm PROM. Amniotic fluid should be checked for meconium and sent for culture/sensitivity. Cord prolapse should be excluded and cervical effacement and dilatation noted.

  b. Exclude chorioamnionitis based on clinical findings. If it is present or suspected to be present, immediate stimulation under broad spectrum antibiotic cover with a view to early delivery is advisable.

  c. If the cervical score is favourable, early induction of labour should be considered as there is little to be gained by an extended period of observation. Increased duration of the latent period increases the risk of maternal and neonatal infection and the minimal risk of cord prolapse.

  d. If the cervical score is not favourable and there is no medical or obstetrical indication for intervention, then expectant treatment is recommended. Spontaneous labour should be awaited for up to 24 hours followed by oxytocic stimulation. If chorioamnionitis develops then labour should be induced promptly. Priming the cervix with local prostaglandins followed 12 – 24 hours later by oxytocin infusion is an alternative approach to the expectant policy in the absence of infection.

e. Any evidence of infection or positive bacterial culture needs antibiotic therapy for the mother and the new born. Prophylactic antibiotics given to the mother in labour if the latent period (PROM to delivery interval) is > 12 hr reduces the incidence of maternal infection. The newborn should be referred to the pediatrician to exclude infection, to be observed for infection and for prophylactic antibiotic therapy.

Preterm PROM (PPROM)

The incidence of preterm PROM in the pregnant population is about 1% (Gibbs and Blanco 1982). However, if elective preterm deliveries, fetal death before labour, and twin pregnancies are excluded, the incidence among women who deliver prematurely ranges between 40% and 60% (Kierse et al 1989). Despite the high prevalence, knowledge of the etiology and pathophysiology of PPROM is limited, and there is a lack of consensus as to how best to manage these patients. Unlike the risks of PROM at term (infection and cord prolapse versus iatrogenic complications of aggressive management), the risks to the preterm infant involve the risks of prematurity if delivered early against infection if there is delay in delivery after rupture of the membranes.

The most common consequence of PPROM is preterm delivery. Irrespective of gestational age, a delay of more than one week will be achieved by less than half the women, ranging from (< 40% when PROM occurs at less than 24 weeks to < 20% when PROM occurs at less than 34 weeks (Keirse et al 1989). It is generally accepted that the principal threat to the fetus in PPROM is from the consequences of prematurity.

Infectious morbidity, mostly due to ascending intrauterine infection, is the second most important hazard for the baby. However unlike PROM which occurs at term, the incidence of amnionitis and perinatal mortality or neonatal sepsis does not appear to increase with increasing duration of PPROM, provided that differences in gestational ages and race are taken into account (Schreiber and Benedetti 1980; Johnson et al 1981; Wilson et al 1982; Vintzileos et al 1986). The infant's ultimate chances of survival are related more to the gestational age at delivery than to the gestational age at rupture of the membrnaes (Taylor and Garite 1984).

Other consequences of PROM in the preterm include increased risks of pulmonory hypoplasia, especially with very preterm PROM, deformities associated with persistent oligohydramnios, placental abruption, umbilical cord complications immediately on PROM and when labour supervenes, as well as mechanical difficulties at caesarean section which may occur due to decreased amniotic fluid and an underdeveloped lower uterine segment.

Assessment

PROM in the preterm period may be associated with a variety of maternal, fetal and obstetric problems which are more common in women delivering preterm than

Flow chart – showing management of PROM at term

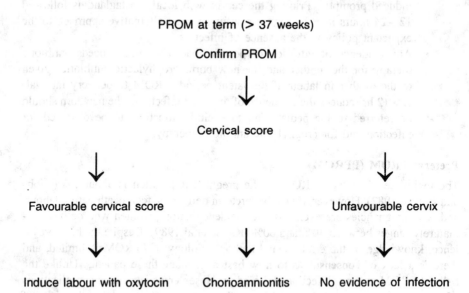

PROM at term (> 37 weeks)

Confirm PROM

↓

Cervical score

Favourable cervical score   Unfavourable cervix

Induce labour with oxytocin   Chorioamnionitis   No evidence of infection

Delivery   Antibiotics and prompt   Expectant treatment for
                induction with oxytocin   12 – 24 hours. OR use
                infusion with the view   of local prostaglandins
                to early delivery   followed 12 – 24 hrs later
                                          by oxytocin infusion.
                                          Observe for infection
                                          and onset of labour

                                          Delivery

in those delivering at term. Careful asseesssment of the fetal and maternal condition should be made before different treatment options are put into practice.

Confirming ROM

It is important to confirm rupture of the membranes, as subsequent management is based on the premise that diagnosis of PPROM has been established. An incorrect diagnosis can subject the patient to the iatrogenic risks of preterm delivery, tocolysis, corticosteroids and caesarean section. The various tests for confirmation of ROM have been mentioned previously.

Establishing the gestational age

Accurate assessment of the fetal gestational age is pivotal in the decision-making process with PPROM. Careful history and physical examination, are often sufficient to date the pregnancy. An ultrasound scan may be helpful, not only to measure fetal parameters, but also to determine the fetal position, to measure liquor volume, and in rare cases, to uncover an unexpected fetal anomaly. Oligohydramnios may distort the measurements of the fetal head and abdomen, and several studies have reported a marked underestimation of fetal weight in PPROM, especially when oligohydramnios is present (Bottoms et al 1987; Asrat and Garite 1991). Other investigators have found no difference in accuracy in the ultrasound estimation of fetal weight in these circumstances (Valea et al 1990; Benaceraff et al 1988). Incorporating the measurement of long bones into formulae for estimation of the fetal weight has improved the predictive value of ultrasonic fetal weight measurements significantly (Asrat and Garite 1991).

Assessing fetal lung maturity

On the basis of gestational age alone, it is possible to identify a fetus that has attained a level of maturity that for practical purposes differs little from the fetus at term. There is also little difficulty in identifying the immature and previable fetus. It is in the fetus which is between these two extremes, most typically between 26 and 34 weeks, that the problems of assessing relative maturity are most difficult.

Fetal pulmonory maturity can be tested by assessing the fetal lung profile from amniotic fluid which can be obtained from the vaginal pool and sent for phosphotidylglycerol analysis. The vaginal pool lecithin : spingomyelin ratio is unreliable as it may be altered by contamination with blood, semen and meconium. Amniotic fluid may also be obtained transabdominally, via amniocentesis, although this is a more invasive procedure, and reports of its success rates in PPROM vary between 50 and 97% (Asrat and Garite 1991).

Even if pulmonary maturity is demonstrated, the necessity for delivering a premature fetus is questionable, because these infants are still prone to other complications of prematurity such as necrotising enterocolitis, intraventricular hemorrhage, and prolonged hospitalisation. The argument in favour of delivering such fetuses is that maternal and perinatal infection may be avoided. Also, when pulmonary maturity is demonstrated, invasive and controversial measures to promote maturity with corticosteroid administration can then be regarded as superfluous. A prospective randomised trial (Cotton et al 1984) showed that amniocentesis for assessing fetal pulmonary maturity could play a beneficial role in the active management of patients who present with PPROM between 32 and 34 weeks gestation. The same view is not shared by many because of the failure in obtaining samples, the invasive nature of the procedure and the tendency to stimulate preterm labour.

Excluding evidence of infection

Any evidence of maternal or fetal infection precludes any treatment option other than immediate delivery of the fetus. Clinical signs of fulminant chorioamnionitis include fever, maternal tachycardia, fetal tachycardia, foul smelling purulent amniotic fluid and a tender uterus. The main aim should be to detect intrauterine infection in its incipient stages, and the earliest clinical signs appear to be a fetal tachycardia and a mild elevation of maternal temperature although both signs are non-specific. Leukocytosis is a reliable but non-specific laboratory marker of on-going infection. Estimation of C-reactive protein in the maternal circulation has been touted for many years as a reliable early sign of intrauterine infection; however this test has not lived up to these hopes in controlled trials (Fisk et al 1991).

When intrauterine infection does develop in PPROM, this is usually from the vagina into the uterine cavity. A high vaginal swab may indicate colonisation of the vagina with organisms pathogenic to the fetus. However care should be taken not to equate colonisation with infection (see below, section on prophylactic antibiotics).

Analysis of the amniotic fluid obtained by amniocentesis is a widely practised method to determine the presence or absence of bacteria in the amniotic cavity. Several authors have documented the statistically significant association of positive Gram stains or cultures from amniotic fluid with subsequent chorioamnionitis and neonatal infection (Mead 1983; Garite and Freeman 1982; Romero et al 1988). However there are problems associated with amniocentesis in PPROM, in that the success rate for obtaining an adequate sample of amniotic fluid may be as low as 50% (Asrat and Garite 1991), and there are the risks of performing the procedure in PPROM where oligohydramnios compounds the complications (such as trauma to the fetus, bleeding, infection, amniotic fluid leakage) associated with this invasive procedure. There is also the possibility that although the initial culture is negative, infection can set in within a short period even prior to when the culture report of the fluid becomes available. In many studies, most women with positive amniotic fluid cultures deliver before the results of the culture are known. The amniotic fluid Gram stain has a high false negative rate showing bacteria in only 50–65% of cases where ultimately the cultures were positive (Asrat and Garite 1991), and this may be related to the colony counts per ml of amniotic fluid. Conversely, bacteria is not always absent in women without infection (Keirse et al 1989). The presence of bacteria in the amniotic fluid obtained by transabdominal amniocentesis has correlated well with the development of amnionitis and postpartum endometritis, but not with fetal and neonatal sepsis (Cotton et al 1984; Vintzileos et al 1986).

The variable success of amniocentesis led several investigators to use biophysical profiles in the evaluation of the fetus for infection in the presence of PPROM (Asrat and Garite 1991; Vintzileos et al 1991). These trials show the fetus to behave differently when intraamniotic infection develops. However the trials are small and as yet there have been no large adequately controlled trials that show that information obtained from biophysical profile testing can be used reliably to predict incipient intrauterine infection.

Prophylactic antibiotics

There is evidence that infection plays a major role in some instances of PPROM, and that infection may be silent or subclinical. Other investigators contend that infection is merely a consequence and not a cause of PPROM (Maxwell 1993). Whichever the case, ascending intrauterine infection after PPROM is a recognised cause of maternal and perinatal mortality and morbidity. The incidence of chorioamnionitis ranges from 4–28% of women with prolonged PROM and the incidence of neonatal infection ranges from 2–19% (Amon et al 1988). If infection is a cause or contributing factor in PPROM or a complication that develops after ROM and triggers the onset of labour, the use of antibiotics may help to arrest infection and postpone labour, which will benefit women and infants.

Results with such managment in individual trials are conflicting (Greenberg and Hankins 1991). Some of these trials are old (Lebherz et al 1963; Brelje et al 1966) and the antibiotics which were utilised are not in use today. However evidence from the meta-analysis of existing randomised trials of antibiotic prophylaxis for PPROM point to a significant reduction in the risk of preterm delivery within one week of entry (Crowley 1994). There is also a significant decrease in maternal and neonatal infection in those treated prophylactically with antibiotics after PPROM. This reduction in neonatal infection coupled with the prolonged latent period between ROM and delivery might be expected to increase neonatal survival and reduce morbidity due to RDS. However no improvement in neonatal survival has been shown. This may be because the benefit of prolonging the latent period in utero may be offset by some other adverse effect such as infection with resistant organisms or fungi. Other confounding factors related to prolongation of pregnancy and infectious complications include oligohydramnios, the gestational age at which PPROM occurs and the use of tocolysis and steroids. It is hoped that a multicentre randomised trial which is in progress (ORACLE) will have sufficient power to assess whether the prolongation of the latent period between rupture of the membranes and delivery improves neonatal morbidity and mortality. In the majority of more recent trials ampicillin (or erythromycin if the patient is allergic to ampicillin) was selected for its broad spectrum activity against genital tract pathogens, and specifically group B hemolytic streptococcus, which is responsible for the majority of fetal and neonatal infections.

Colonisation of the vagina with organisms such as group B sterptococcus, E coli and bacteroides does not mean that intrauterine infection will occur. Disease secondary to infection with group B streptococcus occurs in only 1–2% of colonised infants and is directly related to the number of sites colonised and the quantity of bacteria recovered from each site (Siegel and McCracken 1981). Infants with birthweights of less than 2,500 g were observed to have a much higher attack rate, 7.9 per 1,000 births compared to 1.9 per 1,000 births of infants weighing 2,500 g or more (Wang and Smaill 1989). However it appears that treatment during pregnancy, unless continued into labour, has only a transient effect on the vaginal flora, and will not influence the rate of infant sepsis. It is quite likely that screening during pregnancy and treatment of carriers may not eliminate the transmission of GBS disease (Anthony 1982). There is also the worry that prolonged treatment with antibiotics may perhaps encourage the growth of resistant strains of bacteria.

The role of prophylactic antibiotics remains controversial in cases of PPROM in the absence of infection. It is of little value to give antibiotics for an indefinite period. However because of recent evidence that prophylactic antibiotics may help to postpone the onset of preterm labour of up to 7 days, it may be wise to give a short course of antibiotics of up to 7 days' duration from the time of PROM and during labour.

Antibiotics are used in the following conditions:

1. Confirmed cases of chorioamnionitis
2. Preclinical or occult infection in the presence of positive culture of micro-organisms from the amniotic fluid.
3. Colonisation of the vagina with Group B streptococci infection (and in these cases antibiotic therapy should be continued through labour).
4. During labour if PROM to delivery interval is $\geq$ 12 hr.

The commonly used antibiotics are ampicillin or erythromycin. Metronidazole can be used in combination to cover anerobes after the delivery of the neonate.

Tocolytics

The rationale for using tocolytics in the presence of PPROM is to forestall delivery, either indefinitely as long as signs and symptoms of fetal distress, chorioamnionitis and other complications are not present, or for a short period of time to permit the action of corticosteroids.

The results of studies on the efficacy of tocolytics in the presence of PPROM are mixed (Harlass 1991). This may be because of the small numbers in most studies, different study populations, different definitions of latent periods, different end points and other confounding variables like whether corticosteroids were administered.

Two small prospective investigations showed prolongation of pregnancy for at least 24 – 48 hrs significantly more often in the treated than in the control group (Christensen et al 1980; Levy and Warsof 1985). However they did not show any significant difference in the incidence of hyaline membrane disease, birthweight or neonatal and maternal infection. Other prospective investigations (Garite et al 1987; Weiner et al 1988) did not show significant prolongation of pregnancy in patients treated with tocolytics. All these studies used beta mimetic drugs or magnesium sulphate for tocolysis.

The prostaglandin synthetase inhibitors and calcium channel blockers are potent uterine relaxants, with mild and reversible maternal and fetal side effects when used in patients in preterm labour with intact membranes. Zuckerman et al (1974) were able to stop uterine contraction in 40 of 50 patients with preterm labour using indomethicin. Of the 50 patients, 13 had ruptured membranes. No significant diffference in tocolysis was demonstrated between patients with intact membranes versus patients with PPROM. The prostaglandin synthetase inhibitors hold promise for effective tocolysis if warranted in PPROM. However it should be remembered that it may cause oliguria and oligohydramnios and if continued for a long period it may affect the fetal circulation with fetal cardiac failure.

From these controlled trials there is no evidence that tocolytics are effective in prolonging pregnancy in the presence of preterm PROM beyond the critical period of 24 hours, whether they are given prophylactically or during preterm labour after PROM (Keirse 1994). Although maternal and fetal infectious morbidity do not appear to be significantly increased with tocolysis compared with controls, care must be used in selecting cases when the use of tocolytics is warranted, in order to minimise the complications associated with the use of these agents in the presence of PPROM.

Infection has to be excluded prior to inhibition of labour as it might be the cause of the onset of labour. Further, tachycardia in the fetus and mother may be due to the tocolytic drug and may mask the tachycardia due to infection. Tocolysis is usually advised for 24 – 48 hrs if steroids are administered, for the steroid effect to take place. Tocolysis should not be used for repeated inhibition of labour in cases of PPROM since it may mask infection.

Corticosteroids

Steroid administration in the presence of PPROM begs two questions: 1) Is steroid administration superfluous because ROM in itself accelerates fetal lung maturity? 2) Is steroid administration hazardous as it increases the risk of maternal and fetal infection in the presence of PPROM, especially if infection is already present as either the cause or result of ROM? There is also the fear that steroids may mask the signs and symptoms associated with chorioamnionitis, thereby causing delay in diagnosis and management.

A review of the literature (Mead 1983) found an approximately equal weight of evidence supporting and refuting the claim that PROM per se accelerates fetal lung maturity. Berkowitz et al (1978) have also presented evidence that the protective effect of PROM, if any, is proportional to the duration of membrane rupture.

Irrespective of any effect PROM itself may have on fetal lung maturity, is the incidence of the respiratory distress syndrome significantly reduced by corticosteroid administration? There are many randomised prospective trials on the use of steroids in patients with PPROM (Eriksen and Blanco 1991). Seven trials incorporated patients with PROM and preterm labour; treatment regimens varied between different trials. Dexamethasone and betamethasone were the two corticosteroids used in most trials, although Iams et al (1985) used hydrocortisone in their treatment arm and Schmidt et al (1984) randomised their treatment group to receive either hydrocortisone or bethamethasone and used tocolytics only in the steroid group. Fetal lung profiles were performed routinely in only seven studies (Taeusch et al 1979; Papageorgiou et al 1979; Garite et al 1981; Schmidt et al 1984; Iams et al 1985; Morales et al 1986; Morales et al 1989) to exclude cases with pulmonary maturity. Treatment was also not uniform in all the studies. The steroid groups were variously treated with tocolytics (Block et al 1977; Garite et al 1981; Morales et al 1986), delivered at 48–72 hrs (Nelson et al 1985; Iams et al 1985) or managed expectantly (Morales et al, 1989). In the majority of the trials, the control groups were treated expectantly.

The meta-anlaysis of trials (Ohlsson 1989; Kierse et al 1989; Crowley 1994) demonstrates that antenatal treatment with steroids significantly decreases the incidence of RDS in neonates born to a mother with PPROM at 28–34 weeks gestation.

A majority of the studies in which information on infectious morbidity was available revealed a significantly higher incidence of endomyometritis after vaginal delivery in the group treated with steroids (Taeusch et al 1979; Garite et al 1981; Schmidt et al 1984; Iams et al 1985). In all the studies, there appeared to be a trend towards an increase in neonatal infectious morbidity, although it did not reach statistical significance. Meta-analysis of the data (Ohlsson 1989; Keirse et al 1989; Crowley 1994) also showed the same trend.

If the babies born after PPROM are examined there appears to be a greater morbidity due to RDS than due to sepsis. In addition, the period when steroids are given can be covered by prophylactic antibiotics. Steroids also have a direct action on the gut epithelium causing proliferation of cells and inducing enzyme production. This appears to have some beneficial action in preventing necrotising enterocolitis in preterm babies. Extensive work is under way on other drugs (for example, thyroid releasing hormone) which can enhance lung maturity but which has little effect on infection. Till these methods are perfected and the use of artificial surfectant becomes universal, the use of steroids is indicated in these cases of PPROM in the absence of infection.

Management of PPROM

The case for immediate stimulation of labour

The rationale for advocating active management of PPROM with immediate stimulation of labour is that infection may supervene if delivery is delayed. Also, sporadic stillbirth may be avoided by earlier delivery after PPROM (Keirse et al 1989). However as discussed above, many authors have found no relationship between the duration of PPROM and either perinatal mortality or neonatal sepsis (Schreiber and Benedetti 1980; Mead 1983; Johnson et al 1981; Daikoku et al 1981).

In Nelson's (1985) study, delivery in the group managed actively was instituted between 24 and 48 hr after PPROM, and in the group managed expectantly women were observed without taking measures to effect delivery or arrest labour when it occurred. The women in the first group received betamimetic drug treatment if labour occurred within the first 24 hours. This study found no significant difference between the results of the two management protocols in terms of maternal sepsis, the route of delivery, birthweight, incidence of respiratory distress syndrome and perinatal mortality. In the second study (Spinnato et al 1987), women were entered if they had PPROM between 25 and 36 weeks of gestation and documented fetal pulmonory maturity. There were 47 patients in this series; 26 were assigned for prompt delivery and 21 for conservative management. In this study, expectant management was associated with a significantly increased risk of maternal infection, but neonatal morbidity and mortality were similar in both groups. The results of these two trials do not suggest that an active management policy gives a better outcome in terms of maternal sepsis, neonatal sepsis, RDS in infants and perinatal death (Keirse et al 1989). Meta-analysis of these studies shows a tendency for a less favourable outcome for the group managed actively.

These conclusions are similar to those of Graham et al (1982). In a retrospective analysis of 109 patietns with PPROM prior to 34 weeks gestation, they found that the immediate induction of labour or delivery for patients with PPROM at less than 32 weeks gestation resulted in a significant increase in perinatal mortality and morbidity; there was a significantly increased incidence of the respiratory distress syndrome, and intracranial hemorrhage in the group managed aggressively, but there was no difference in the incidence of neonatal sepsis in both groups.

Three trials (Garite et al 1981; Nelson et al 1985; Iams et al, 1985) compared steroid administration followed by active measures to effect delivery with an expectant policy that included neither corticosteroid nor active measures to effect delivery. Meta-analysis of the three trials (Keirse et al 1989) showed no statistically significant difference in the incidence of respiratory distress syndrome between the two policies.

The case for expectant management

From the clinician's point of view, PPROM is a clinical dilemma because the dangers of preterm delivery must be weighed against the risk of maternal or neonatal sepsis. Considering that the expectant management of PPROM does not appear to have significantly increased adverse effects on the incidence of maternal or neonatal sepsis (Daikoku et al 1981; Johnson et al 1981; Wilson et al 1982; Mead 1983; Veille 1988) and that the neonatal outcome is more often related to maturity at delivery rather than to the time of rupture of the membranes, an expectant management policy is practised. It is hoped that sufficient time will pass for the fetus to become mature, although only 20% of patients with PPROM in the preterm period fail to labour spontaneously within seven days (Mead 1983; Spinnato et al 1987). Expectant management in PPROM did not have adverse effects on the incidence of maternal or neonatal infection but was relatively ineffectual in achieving significant extension of time in utero (Mead 1983; Schreiber and Benedetti 1980; Wilson et al 1982); the earlier the PROM, the longer the latency period (Johnson et al 1981; Wilson et al 1982; Veille 1988). For the woman who is not in labour, is not infected, and shows no evidence of fetal distress or other fetal or maternal pathology, continuation of the pregancy is likely to be more beneficial than harmful (Keirse 1989; Crowely 1994).

Fetal surveillance

When a patient with PPROM is managed expectantly, fetal surveillance must be guided by the awareness of the complications which are known to occur frequently after PPROM. They include infection, cord prolapse, cord compression, abruptio placentae, fetal deformities and pulmonary hypoplasia.

The clinical assessment of incipient infection has been dealt with previously. Analysis of the amniotic fluid by amniocentesis and assessment of the fetal biophysical profile have been discussed as methods to identify early infection in the fetus for those at risk for developing sepsis. These methods are used sparingly and much larger trials need to be performed before they are adopted for routine use.

Umbilical cord prolapse may occur at any time after PPROM. Any change in the clinical situation, like an increased leakage of the amniotic fluid or onset of uterine contractions should alert the clinician to look out for cord prolapse. Cardiotocography may indicate cord compression due to prolapse and careful ultrasound examination may be useful in detecting loops of the cord below the presenting part and the possibility of cord prolapse.

Umbilical cord compression occurs due to loss of the cushioning effect of the amniotic fluid. The incidence of severe decelerations of the fetal heart rate is directly related to the degree of oligohydramnios (Moberg et al 1984; Vintzileos et al 1985). Regular and frequent cardiotocography is needed, parhaps on a daily basis, for a duration of one to two hours in order to observe the effect of the Braxton-Hicks contractions. When uterine contractions suggestive of the onset of labour are reported by the patient it is wise to perform cardiotocography to observe the probability of cord compression.

Fetal postural deformities may occur when prolonged rupture of the membranes occurs and there is severe oligohydramnios for several weeks. These deformities are mainly postural/compressional and are generally reversible to a major extent after delivery. They comprise facies characterised by lowset flattened ears, a sloping tip of the nose, a sloping chin, and deformities of the extremities consisting of edematous spadelike hands and flexion contractures at the elbows, knees or feet. These deformities appear to be highly correlated to lethal pulmonary hypoplasia (Richards 1991).

Fetal pulmonary hypoplasia is a complication associated with very high perinatal mortality and morbidity. The severity of hypoplasia is dependent on the severity of oligohydramnios, the duration of the oligohydramnios and the gestational age at which PPROM occurs. The risk appears to be largest when amniotic fluid leakage occurs in the first half of the second trimester and results in the absence of amniotic fluid for several weeks. Small studies have been published associating the absence of fetal breathing movements and other ultrasound parameters with pulmonary hypoplasia (Blott et al 1987; Moessinger et al 1987; Nimrod et al 1988). The results vary and much work has to be done before reliable conclusions can be drawn with regard to the risk of pulmonory hypoplasia and its prediction.

The accumulation of amniotic fluid is an important prognostic factor for a decreased incidence of infection, preterm labour, abruptio placentae and postural deformities. A quantitative assessment of amniotic fluid by ultrasound measurement of the Amniotic Fluid Index (Phelan et al 1987), may be useful in identifying women and their fetuses who are less at risk with expectant management.

Amnioinfusion

In recent years, amnioinfusion has been used both antenatally and in labour in patients with PROM, in order to augment the amniotic the fluid volume.

In the antepartum period amnioinfusion, and at times peritoneal infusion, have been used to improve ultrasound visualisation of the fetus when there is oligohydramnios (Stringer et al 1990; Arulkumaran and Rodeck 1991), and also to confirm membrane rupture if present (Gembruch and Hansmann 1988). Amnioinfusion has also been advocated in the antenatal period, not only to decrease the incidence of cord compression and fetal distress, but also to relieve the risk of postural deformities, fetal pulmonary hypoplasia, infection and early labour (Biswas and Arulkumaran 1991). In a small uncontrolled series of ten patients with PPROM and oligohydramnios who were managed conservatively, Imanaka et al (1989) used an indwelling cervical catheter with a cervical plug to infuse normal saline into the amniotic cavity. They were able to enlarge the amniotic cavity enough to provide a favourable intrauterine environment for the fetus to breathe and move freely. The cervical plug prevented subsequent leakage of infused fluid during the subsequent latent period. A recent series of nine cases (Fisk et al 1991) suggests that serial transabdomimnal saline amnioinfusion may partially prevent pulmonary hypoplasia and improve fetal salvage rates in cases of PPROM with severe oligohydramnios in the second trimester. Fibrin adhesion treatment has been used in cases of PPROM between 15 weeks and 32 weeks (Anger 1986; Genz 1986), in order to interrupt the passage of amniotic fluid and to increase the chances of spontaneous repair of the fetal membranes. Theoretically, fibrin sealing may also prevent infection ascending through the cervical canal.

Nageotte et al (1985) assessed the effect of intrapartum amnioinfusion in patients with preterm PROM. This randomised controlled trial showed the advantages that prophylactic amnioinfusion in PPROM had in reducing the incidence of and severity of variable decelerations, and establishing a better umbilical cord arterial and venous pH in the study group compared with the control. There was also a trend in the control group towards a higher caesarean section rate for fetal distress.

As with all new clinical techniques, the use of this approach both in the antepartum period and in labour should be restricted to randomised trials to define clearly the potential benefits and possible adverse effects for the mother and fetus (Hofmeyer 1992) before it is recommended for general use.

A protocol for the management of PPROM

PPROM needs a conservative approach in the absence of any complication, to prevent the hazard of prematurity. PPROM should be managed according to the period of gestation and is discussed below.

PPROM between 34 and 37 weeks

In this group of women fetal lung maturity is not a problem. Unnecessary induction of labour in the absence of any complication can result in abdominal operative delivery for failed induction, as the cervical score is usually poor at this period of gestation. If the woman goes into labour, it should not be inhibited and she should be allowed to deliver vaginally. If signs and symptoms of chorioamnionitis appear, labour should be induced with appropriate care aiming for early delivery. In the absence of any obstetrical or medical complications, expectant treatment is advised and is described in the following section.

PPROM between 28 and 34 weeks

The greatest risk in this group is that of prematurity and its associated complications. The danger of preterm delivery must be weighed against the risks of maternal or neonatal sepsis. In the absence of any complication, this group needs conservative or expectant treatment. This type of management does not have a significant increase in adverse outcome in terms of the incidence of maternal or neonatal sepsis compared with complications of prematurity. Neonatal outcome is more related to maturity at delivery with a better outcome when the maturity is greater despite a long PROM to delivery interval.

Expectant or conservative treatment

*   Women with PPROM are better admitted to a tertiary care institution where facilities for neonatal intensive care is available.

* Sterile speculum examination should be done to confirm rupture of the membranes, to assess effacement and dilatation of the cervix, the presence of meconium in the amniotic fluid and cord prolapse.
* Chorioamnionitis should be excluded on admission and the patient monitored closely for early evidence of infection in order to terminate the pregnancy.
* Bed rest is advised and a sterile sanitary pad given to observe the amount, colour, and smell of liquor. Maternal vital signs of pulse, temperature and evidence of uterine tenderness should be watched every 4 – 6 hours.
* Total and differential white blood cell counts can be done twice weekly and whenever there is any suspicion of chorioamnionitis.
* Fetal monitoring by daily fetal movement chart, auscultation of the fetal heart rate, CTG, or biophysical profile by ultrasound should be undertaken based on the facilities available. The frequency of testing will depend on the clinical situation but some form of monitoring should be carried out daily to ascertain the fetal condition.
* If the amniotic fluid can be collected it should be sent for microscopic examination, culture and sensitivity test and for L:S ratio.
* In the absence of any complications, pregnancy is usually prolonged till 37 weeks.
* Dexamethosone 12 mg is given in two doses 12 hours apart after ruling out infection.
* If the patient goes into labour within 24 hours of administering steroids, labour can be inhibited by tocolytics for 24 hours provided infection is ruled out.
* If chorioamnionitis develops then labour should be induced under the cover of broad spectrum antibiotics, and early recourse to delivery taken to avoid septic complications to the mother and the neonate.
* Caesarean section becomes the choice for delivery of the fetus in the presence of a poor cervical score and chorioamnionitis.

PPROM before 28 weeks (previable)

This category creates a unique set of circumstances. Despite advances in the neonatal intensive care of the extremely premature, survival in this group is poor. The major risks to the fetus are postural deformities and lung hypoplasia (if PPROM was < 24 weeks) due to prolonged oligohydramnios. Some of these fetuses may reach the period of viability.

Considering the low likelihood of reaching a viable gestational age, the expense and possible sequelae involved in delivering a very premature baby, the prolonged maternal rest necessary and the risk of maternal infection, termination of pregnancy may be offered to those women who have ROM prior to 24 weeks. If the mother is not in favour of termination, her wish should be respected. In the absence of infection these patients should be managed expectantly.

Although most of these women are managed in institutions the role of prolonged hospitalisation is debatable. It may be adequate if she takes bed rest at home with the proviso she comes to hospital if she feels unwell, has fever, uterine pain, foul smelling discharge or absent fetal movements. Sexual activity should be avoided for the fear of introducing infection. Monitoring may be better in a hospital

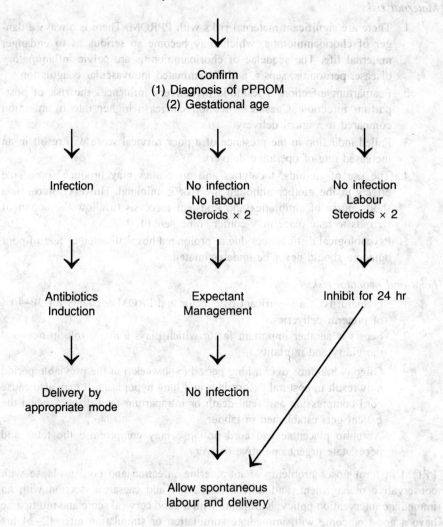

Flow chart showing management of PPROM

History of PROM 28 – 34 weeks

↓

Confirm
(1) Diagnosis of PPROM
(2) Gestational age

| Infection | No infection
No labour
Steroids × 2 | No infection
Labour
Steroids × 2 |

| Antibiotics
Induction | Expectant
Management | Inhibit for 24 hr |

| Delivery by
appropriate mode | No infection |

Allow spontaneous
labour and delivery

set up provided it is acceptable to the woman and it is felt to be safer. Diagnosis of fetal death or onset of infection need prompt delivery.

If she wishes to terminate the pregnancy prior to 24 weeks it can be achieved by administering prostaglandins intravenously or by ripening the cervix with prostaglandin vaginal pessaries followed by oxytocin infusion.

Complications of PPROM

Maternal risks

1. There are significant maternal risks with PPROM. There is always a danger of chorioamnionitis, which may become so serious as to endanger maternal life. The sequelae of chorioamnionitis are pelvic inflammatory disease, peritonitis, sepsis, and disseminated intravascular coagulation.
2. Postpartum infection: The mode of delivery influences the risk of postpartum infection. Caesarean section carries a higher rate of infection compared to vaginal delivery.
3. Failed induction in the presence of a poor cervical score will result in an increased rate of operative delivery.
4. The use of steroids, tocolytics and antibiotics may produce some side effects in the mother although the risk is minimal. However steroids, a short course of antibiotics and transient tocolysis to allow the action of steroids to take place may confer some benefit.
5. Psychological disturbances due to prolonged hospitalisation or fear of poor outcome should never be underestimated.

Fetal and neonatal risks

1. Prematurity is a significant risk factor and PROM accounts for 30–40% of preterm deliveries.
2. Sepsis is another important factor which plays a major role in neonatal morbidity and mortality.
3. Oligohydramnios over a long period (> 4 weeks) in the previable period may result in postural deformities and lung hypoplasia. It may also cause cord compression and fetal death or intrapartum fetal distress when the patient gets established in labour.
4. Abruptio placentae and cord prolapse may compromise the fetus and necessitate urgent operative delivery.

PROM at term poses problems of intrauterine infection and cord prolapse with conservative management, and failed stimulation and caesarean section with an immediate intervention policy. Nulliparae with a good cervical score and multiparae have a good outcome with immediate stimulation or stimulation after 12–24 hrs of conservatism. Nullipare with a poor cervical score do not fare well with immediate stimulation or after 12–24 hrs of conservatism. Use of vaginal prostaglandins in this group for 8 hours followed by oxytocin stimulation does not appear to offer better results and a longer interval between prostaglandin insertion and oxytocic titration needs further study. Signs of infection on admission or subsequently warrants broad spectrum antibiotic therapy and early delivery.

Management of PPROM has to be stratified according to different gestations. Those beyond 34 weeks can be managed expectantly as active intervention leads to an increased operative delivery rate. Those between 26 and 34 weeks appear to benefit by the use of corticosteroids, a short course of antibiotics and if necessary 24 hr of tocolysis to allow the action of steroids. Subsequent prophylactic or therapeutic tocolysis is not beneficial and may be fraught with problems. Streptococci or gono-cocci identified on swabs warrants therapy and the use of antibiotics in labour reduces the incidence of maternal infection. Those under 26 weeks may benefit by the use of fibrin sealant therapy or repeated amnioinfusion to prevent pulmonary hypoplasia but these therapies are still experimental. More work needs to be done to identify the etiology and prevention of PROM especially in the preterm period.

References

Allen Steven R 1991. Premature rupture of membranes. *Clin Obstet Gynecol* 34(4): 685-693.

Amon E, Lewis SV, Sibai BM, Villar MA, Arheart KL 1988. Ampicillin prophylaxis in preterm premature rupture of the membranes: A prospective randomized study. *Am J Obstet Gynecol* 159:539-543.

Anger H 1986. Fibrin sealing in premature rupture of membranes in pregnancy. In: Schlag G, Redl H, eds. Gynecology and Obstetrics - Urology, Vol 3. Berlin: Springer-Verlag, pp 95-97.

Anthony Bascom 1982 Carriage of Group B Streptococci during pregnancy: a puzzler. *J Infect Dis* 145(6): 789-793.

Arulkumaran S, Gibb DMF, TambyRaja RL et al 1985. Rising caesarean section rates in Singapore. *Sing J Obstet Gynecol* 16: 5.

Arulkumaran S, Khashoggi YT, Thavarasah AS, Ratnam SS 1988. Obstetric outome of overnight conservative and immediate stimulation policies for premature rupture of membranes. *Sing J Obstet and Gynecol* 19(3): 163-168.

Asrat Tamerou, Garite Thomas J 1991. Management of preterm premature rupture of membranes. *Clin Obstet Gynecol* 34(4): 730-741.

Benacerraf BR, Gelman R, Frigoletto FD 1988. Sonographically estimated fetal weights: accuracy and limitation. *Am J Obstet Gynecol* 159: 1118-1121.

Berkowitz RL, Kantor RD, Bech GT, Warshaw JB 1978. The relationship between premature rupture of the membranes and the respiratory distress syndrome. *Am J Obstet Gynecol* 131: 503-508.

Beyduin SN, Yasin SY 1986. Premature rupture of the membranes before 28 weeks: Conservative management. *Am J Obstet Gynecol* 155: 471-479.

Biswas A, Arulkumaran S 1991. Pulmonary hypoplasia. *Sing J Obstet Gynecol* 22(3): 147-155.

Block Mary F, Kling O Ray, Crosby Warren M 1977. Antenatal glucocorticoid therapy for the prevention of respiratory distress syndrome in the premature infant. *Obstet Gynecol* 50(2): 186-190.

Blott M, Nicolaides KH, Gibb D et al 1987. Fetal breathing movements as predictor of favourable pregnancy outcome after oligohydramnios due to membrane rupture in second trimester. *Lancet* 2: 129-131.

Bottoms SF, Ulch RA, Zador IE, Sokol RJ 1987. Clinical interpretation of ultrasound measurements in preterm pregnancies with premature rupture of the membranes. *Obstet Gynecol* 69: 358-362.

Brelje MC, Maltreider DF, Kassir L 1966. The use of vaginal antibiotics in premature rupture of the membranes. *Am J Obstet Gynecol* 94: 889-897.

Caspi E, Schreyerf, Weinraub Z, Lifshitz Y, Goldberg M 1981. Dexamethasone for prevention of respiratory distress syndrome: multiple perinatal factors. *Obstet Gynecol* 57(1): 41-47.

Christensen KK, Ingemarsson I, Leideman T, Solum H, Svenningsen N 1980. Effect of ritodrine on labor after premature rupture of the membranes. *Obstet Gynecol* 55(2): 187-190.

Chua S, Arulkumaran S, Kurup A, Anandakumar C et al 1991. Does prostaglandin confer significant advantage over oxytocin infusion for nulliparas with prelabour rupture of membranes at term? *Obstet Gynecol* 77(5): 664-667.

Chua S, Arulkumaran S, Sailesh Kumar S, Selamat N, Ratnam SS 1995. Prelabour rupture of membranes to delivery interval related to incidence of maternal and neonatal infection. *Asia-Oceania J Obstet Gynecol* 21: 367-72.

Chua S, Arlkumaran S, Yap C, Selamat N, Ratnam SS 1995. Premature rupture of membranes in nulliparas at term with unfavourable cervices: A double-blind randomised trial of prostaglandin and placebo. *Obstet Gynecol* In press.

Chung T, Rogers MS, Gordon H, Chang A 1992. Prelabour rupture of membranes at term and unfavourable cervix; a randomised placebo-controlled trial on early intervention with intravaginal prostaglandin E_2 gel. *Aust NZ J Obstet Gynecol* 32:25-27.

Conway DI, Prendiville WJ, Morris A et al 1984. Management of spontaneous rupture of the membranes in the absence of labor in primigravid women at term. *Am J Obstet Gynecol* 150(8): 947-951.

Cotton David B, Hill Lyndon M, Strassner Howard T et al 1984. Use of amniocentesis in preterm gestation with ruptured membranes. *Obstet Gynecol* 63(1): 38-43.

Crowley P 1994. Antibiotics for preterm prelabour rupture of membranes, 5 May 1994. In: Enkin MW, Kerise MJNC, Renfrew MJ, Neilson JP, eds. Pregnancy and Childbirth Module. 'Cochrane Database of Systematic Reviews': Review 04391. Published through Cochrane Updates on Disk. Oxford: Update Software 1994, Disk Issue 1

Crowley P 1994. Corticosteriods after preterm prelabour rupture of membranes. In: Enkin MW, Kerise MJNC, Renfrew MJ, Neilson JP, eds. Pregnancy and Childbirth Module. 'Cochrane Database of Systematic Reviews': Review No. 04395, 5 May 1994. Published through Cochrane Updates on Disk, Oxford: Update Software 1994, Disk Issue 1

Crowley P 1994. Elective delivery after preterm prelabour rupture of membranes. In: Enkin MW, Keirse MJNC, Renfrew MJ, Neilson JP, eds. Pregnancy and Childbirth Module. 'Cochrane Database of Systematic Reviews': Review No. 04473, 5 May 1994. Published through 'Cochrane Updates on Disk, Oxford: Update Software, 1994, Disk Issue 1

Daikoku NH, Kaltreider DF, Johnson TRB et al 1981. Premature rupture of membranes and preterm labor: Neonatal infection and perinatal mortality risks. *Obstet Gynecol* 58(4): 417-425

Duff Patrick, Huff Robert W, Gibbs Ronald S 1984. Management of premature rupture of membranes and unfavorable cervix in term pregnancy. *Obstet Gynecol* 63(5): 697-702.

Duncan SLB, Beckley S 1992. Prelabour rupture of the membranes - why hurry? *Br J Obstet Gynecol* 99: 543-545.

Eckman-Ordeberg G, Uldbjerg N, Ulmsten U 1985. Comparison of intravenous oxytocin and vaginal prostaglandin E_2 gel in women with unripe cervixes and premature rupture of the membranes. *Obstet Gynecol* 66(3): 307-310.

Eriksen Nancy L, Blanco Jorge D 1991. The role of corticosteroids in the management of patients with preterm premature rupture of the membranes. *Clin Obstet Gynecol* 34(4): 694-701.

Fisk NM, Ronderos-Dumit D, Soliani A, Nicolini U, Vaughan J, Rodeck CH 1991. Diagnostic and therapeutic transabdominal amnioinfusion in oligohydramnios. *Obstet Gynecol* 78: 270-8.

Garite Thomas J 1985. Premature rupture of the membranes: The enigma of the obstetrician. *Am J Obstet Gynecol* 151(8): 1001-1005.

Garite Thomas J, Keegan Kirk A, Freeman Roger K, Nageotte Michael P 1987. A randomised trial of ritodrine tocolysis versus expectant management in patients with premature rupture of membranes at 25 to 30 weeks of gestation. *Am J Obstet Gynecol* 157(2): 388-393.

Garite Thomas J, Freeman Roger K, Linzey E Michael et al 1981. Prospective randomised study of corticosteroids in the management of premature rupture of the membranes and the premature gestation. *Am J Obstet Gynecol* 141(5): 508-515.

Garite Thomas J, Freeman Roger K 1982. Chorioamnionitis in the preterm gestation. *Obstet Gynecol* 59(5): 539-545.

Gembruch U, Hansmann M 1988. Artificial instillation of amniotic fluid as a new technique for the diagnostic evaluation of cases of oligohydramnios. *Prenat Diagn* 8: 33-45.

Genz H-J 1986. Fibrin sealing in premature rupture of the membranes. In: Schlag G and Redl H, eds. Gynecology and Obstetrics - Urology, Vol. 3. Berlin: Springer-Verlag, pp 98-102.

Gibbs Ronald S, Blanco Jorge D 1982. Premature rupture of the membranes. *Obstet Gynecol* 60(6): 671-679.

Graham R Leon, Gilstrap III Larry C, Hauth John C et al 1982. Conservative management of patients with premature rupture of fetal membranes. *Obstet Gynecol* 59(5): 607-610.

Granstrom Lena, Ekman Gunvor, Ulmsten Ulf 1987. Cervical priming and labor induction with vaginal application of 3 mg PGE_2 in suppositories in term pregnant women with premature rupture of amniotic membranes and unfavorable cervix. *Acta Obstet Gynecol Scand* 66: 429-431.

Grant John, Keirse Marc JNC 1989. Prelabour rupture of the membranes at term. In: Iain Chalmers, Murray Einken, Keirse MJNC, eds. Effective Care in Pregnancy and Childbirth. Oxford: Oxford University Press, pp 1112-1117.

Grant John M, Serle Elisabeth, Mahmood Tahir et al 1992. Management of prelabour rupture of the membranes in term primigravidae: report of a randomised prospective. *Br J Obstet Gynecol* 99: 557-562.

Gravett Michael G, Hummel Deborah, Eschenbach David A, Holmes King K 1986. Preterm labor associated with subclinical amniotic fluid infection and with bacterial vaginosis. *Obstet Gynecol* 67(2): 229-237.

Greenberg Rosemary T, Hankins Gary DV 1991. Antibiotic therapy in preterm premature rupture of membranes. *Clin Obstet Gynecol* 34(4): 742-750.

Gunn GC, Mishell DR, Morton DG 1970. Premature rupture of the fetal membranes - A review. *Am J Obstet Gynecol* 106: 469-483.

Hannah ME 1993. Active management of prelabour rupture of membranes at 37+ weeks. In: Enkin MW, Keirse MJNC, Renfrew MJ,

Neilson JP, eds. Pregnancy and Childbirth Module. 'Cochrane Database of Systematic reviews': Review No. 03272, 24 March 1993. Published through Cochrane Updates on Disk, Oxford: Update Software 1993, Disk Issue 2.

Hannah MSE 1993. Prostaglandins vs oxytocin for prelabour rupture of membranes at 37+ weeks. In: Enkin MW, Keirse MJNC, Renfrew MJ, Neilson JP, eds. Pregnancy and Childbirth Module. 'Cochrane Database of Systematic Reviews': Review No. 03273, 24 March 1993. Published through Cochrane Updates on Disk, Oxford: Update Software 1993, Disk Issue 2.

Hannah ME 1993. Prostaglandins vs oxytocin for prelabour rupture of membranes at 34+ weeks. In Enkin MW, Keirse MJNC, Renfrew MJ, Neilson JP, eds. Pregnancy and Childbirth Module 'Cochrane Database of Systematic Reviews': Review No. 07152, 22 April 1993. Published through Cochrane Updates on Disk, Oxford: Update Software, 1994, Disk Issue 1.

Harlass Frederick E 1991. The use of tocolytics in patients with preterm premature rupture of the membranes. *Clin Obstet Gynecol* 34(4): 751-758.

Hauth John C, Cunningham Gary F, Whalley Peggy J 1977. Early labor initiation with oral PGE$_2$ after premature rupture of the membranes at term. *Obstet Gynecol* 49(5): 523-526.

Hofmeyr GJ 1992. Amnioinfusion: a question of benefits and risks. *Br J Obstet Gynecol* 99: 449-451.

Iams Jay D, Talbert Madonna L, Barrows Holly, Sachs Larry 1985. Management of preterm prematurely ruptured membranes: A prospective randomised comparison of observation versus use of steroids and timed delivery. *Am J Obstet Gynecol* 151: 32-38.

Imanaka Motoharu, Ogita Sachio, Sugawa Tadashi 1989. Saline solution amnioinfusion for oligohydramnios after premature rupture of the membranes. *Am J Obstet Gynecol* 161: 102-106.

Johnson John WC, Niebyl Jennifer R, Johnson Timothy RB et al 1981. Premature rupture of the membranes and prolonged latency. *Obstet Gynecol* 57(5): 547-556.

Johnson MM, Sanchez-Ramos L, Vaughn AJ et al 1990. Antibiotic therapy in preterm premature rupture of membranes: A randomised, prospective, double-blind trial. *Am J Obstet Gynecol* 163(3): 743-747.

Kappy Kenneth A, Cetrulo Curtis L, Knuppel Robert A et al 1979. Premature rupture of the membranes: A conservative approach. *Am J Obstet Gynecol* 134(6): 655-661.

Kappy Kenneth A, Cetrulo Curtis L, Knuppel Robert A et al 1982. Premature rupture of the membranes at term: A comparison of induced and spontaneous labors. *J Reprod Med* 27(1): 29-33.

Keirse MJNC, Ohlsson Arne, Treffers and Kanhai Humphrey HH 1989. Prelabour rupture of the membranes preterm. In: Iain Chalmers, Murray Fenkin, MJNC Kriese, eds. Effective

Care in Pregnancy and Childbirth. Oxford: Oxford University Press, pp 666-693.

Keirse MJNC 1994. Tocolytic treatment during preterm labour after PROM. In: Enkin MW, Keirse MJNC, Renfrew MJ, Neilson JP, eds. Pregnancy and Childbirth Module. 'Cochrane Database of Systematic Reviews': Review No. 04397 22 April 1993. Published through 'Cochrane Updates on Disk', Oxford: Update Software, Disk Issue 1.

Keirse MJNC 1994. Betamimetics after preterm labour after PROM. In: Enkin MW, Keirse MJNC, Renfrew MJ, Neilson JP, eds. Pregnancy and Childbirth Module. 'Cochrane Database of Systematic Reviews': Review No. 04396 22 April 1993. Published through 'Cochrane Updates on Disk', Oxford: Update Software, Disk Issue 1.

Koh KS, Chan FH, Monfared AH, Ledger WJK, Paul RH 1979. The changing perinatal and maternal outcome in chorioamnionitis. *Obstet Gynecol* 53: 730-734.

Lange Askel P, Secher Niels J, Nielsen Folmer Hassing, Pederson Gunnar Thomsen 1981. Stimulation of labor in cases or premature rupture of the membranes at or near term. *Acta Obstet Gynecol Scand* 60: 207-210.

Lanier RL, Scarborough RW, Fillingim DW, Baker RE 1965. Incidence of maternal and fetal complications associated with rupture of the membranes before onset of labour. *Am J Obstet Gynecol* 93: 398-404.

Lebherz TB, Hellman LP, Madeling R et al 1963. Double-blind study of premature rupture of the membranes. *Am J Obstet Gynecol* 87: 218-225.

Levy DL, Warsof SC 1985. Oral ritodrine and preterm premature rupture of membranes. *Obstet Gynecol* 66: 621-623.

Lonky Neal M, Hayashi Robert H 1988. A proposed mechanism for premature rupture of membranes. *Obstet Gynecol Surv* 43(1): 22-28.

Magos AL, Noble MCB, Wong T Ten Yuen, Rodeck CH 1983. Controlled study comparing vaginal prostaglandin E$_2$ pessaries with intravenous oxytocin for the stimulation of labour after spontaneous rupture of the membranes. *Br J Obstet Gynecol* 90: 726-731.

Mahmood TA, Dick MJW, Smith NC, Templeton AA 1992. Role of prostaglandin in the management of prelabour rupture of the membranes at term. *Br J Obstet Gynecol* 99: 112-117.

Maxwell GL 1993. Preterm premature rupture of membranes. *Obstet Gynecol Surv* 576-83.

Mead PB 1983. Premature rupture of the membranes. In: Chiswick MC. ed. Recent Advances in Perinatal Medicine, Vol 1. London: Churchill Livingstone, pp 77-94.

Moberg LJ, Garite TJ, Freeman RK 1984. Fetal heart rate patterns and fetal distress in patients with preterm premature rupture of membranes. *Obstet Gynecol* 64(1): 61-64.

Moessinger AC, Fox HE, Higgins A et al 1987. Fetal breathing movements are not a reliable predictor of continued lung development in pregnancies complicated by oligohydramnios. *Lancet* 2: 1297-1299.

Morales Walter J, Diebel Donald, Lazar Arnold J, Zadrozny Deborah 1986. The effect of antenatal dexamethasone administration on the prevention of respiratory distress syndrome in preterm gestations with premature rupture of membranes. *Am J Obstet Gynecol* 154(3): 591-595.

Morales Walter J, Angel Jeffrey L, O'Brien William F, Knuppel Robert A 1989. Use of ampicillin and corticosteroids in premature rupture of membranes: A randomised study. *Obstet Gynecol* 73(5): 721-726.

Nageotte Michael P, Freeman Roger K, Garite Thomas T, Dorchester Wendy 1985. Prophylactic intrapartum amnioinfusion in patients with preterm premature rupture of membranes. *Am J Obstet Gynecol* 153: 557-562.

Naeye Richard L 1982. Factors that predispose to premature rupture of the fetal membranes. *Obstet Gynecol* 60(1): 93-98.

Naeye Richard, Peters Ellen C 1980. Causes and consequences of premature rupture of fetal membranes. *Lancet* 1: 192-194.

Nelson Lewis H, Meis Paul J, Hatjis Christos G et al 1985. Premature rupture of membranes: A prospective, randomised evaluation of steroids, latent phase and expectant management. *Obstet Gynecol* 66(1): 55-58.

Nimrod C, Nicholson S, Davies D, Harder J et al 1988. Pulmonary hypoplasia testing in clinical obstetrics. *Am J Obstet Gynecol* 158: 277-280.

Ohlsson Arne 1989. Treatment of preterm premature rupture of the membranes: A meta-analysis. *Am J Obstet Gynecol* 160(4): 890-906.

Papageorgiou Apostolos N, Desgranges Marie F, Masson Michel et al 1979. The antenatal use of betamethasone in the prevention of respiratory distress syndrome: A controlled double-blind study. *Pediatrics* 63(1): 73-79.

Phelan JP, Ahn MO, Smith CV, Rutherford SE, Anderson E 1987. Amniotic fluid index measurements during pregnancy. *J Reprod Med* 32: 601-604.

Ray DA, Garite TJ 1992. Prostaglandin E₂ for induction of labour in patients with premature rupture of membranes at term. *Am J Obstet Gynecol* 166: 836-43.

Richards Douglas S 1991. Complications of prolonged PROM and oligohydramnios *Clin Obstet Gynecol* 34(4): 759-768.

Robson MS, Turn MJ, Stronge JM, O'Herlihy 1990. Is amniotic fluid quantitation of value in the diagnosis and conservative management of prelabour rupture of membranes at term? *Br J Obstet Gynecol.* 97:324-328.

Romero Roverto, Emamian Mohamed, Quintero Ruben et al 1988. The value and limitations of the Gram stain examination in the diagnosis of intraamniotic infection. *Am J Obstet Gynecol* 159(1): 114-119.

Russel KP, Anderson GV 1962. The aggressive management of rupture membranes. *Am J Obstet Gynecol* 83: 930-937.

Rydhstrom H, Arulkumaran S, Ingemarsson I et al 1986. Premature rupture of the membranes at term: Obstetric outcome with oxytocin stimulation in relation to parity and cervical dilatation at admission. *Acta Obstet Gynecol Scand* 65.

Rydhstrom Hakan, Ingemarsson Ingemar 1991. No benefit from conservative management in nulliparous women with premature rupture of the membranes (PROM) at term: A randomised study. *Acta Obstet Gynecol Scand* 70: 543-547.

Schreiber J, Benedetti T 1980. Conservative management of preterm premature rupture of the fetal membranes in a low socioeconomic population. *Am J Obstet Gynecol* 136: 92-96.

Shubeck F, Benson RC, Clark WW et al 1966. Fetal hazard after rupture of the membranes. *Obstet Gynecol* 28: 22-31.

Siegel Jane D, McCracken George H 1981. Sepsis Neonatorum. *N Engl J Med* 304(11): 642-647.

Spinnato JA, Shaver DC, Bray EM, Lipshitz J 1987. Preterm premature rupture of the membranes with fetal pulmonary maturity present: A prospective study. *Obstet Gynecol* 69: 196-201.

Taeusch William H, Frigoletto Frederic, Kitzmiller John et al 1979. Risk of respiratory distress syndrome after prenatal dexamethasone treatment. *Pediatrics* 63(1): 64-72.

Taylor O, Garite TJ 1984. Premature rupture of membranes before fetal viability. *Obstet Gynecol* 64: 615-620.

Valea FA, Watson WJ, Seeds JW 1990. Accuracy of ultrasonic weight prediction in the fetus with preterm premature rupture of membranes. *Obstet Gynecol* 75: 183-185.

Van der Walt D, Venter PF 1989. Management of term pregnancy with premature rupture of the membranes and unfavourable cervix. *SAMJ* 75: 54-56.

Veille JC 1988. Management of preterm premature rupture of membranes. *Clin Perinatol* 15(4): 851-863.

Vintzileos Anthony M, Campbell Winston A, Rodis John F 1991. Antepartum surveillance in patients with preterm PROM. *Clin Obstet Gynecol* 34(4): 779-793.

Vintzileos AM, Campbell WA, Nochimson DJ, Weinbaum PJ 1985. Degree of oligohydramnios and pregnancy outcome in patients with premature rupture of the membranes. *Obstet Gynecol* 66: 162.

Vintzileos AM, Campbell WA, Nochimson DJ et al 1986. Fetal biophysical profile versus amniocentesis in predicting infection in preterm premature rupture of the membranes. *Obstet Gynecol* 68: 488-494.

Wang Elaine, Smaill Fioma 1989. Infection in pregnancy. In: Iain Chalmers, Murray Enkin, Marc JNC Keirse, eds. Effective Care in Pregnancy and Childbirth. Oxford: Oxford University Press, pp 534-564.

Wagner Michael V, Chin Victor P, Peters Christyne J et al 1989. A comparison of early and delayed induction of labor with spontaneous rupture of membranes at term. *Obstet Gynecol* 74(1): 93-97.

Webb GA 1967. Maternal death associated with premature rupture of the membranes. *Am J Obstet Gynecol* 98: 594-601.

Weiner CP, Renk K, Klugman M 1988. The therapeutic efficacy and cost-effectiveness of aggressive tocolysis for premature labor associated with premature rupture of the membranes. *Am J Obstet Gynecol* 159: 216-222.

Westergaard JG, Lange AP, Pedersen Thomsen G, Secher NJ 1983. Use of oral oxytocics for stimulation of labor in cases of premature rupture of the membranes at term. *Acta Obstet Gynecol Scand* 62: 111-116.

Wilson Joan C, Levy Donald L, Wilds Preston Lea 1982. Premature rupture of membranes prior to term: consequences of nonintervention. *Obstet Gynecol* 60(5): 601-606.

Yoder PR, Gibbs RS, Blanco ID et al 1983. A prospective, controlled study of maternal and perinatal outcome after intra-amniotic infection at term. *Am J Obstet Gynecol* 145: 695-701.

Zuckerman Henryk, Reiss Uziel, Rubinstein Igal 1974. Inhibition of human premature labor by indomethacin. *Obstet Gynecol* 44(6): 787-792.

16

Preterm Labour

M Choolani
C Anandakumar

Preterm labour remains one of the last frontiers of present day obstetric practice. Prematurity has always been a principal contributor to perinatal mortality and morbidity. Now that advances in infectious diseases, prenatal diagnosis and neonatology have reduced morbidity from other conditions, prematurity is assuming increasing prominence. This is true also because of the increased number of preterm births associated with multiple pregnancies in infertility programmes, the moral, ethical and legal dilemmas that surround the issue of viability and the gestational age at which to initiate active resuscitative measures; and additionally, of the cost involved. So far, improvements in the care of the premature neonate have come from specialists in neonatology. However a real reduction in preterm delivery rates will only take place through an improved understanding of the physiology of labour, the identification of the patient at risk of preterm labour (PTL), the prediction and prevention of its occurrence, early detection of its onset and effective tocolysis. So far, the science has been inadequate on all counts.

In the past, the term *premature* was used to describe babies born before 37 completed weeks as well as those with a birthweight below 2,500 g. This definition is at best confusing and at worst, misleading. Many term babies weigh less than 2,500 g. It is much clearer to speak of birthweight or gestational age separately. The World Health Organisation's (WHO) recommendation is that infants delivered prior to 37 completed weeks (< 259 days) from the first day of the last normal menstrual period be defined as preterm and those with birthweights below 2,500 g be classified as low birthweight. Preterm labour would then be defined as the initiation of regular painful contractions that occur usually with increasing frequency and intensity associated with progressive cervical changes of effacement and dilatation culminating (unless inhibited) in the delivery of a preterm infant (WHO 1969, Anderson 1977).

The lower limit of this definition is less clearly defined: it will be that gestational age thought to correlate with fetal viability. In the USA, this is often taken as 20 weeks. In Singapore, as in the UK, for legal purposes viability is defined as any gestation carried beyond 28 weeks (196 days) but fundamental to the issue of viability is the gestation at which the fetus is thought to be 'capable of being born alive' and the capacity to sustain such life without undue morbidity or mortality. A Royal College of Obstetricians and Gynecologists (RCOG) Working Party (Beard 1985) recommended, based upon survival figures of highly preterm babies in the UK neonatal units, that the gestational age after which a fetus is considered viable should be changed from the limit of 28 weeks (196 days) to 24 weeks (168 days). This change would make clearly definable the legal limits of termination in Singapore, which is up to 24 weeks. FIGO defines it as 22 weeks above which the fetus is thought to be viable. These changes would create an intrinsic consistency in medical thought. The salvage rates for these widely preterm babies would vary from country to country and from institution to institution. The obstetric practice of that institution or country then would be dictated by the salvage rates of their own neonatal teams.

Incidence

The true incidence of preterm labour is difficult to establish. Confounding factors include fundamental problems such as inaccurate computation of dates, establishing the diagnosis of preterm labour, the difference in the incidence of preterm labour and preterm birth either due to spontaneous delay or tocolysis, and the lack of differentiation, especially in the older data, between preterm births and low birth-weight growth-retarded infants. The incidence in developed countries lies between 5 and 10 per cent of all births (Rush 1979; New Zealand Health Statistics Report 1978). Figures from the USA must be interpreted with caution since their lower limit for viability (and PTL) is usually taken as 20 weeks (114 days). In Singapore, the incidence of preterm births is about 6% (TambyRaja 1991).

Consequences of preterm birth

Preterm births account for the majority of perinatal deaths amongst infants born without any congenital anomalies. Not long ago, as many as 85% of neonatal deaths in structurally normal infants have been shown to be due to preterm delivery (Rush 1979). Since 1975, however improvements in obstetric and neonatal care have dramatically improved the survival outcomes of preterm infants. Most tertiary referral neonatal centres can boast of close to 100% survival for infants born after 32 weeks in those centres. In fact some even report astounding figures at the threshold of viability (Table 1) (Yu et al 1986). These figures are not representative of survival rates at most other centres (Powell et al 1986) and each neonatal unit should attempt to establish local data that would help the obstetricians counsel their patients appropriately. Mortality data provided to patients must include perinatal and neonatal mortality and an additional 15% of deaths that occur past the first month from broncho-pulmonary dysplasia, necrotising enterocolitis and sudden infant death syndrome (Yu et al 1984). This additional post-neonatal mortality is especially high in preterm births before 30 weeks.

Table 1: Survival rates of preterm live births by gestational age at birth

Gestational Age	Survival (%)
28	72
26	56
24	33

Although survival figures continue to improve, the consequences of preterm birth on perinatal, neonatal and long-term morbidity are of concern. Table 2 describes the list of possible untoward risks of preterm delivery on the newborn. With the decreasing size of the family in developed countries, emphasis is shifting from mere survival of the preterm neonate to heightened expectations for the quality of life. Cerebral palsy is commonest in survivors of lower gestational ages: 2.1% after 34 weeks, 6.1% at 31–34 weeks and 15.3% at 25–30 weeks (Powell et al 1986).

The birth of a preterm infant is socially, emotionally, physically and financially taxing for parents. Some of these costs are tangible while others remain unmeasurable. Prolonged hospitalisation of the neonate can adversely affect parent-infant bonding (Taylor and Hall 1979). Many experience typical negative responses of denial, guilt, anger and depression before coming to terms with the event. There is also the issue of the financial implications of a preterm delivery, whether this cost is borne by the parents or the state. Such costs have been estimated in the USA and in UK (Sandhu et al 1986; Newns et al 1984; Boyle et al 1983; Morrison 1990). The initial and long-term medical costs are so heavy that questions have been asked about the potential benefits to the state from the future earnings of the survivors!

Table 2:   Risks to the preterm infant

birth asphyxia	iatrogenic induced complications, for example, retrolental fibroplasia
respiratory distress syndrome (RDS)	sensorineural deafness
apnoea of prematurity	developmental delay
jaundice	reduced growth potential
hemorrhage	recurrent respiratory infections
impaired thermal homeostasis (cold stress)	learning difficulties
metabolic problems: hypoglycemia/hypocalcemia	social: enforced separation of mother and baby
sepsis	sudden infant death syndrome (SIDS)
feeding difficulties	blindness
intraventricular/periventricular/ intracerebral hemorrhage (IVH/PVH)	child abuse
patent ductus arteriosus (PDA)	
necrotising enterocolitis (NEC)	

Etiology and pathophysiology

According to Eastman (1947) 'only when the factors causing prematurity are clearly understood, can any intelligent attempt at prevention be made'.

The etiology and the pathophysiology of term and preterm labour have been subjects of intense research over the past two decades. Research has been focused on the control of uterine contractions and the regulation of cervical softening and dilatation. Our understanding remains unclear because of the fragmentary nature of studies based upon animal and human models. Although described in detail in Chapter 1, the discussion below summarises the current thoughts on the initiation and maintenance of labour. Understanding the physiology and endocrinology of labour will help us develop and use pharmacologically appropriate agents that can prevent or abort preterm labour.

The animal model   In the sheep, the fetus plays a fundamental role in the physiological onset of labour (Liggins 1977). It is thought that hypothalamic corticotrophin releasing hormone (CRH) acts to release adrenocorticotrophin (ACTH) which in turn leads to fetal adrenal maturation and the secretion of cortisol. Cortisol acts as a crucial link, modifying placental progesterone production and leading to the classical rise of the oestrogen:progesterone (E:P) ratio in maternal plasma, the endometrium and myometrium; this is associated with prostaglandin release and probably the onset of labour (Challis and Brooks 1989; Challis and Olson 1988).

The human model   In the human, control of parturition is probably achieved by a complex integration of endocrine, paracrine and autocrine mechanisms. The place of para- and autocrine mechanisms by way of prostaglandin biometabolism seems to be of central importance. The primary signal that initiates the labour cascade remains a mystery but it appears that the fetal pituitary-adrenal axis needs to be intact (Price et al 1971; Honnebier and Swaab 1973). The role of oxytocin and oxytocin-prostaglandin interactions is still unclear (Casey and MacDonald 1988; Fuchs et al 1982; Roberts et al 1976). Prostaglandins, both PGE_2 and $PGF_{2\alpha}$, are synthesised de novo in the amnio-chorio-decidual complex. Control of the prostaglandin biosynthetic pathway could be achieved by regulating singly or in combination its three key enzyme complexes (Mitchell 1986): the phospholipases, PGH_2 synthase enzyme complex (PGHS) or 15-hydroxyprostaglandin dehydrogenase (PGDH). Differential production of each compound in different segments may be a key in the balance between uterine quiescence and activity (Lundin-Schiller and Mitchell 1990; Skinner and Challis 1984). Such evidence strongly suggests that most likely it is the decidua that produces the uterotropins of labour. Decidual activation is probably the penultimate event in the initiation of human labour.

Epidemiology and risk factors

While further inroads are being made into the etiology of PTL, the presently recognised epidemiological associations and risk factors help to identify women who may be at risk of developing PTL. Such women deserve closer antenatal supervision as early diagnosis affords a better prospect of inhibition and appropriate management.

1.   *Maternal biodata and socioeconomic status*

Mothers below the age of 20 or above the age of 35 in their first pregnancy, those who weigh under 50 kg, Indian women, single women, women who smoke cigarettes and those who abuse cocaine are at an increased risk of preterm labour (Bakketeig and Hoffman 1981; Fredrick and Anderson 1976; Meyer and Tonascia 1977; Neerhof et al 1989). Careers which involve considerable physical fatigue or high psychological stress are also associated with increased preterm births (Papiernik and Kaminski 1974). In general, mothers from lower socioeconomic classes tend to be less educated, be involved in manual work and not have satisfactory general health and antenatal care (Kaltreider and Kohl 1980; Schwartz 1962). It remains controversial whether coitus during the second half of pregnancy increases the risk of preterm delivery. Therefore restriction of sexual activity is not generally advised during pregnancy unless there is a previous or current history of preterm labour, PROM or other strong risk factors.

2. *Reproductive history*

Previous preterm delivery.   This perhaps has the strongest association and is a risk marker for preterm delivery in the index pregnancy. The risk of a recurrent preterm labour in the index pregnancy after a single preterm labour is reported as being variously between 15 and 30 per cent (Keirse et al 1978). Though not without some design difficulties in the Norway study (Bakketeig and Hoffman 1981) of birth registration data, the results summarised in Table 3 provide a good practical working guide for the counselling of patients.

Table 3:   Risk of preterm birth in subsequent pregnancy

First birth	Second birth	Subsequent risk of preterm birth (%)
Not preterm		4.4
Preterm		17.2
Not preterm	Not preterm	2.6
Preterm	Not preterm	5.7
Not preterm	Preterm	11.1
Preterm	Preterm	28.4

Previous abortions   First trimester abortions appear to have no predictive value for preterm births (Keirse et al 1978). Second trimester miscarriages or stillbirths on the other hand are definite risk factors for subsequent preterm births (Rush 1979).

Cervical incompetence   Cervical incompetence may be due to an inherent defect in the cervical 'sphincter' mechanism, uterine abnormalities, prior trauma to the cervix as in cone biopsy or excessive dilatation at induced abortions. It is an uncommon cause of preterm labour (Savarese and Chang 1964; Weber and Obel 1979).

Uterine anomalies   Congenital uterine anomalies are known to predispose to preterm labour and birth. Up to 15% of all preterm births are known to be associated with uterine anomalies. Conversely, of all gravidae with known uterine anomalies, the incidence of preterm labour varies from as little as 4% in patients with a septate uterus to as much as 80% amongst those with a bicornuate bicollis uterus (Heinonen et al 1982). The T-shaped uterus that may be present in women exposed in utero to diethylstilbesterol (DES) is associated with an increased risk of preterm labours (Herbst et al 1980).

3. *Pregnancy complications*

Pregnancies complicated by congenital abnormalities (Honnebier and Swaab 1973), intrauterine fetal demise, antepartum hemorrhage (Roberts 1970) and uterine overdistension from multiple pregnancies or polyhydramnios (Kirbinen and Jouppila 1978) are often associated with preterm labour. Almost any maternal illness may be associated with preterm labours and deliveries; some of these may indeed be iatrogenically induced labour in the interest of the mother or fetus. Endotoxins have, in experimental studies, been shown to stimulate myometrial activity (Creasy 1989). Systemic infections like bacterial pneumoniae, acute pyelonephritis and appendicitis may release endotoxins and therefore initiate preterm labour. Asymptomatic bacteriuria appears to be associated with preterm births only in the presence of renal disease or acute pyelonephritis (Kincaid-Smith 1968). Abdominal surgery during the second half of pregnancy is associated with increased uterine activity and preterm labour. Intrauterine infections by different viruses, bacteria, chlamydia and protozoa may incite preterm labour.

Diagnosis of preterm labour

Early and accurate diagnosis of preterm labour is crucial to the management of this condition: yet, diagnosing preterm labour is not easy and judging whether it will culminate in a preterm birth is even harder. A working criteria used to diagnose preterm labour are summarised in Table 4. The cervical changes required to make the diagnosis include either a cervical dilatation of 2 cm or an effacement of 80% on initial evaluation of the cervix or documented cervical change by the same examiner on two successive examinations a few hours apart.

Table 4: A working criteria that is used for the diagnosis of preterm labour

Gestation:	**28-37 weeks**	
Contractions:	**4 in 20 min**	**or 8 in 60 min**
	and	
(i) Membranes:	Ruptured	
	or	
(ii) Membranes:	Intact	with cervical changes

The problem with the diagnosis of preterm labour is the difficulty in identifying 'true' from 'false' labour. This problem is no different from that encountered in term labours except that in the preterm situation, the cost of a 'wait-and-see' attitude could mean the difference between effective tocolysis and failed tocolysis and a preterm birth. On the other hand, an aggressive policy of tocolysis may subject many mothers to the unnecessary risks of potentially harmful tocolytics. Placebo controlled trials indicate that as many as 50% of women presenting with threatened preterm labour may be in false labour. In order to improve the accuracy of the diagnosis, different methods have been tried. In Castle and Turnbull's (1983) work, the cessation of fetal breathing movements correlated well with delivery within 48 hours but the presence of breathing movements did not preclude preterm delivery. Others have measured prostaglandin F metabolite in patients with threatened preterm labour (Weitz et al 1986). However none of these methods have been shown to significantly improve the ability to diagnose preterm labour early or to identify cases likely to end in preterm delivery.

Management of preterm labour

1. *Initial evaluation*

At the outset, efforts must be taken to determine the gestational age accurately. The next step is to establish the diagnosis of preterm labour. The issues that remain include searching for treatable conditions contributing to preterm labour and the suitability of the index patient for tocolysis and steroid administration. If there is evidence of bacteriuria or overt urinary tract infection, antibiotics should be initiated. Cervical cultures using a sterile speculum examination should be performed and treatment instituted if an infection is demonstrated. If the patient is febrile, the source of the infection should be sought and antipyretic and antibiotic therapy initiated. Some authors recommend amniocentesis to look for bacteria; this however is not a universal practice. Once the patient is thought to be 'eligible' for tocolysis, the immediate issue is to identify those in whom tocolysis may be contraindicated for various reasons (Table 5). There are a few conditions in which tocolysis is

Table 5:   Contraindications to the inhibition of preterm labour

---

Absolute contraindications

    chorioamnionitis
    fetal death
    lethal fetal congenital anomaly
    any maternal or fetal complication that by itself warrants immediate delivery

Relative contraindications

    gestational age > 34 weeks
    fetal weight > 2 kg
    pre-eclampsia, uncontrolled diabetes, hyperthyroidism, cardiac disease
    fetal intrauterine growth retardation
    fetal distress
    vaginal bleeding (placenta previa, abruptio placentae: depends on
    severity and cause)

Contraindications to specific tocolytics

    Described in text

---

absolutely contraindicated but in the majority of cases there is usually no contra-indication or only a relative one. In cases where there may be a relative contrain-dication, its risk must be weighed against that of neonatal mortality and morbidity. Occasionally choosing the appropriate tocolytic may modify the risk:benefit ratio in an individual case. For example, magnesium sulphate or nifedipine may prove a better choice (than a β-agonist) in cases of severe diabetes or cardiac disease. Mild vaginal bleeding from a placenta previa or placental abruption associated with early preterm labour might benefit from a short-acting single bolus dose of a beta mimetic drug as opposed to inhibition with infusion of the same drug which is contraindicated in the presence of APH. Individualisation of treatment is the key.

2. *Tocolysis: the pharmacological inhibition of preterm labour*

The pharmacologic agents currently used include β-adrenergic agonists, magnesium sulphate, prostaglandin synthase inhibitors, calcium channel blockers and nitric ox-ide donors. These agents act at different points in the contraction pathway of uterine smooth muscle. Ethanol as a tocolytic has fallen out of favour and is hardly used now because alternative effective therapy is available. Sedatives and narcotics are generally no longer used as 'tocolytic'. They may be useful in false labour but should the fetus deliver in a few hours after onset, there may be neonatal respiratory depression.

β-adrenergic agonists: pharmacology and mechanism of action.   Most insti-tutions presently use β-adrenergic agonists like salbutamol, ritodrine, terbutaline, hexoprenaline, orciprenaline, isoxipurine and fenoterol for tocolysis. The activity of these agents as tocolytics depends upon modifications to the basic epinephrine (adrenaline) structure. A large alkyl group is added to the ethylamine side chain and hydroxyl groups to the 3,.5 positions of the benzene ring. This modification maximises β_2-adrenergic effects; all the agents have some β_1-adrenergic effects. Bioavailability is much better by the intravenous route than the oral route. After oral administration, the bioavailability is approximately 30% of the intravenous route. The clearance of the drug appears different from the clearance of the endo-genous catecholamines. These agents appear to be excreted unaltered or as conjugates through the kidney. The half-life pattern after a single bolus intravenous or oral dose takes the shape of a hyperbolic curve with initial rapid decay followed by a protracted phase of slower clearance.

The β-adrenergic agonists interact on the myometrial cell membranes with the β_2-adrenergic receptors and the agonist-receptor complex activates adenylate cyclase. This then increases intracellular cyclic adenosine monophosphate. The latter activates protein kinase which then has synergistic effects: it phosphory-lates membrane proteins on the sarcoplasmic reticulum to decrease intracellular calcium and inhibits myosin light-chain kinase to prevent contraction.

Dosage and administration   There are three key steps in the safe administra-tion of this potentially 'dangerous' drug: first, the preparation and assessment prior to administration; next, the administration according to specified guidelines; and lastly, the close monitoring of the mother (and fetus) throughout the duration of administration.

After excluding specific contraindications to β-adrenergic agonists like maternal cardiac disease or severe hypertension, the mother is placed in the left lateral position. An intravenous access is established. Baseline measurements of the maternal pulse, respiratory rate, blood pressure and urine output are charted. Fetal heart rate activity and uterine contractions are monitored by continuous external cardiotocography. Baseline hematological investigations like a full blood count and serum potassium and glucose estimation are useful (Gonik and Creasy 1986).

The drug should be administered via a calibrated infusion pump. It has been suggested that the incidence of pulmonary edema might be lower if the β-adrenergic agonist is diluted in 5% dextrose in water rather than isotonic saline (Philipsen et al 1981). In the presence of significant hyperglycemia, it may be appropriate to use half-strength normal saline. The drug is initially infused at the lowest recommended dose for that agent and gradually increased every 10–30 minutes until either adequate tocolysis is achieved or maternal side effects supervene. The drug should probably not be increased any further when the maternal pulse rate reaches 130 to 140 beats per minute or when the systolic blood pressure falls below 90 mm Hg or 20 to 30 mm from preinfusion BP.

During the infusion, maternal vital signs, uterine activity and fetal heart rate should be monitored at 15–30 minute intervals. The mother's intake and output should be measured diligently, taking care not to overinfuse her. Her lungs should be auscultated at regular intervals (every 4–6 hours) for evidence of early pulmonary edema. The serum potassium and glucose estimations should be repeated every 4–6 hours.

Once uterine contractions are satisfactorily inhibited, the infusion dose is tailed down and finally a maintenance infusion of the tocolytic at the lowest dose is continued for the next few hours. Prior to cessation of the infusion, an alternate form of the therapy is instituted: intramuscular, subcutaneous and oral forms have all been tried. Initiating oral therapy about 2 – 4 hours prior to the cessation of intravenous therapy proves quite satisfactory. There is a close correlation between the maternal pulse and serum β-adrenergic agonist levels (Post 1977) and maintaining a mild tachycardia whilst on oral therapy probably indicates some uterine effect. It is probable however that tachyphylaxis of both the maternal heart rate response and uterine relaxation occurs with continuous exposure to the tocolytic agent (Caritas et al 1983; Ke et al 1984). This may be by down-regulation of the β_1- and β_2-adrenergic receptors.

Side effects   The side effects of β-agonists occur primarily from their extra-uterine effects on sites with β_1- and β_2-adrenergic receptors. Table 6 lists the physiological effects of β_1- and β_2-adrenergic receptors and will make understanding of the side effects much clearer. Each of the significant side effects is then discussed in more detail. Serious side effects of tocolytic therapy with β-agonists include cardiovascular side effects like hypotension, cardiac arrhythmias, myocardial ischemia and pulmonary edema. The altered cardiovascular physiology of pregnancy and labour (increased plasma volume and cardiac output) probably contributes to some of these adverse side effects of β-adrenergic tocolytics.

Table 6: Physiological effects of β_1- and β_2-adrenergic receptors

System	β_1-Receptor effects	β_2-Receptor effects
cardiac	↑ heart rate ↑ stroke volume ↑ cardiac output	↓ vascular tone ↓ mean arterial pressure
metabolic	↑ intracellular potassium ↑ lipolysis, ketones	↑ glycogenolysis ↑ insulin release
bowel	↓ bowel motility	
kidney		↑ renin output ↓ urine output
lungs		↓ bronchiolar tone
uterus		↓ uterine activity

Maternal side effects

Sinus tachycardia is present in all patients.

Mild palpitations occur in up to a third of the patients. These resolve upon tailing off of the intravenous infusion.

Flushing occurs in up to 15% of patients.

Restlessness, agitation, anxiety, headaches, tremor, chest tightness, nausea and vomiting may occur in some patients. Rarely, patients may suffer paralytic ileus or dermatitis (Horowitz and Creasy 1978).

Hypotension can occur as a consequence of peripheral vasodilatation. This potential problem is compensated for by the physiologic increased cardiac output of pregnancy and the β_1-adrenergic effects of increasing the heart rate and stroke volume and thus the cardiac output (Bieniarz et al 1974). The tendency therefore is for the systolic pressure to rise and the diastolic pressure to fall, increasing the pulse pressure (Bieniarz et al 1974).

Cardiac arrhythmias occur in up to 2% of patients on intravenous infusion therapy. They are usually asymptomatic and of the junctional and ventricular ectopic variety. They resolve upon cessation of therapy (Benedetti 1983). They are more likely to occur in those with undetected cardiac problems.

Myocardial ischemia appears to be a function of maternal tachycardia above 120 beats per minute (Benedetti 1983; Ying and Tejani 1982). Cardiac enzymes (creatinine phosphokinase isoenzyme MB) do not confirm myocardial damage. Increased blood volume has been found to be the contributing factor as salbutamol infusion in a woman who had myocardial strain during pregnancy did not lead to the same problem in a nonpregnant state (Arulkumaran et al 1986).

Pulmonary edema is one of the more serious adverse side effects of intravenous β-mimetic therapy. How frequently it occurs, which drug is more likely to cause it and whether the method of administration matters significantly is still a matter of serious research (Katz et al 1981; Ingermarsson et al 1985). It can be prevented by cautious and judicious administration of the drug and can be reversed by cessation of the therapy and appropriate treatment if recognised early. It may progress to the adult respiratory distress syndrome if it is not recognised early and appropriate treatment instituted. It is unusual for this complication to occur within the first 24 hours of carefully instituted intravenous β-mimetic therapy (Creasy 1989; Katz 1981). The pathophysiology of the condition is unclear but probably related to a constellation of interacting factors: a high output state associated with pregnancy and in particular with multiple pregnancies, a maternal heart rate above 130 beats per minute and maternal anemia below 9 g/dl; fluid retention and overload that may in part be iatrogenic especially if isotonic solutions are used, and in part due to the stimulation of the renin-aldosterone system and the antidiuretic hormone by the β-mimetic that leads to a decrease in the urinary output and a decrease in colloid osmotic pressure (Ingemarsson and Arulkumaran 1985); and finally, capillary endothelial leakage that is generally seen in pregnancy. The use of corticosteroids has been implicated as another predisposing factor for the development of pulmonary edema but in fact the mineralocorticoid activity in these drugs is small and their association is more likely casual rather than causal to the condition (Robertson et al 1981).

Maternal deaths have been reported in association with β-adrenergic agonist tocolysis. In particular they occur in patients with unrecognised underlying cardiac disease or myocarditis. The penultimate event could be pulmonary edema (Kubli 1977).

The elevation of intracellular cAMP in the liver as a result of β_2-receptor stimulation leads to gylcogenolysis and therefore maternal hyperglycemia. This elevation of the blood glucose level occurs quite rapidly, begins to decline after its peak and persists for a as yet unquantified period of time, possibly even beyond 24 hours (Young et al 1983). The maternal insulin level too rises. This is in response to both a direct effect of the stimulation of β_2-receptors in the pancreas (and cAMP rise) and in response to maternal hyperglycemia (Lipshitz and Vinik 1978). The blood sugar levels usually do not exceed 10 mmol/L (180 mg/dl) and generally, exogenous insulin is unnecessary. These acute alterations in the carbohydrate metabolism are usually of little consequence in a normal patient but there are exceptions. In the insulin-dependent diabetic and rarely even in non-diabetics, ketoacidosis may ensue (Thomas et al 1977b; Steel and Parboosingh 1977; Mordes et al 1982; Leopold and McEvoy 1977). Long term oral therapy with terbutaline but not the other β_2-mimetics has been reported to be associated with altered glucose tolerance (Main et al 1987). The lactate that is produced by muscle glycogenolysis rarely causes maternal acidosis probably because of the concomitant respiratory alkalosis that exists in pregnancy.

Maternal hypokalemia is a constant finding in most patients on β-mimetic tocolytic therapy (Schreyer et al 1979). This effect is partly a function of the concomitant hyperglycemia and hyperinsulinemia that drives the potassium into the intracellular compartment and possibly also partly a direct effect of β-adrenoreceptor stimulation (Cano et al 1985). The serum potassium may fall below 3 mmol/L. The hypokalemia is transient, usually not warranting any treatment and often normalising within 24 hours (Young et al 1983; Kirkpatrick et al 1980). The electrocardiogram remains normal unless other effects of tachycardia or myocardial ischemia supervene (Thomas et al 1977a).

Fetal and neonatal side effects   Apart from hexoprenaline, the other β-adrenergic agents cross the placenta. Their exact pharmacokinetics is not clearly understood in humans and the effects on animal models do not seem to be equivalent to those in the human model. In the fetus, there can be mild tachycardia with moderate infusion rates (Unbehaun 1974; Ingermarsson 1976). In the neonate, hypoglycemia, hypotension, hypocalcemia, ileus and death have been reported with the use of isoxsuprine (Brazy and Pupkin 1979; Epstein et al 1979). With the other agents, the principal neonatal problem appears to be hypoglycemia and an estimation of the infant's blood sugar level soon after birth is essential especially if delivery takes place within 48 hours of tocolysis. No long term adverse effects have been established in children exposed in utero to β-mimetic tocolytic therapy (Freysz et al 1977; Hadders-Algra et al 1986).

Efficacy β-adrenergic agonists are effective in postponing delivery albeit for a short duration. In themselves they have not been shown to be beneficial for the fetus or neonate (Canadian preterm labour investigation group 1992) but they buy the fetus some time within the intrauterine environment during which useful measures may be initiated. These may be in the form of corticosteroid administration to promote fetal lung maturity, in utero transfer to a facility with an adequate neonatal set up or just more time to improve the overall chances of intact infant survival.

Magnesium sulphate

Magnesium sulphate has been used extensively in pre-eclampsia but there is presently a mounting interest on both sides of the Atlantic in the use of this drug as a tocolytic agent.

Pharmacology and mechanism of action The active agent is magnesium cation (Mg^{++}). It has been recognised for a long time now that magnesium has a inhibitory capacity upon myometrial contractility (Hall et al 1959). The precise mechanism is unclear but it is likely that magnesium uncouples the depolarisation-contraction couplings (Harbert et al 1969). It is thought that at depolarisation of the myometrial cell, magnesium competes with calcium for entry into the cell. So, there is less intracellular free calcium (Ca^{++}) to participate in the actin-myosin interaction during the smooth muscle contraction. Magnesium is also known to affect neural transmission by modifying acetylcholine release and sensitivity at the motor end-plate. The drug is rapidly cleared by the kidneys (Cruikshank et al 1981). Its activity on different organ systems is dose dependent: myometrial contractility is inhibited at a maternal serum level between 5 and 8 mg/dl; deep tendon reflexes may be lost at a concentrations of 9 to 13 mg/dl; and respiratory depression may occur at or above 14 mg/dl (Petrie 1981).

Dosage and administration In addition to all the precautions, preparations and monitoring described under β-adrenergic agonists, three special measures need to be taken when administering magnesium sulphate. These include the measurement of serum magnesium levels at 6 hourly intervals, regular 2 to 4 hourly monitoring of the patient's deep tendon reflexes (DTR) and keeping ready available vials of calcium gluconate as an antidote to reverse any serious toxic effects of the magnesium. An intravenous loading dose of 4 g is administered over 20 min followed by a maintenance dose of 4 g/hr. If the contractions are successfully inhibited, the infusion is tapered to 2 g/hr for the next 12 – 24 hours. Most authors would pre-scribe oral β-mimetics as maintenance but some have described the availability of oral magnesium supplement (Martin et al 1987). If there is no response to the initial infusion, the dose may be increased gradually every half hour or so by 0.5 g/hr until a maximum dose rate of 6 g/hr or a maximum serum magnesium concentration of 8 mg/dl is reached.

Side effects

Maternal side effects   Most studies have been done on patients with severe pregnancy-induced hypertension. A bolus infusion of 4 g of magnesium sulphate brought about a mild lowering of the mean arterial blood pressure with mild tachy-cardia. There was no significant drop in diastolic blood pressure, no depression of myocardial workload and no effect on oxygen transport or consumption (Cotton et al 1984). The peripheral vasodilatation caused by magnesium sulphate causes flushing, warmth and headaches. Nausea, dizziness, lethargy and chest tightness can occur especially during the bolus dose. Pulmonary edema has been reported in patients on concomitant magnesium sulphate and corticosteroid therapy (Elliott et al 1979; Elliott 1984) so the cautions described for β-adrenergic agonists must hold. Hypocalcemia occurs with increases in maternal serum magnesium levels from an increased urinary excretion (Cruikshank et al 1981). Mostly asymptomatic, this hypocalcemia may produce symptoms occasionally (Savory and Monif 1971). Parathormone levels increase but phosphate and calcitonin levels remain unchanged. Maternal body temperature may fall by 0.5°C, potentially masking a chorioam-nionitis (Parsons et al 1987). Levels of 15 to 18 mg/dl may cause respiratory depression and levels above this may lead to cardiac arrest and death (Caritas et al 1979). Adequate monitoring of deep tendon reflexes, maternal serum magnesium levels and standby of an effective antidote (calcium gluconate) should prevent any undesired side effects.

Fetal and neonatal side effects   Magnesium ions cross the placenta easily into the fetal circulation (Cruikshank et al 1979). The clearance in the fetus appears to be slower than the time the mother takes which is up to 4 days, to eliminate excess magnesium. In general, most infants are born with no neonatal depression (Green et al 1983). However if the umbilical cord magnesium sulphate concentration is above 4 mg/dl, it is possible to have depressed respiratory and motor activity in the neonate (Lipshitz and English 1967). In fact, infants born during or shortly after maternal tocolytic treatment are not uncommonly drowsy, limp and have low calcium levels (Petrie 1981).

Efficacy   This has yet to be established with certainty. Thus far the trials have been either observational or have been made in comparison with β-mimetic to-colytics. Steer and Petrie (1977) found that magnesium sulphate was superior to ethanol but only marginally effective if the cervical dilatation exceeded 1 cm. Miller and colleagues (1982) showed it to be at least as effective as terbutaline with fewer adverse cardiovascular effects but the numbers in the trial were small. Elliott (1984) and Wilkins and co-workers (1986) demonstrated reasonable efficacies but the trials lacked the power of design. Problems with study design and reporting also exist in the studies by Parsons et al (1987) and Tchilinguirian et al (1984) and so far the results are inconclusive. Some authors have attempted a cocktail of β-agonists and magnesium sulphate but this approach may be hazardous with cumulative side effects (Hatjis et al 1984; Ferguson et al 1984). Keirse et al (1989) recommend that 'where it is still in use for the inhibition of preterm labour, it should be phased out' except perhaps in the context of a well-designed, well-conducted, well-reported, randomised, placebo-controlled trial made in the interest of bringing the debate to rest.

Prostaglandin synthetase inhibitors (PGSI)

Pharmacology and mechanism of action   The section on pathophysiology describes the significant role of prostaglandins in the initiation of preterm labour. Based on this the role of cyclo-oxygenase inhibitors seems obvious (Zuckerman et al 1974). Both aspirin and other non-steroidal anti-inflammatory agents (NSAIDs) like indomethacin inhibit the cyclo-oxygenase system. Naproxen, flufenamic acid, aspirin and indomethacin have all been used to treat preterm labour but indomethacin has been most widely used. Aspirin is generally not recommended as a tocolytic as it binds irreversibly to platelet cyclo-oxygenase and may be associated with maternal and fetal hemorrhage peripartally (Stuart et al 1982). Indomethacin has been shown in vitro studies to abolish spontaneous contractions of myometrial strips (Garrioch 1978). The drug is absorbed both orally and rectally with plasma levels peaking within two hours. It remains extensively protein-bound and is excreted unchanged. Its serum half-life is two hours. Indomethacin readily crosses the placenta.

Dosage and administration   The specific contraindications for the use of PGSIs include a history of peptic ulcer disease, coagulation disorders, drug induced asthma and hepatic or renal insufficiency. There are no studies with controlled data to indicate what optimal dose of indomethacin will most effectively inhibit preterm labour with the minimum of side effects. Most authors appear to use up to 200 mg initially in divided doses followed by 100 mg daily in divided doses. In view of the short half-life of the drug, it is more likely to keep the uterus quiescent when given in 4 – 8 hourly doses (Keirse 1981). In our experience, 25 mg given 3 times a day orally seems to be quite adequate and effective. Generally 1–3 mg/kg maternal body weight per day is recommended in divided doses. Again the duration of treatment has not been established (Van Kets et al 1979). A reasonable line of management would be to give the therapy with the aim of achieving as much time as possible for reasonable fetal maturity (approximately 32 weeks), while regularly monitoring the mother and fetus for evidence of untoward side effects.

Side effects

Maternal side effects   Gastrointestinal side effects commonly associated with NSAID use can be kept to a minimum by taking the drug with meals or when needed with antacid. Rarely, postpartum hemorrhage may be associated with indomethacin use (Reiss et al 1976).

Fetal and neonatal side effects   Concern has been raised about the effects of indomethacin on the fetal and neonatal circulation: narrowing of the fetal ductus arteriosus, primary pulmonary hypertension and persistent fetal circulation. These effects appear to be related to the use of indomethacin in high doses for prolonged periods of time and close to term. The ductus itself appears to become more sensitive to PGSIs beyond 32 weeks of gestation (Goudie and Dossetor 1979; Csaba et al 1978). Careful fetal surveillance with echocardiographic techniques can identify abnormal flow patterns across the ductus when it starts to narrow; prompt cessation of therapy reverses this untoward trend (Moise et al 1987).

Indomethacin therapy is associated with decreased fetal urine excretion and oligohydramnios (Cantor et al 1980). Occasionally the oligohydramnios is associated with fetal death (Itskovitz et al 1980). Short-term therapy (less than 48 hours) with indomethacin used before 34 weeks did not appear to cause any adverse side effects (Niebyl and Witter 1986; Dudley and Hardie 1985).

Efficacy   Indomethacin has been shown to be extremely effective in inhibiting preterm labour (Higby et al 1993; Norton et al 1993). However it cannot be recommended for routine use till more large randomised controlled trials are conducted. Meanwhile, it can be used on a limited scale with careful surveillance for fetal effects and for short durations. It is especially useful in situations associated with polyhydramnios.

Calcium channel blockers

Agents that block the influx of calcium into the uterine smooth muscle cell inhibit uterine contractility by diminishing the free intracytoplasmic calcium. Verapamil and nifedipine are two such drugs. Verapamil has an independent effect on atrioventricular conduction, nifedipine much less so. Though known to be effective in small scale trials (Andersson 1977; Ulmsten et al 1980; Read and Wellby 1986), their role in tocolysis for preterm labour has yet to be defined with certainty (Higby et al 1993).

Diazoxide

Diazoxide is a potent antihypertensive. It has an inhibitory effect on smooth muscle through the adenyl cyclase pathway similar to β-mimetics. Like β-mimetics it causes a decreased peripheral resistance, accelerated heart rate and increased cardiac output. Although popular in some centres (Adamsons and Wallach 1984), diazoxide is not commonly used as a tocolytic in most places because of its diabetogenic potential, its propensity to cause profound hypotension and the availability of safer alternatives.

Ethanol

While it was the first widely used tocolytic especially in the United States (before β-mimetics became approved for tocolysis), the use of ethanol in the inhibition of preterm labour is now only of historical interest. Ethanol is thought to act both centrally and peripherally to inhibit uterine contractions. Centrally it acts on the posterior pituitary to decrease oxytocin and antidiuretic hormone release (Fuchs and Fuchs 1981). Peripherally it appears to blunt the response of the myometrium to exogenous and endogenous oxytocics (Mantell and Liggins 1970). Intravenous ethanol infusion can be quite toxic and extremely close supervision is necessary. The mother can suffer intoxication, headache, vomiting, disorientation, diuresis, dehydration, hypoglycemia, lactic acidosis and aspiration pneumonia. The lactic acidosis on occasion may become severe and life-threatening if multiple courses of ethanol are used (Ott et al 1976). In patients obtunded from inebriation, vomiting may lead to aspiration (Greenhouse et al 1969). Ethanol readily crosses the placenta; the fetal blood levels approximate the mother's. Since the neonate's ability to metabolise and clear the alcohol is poorer than the mother's, the effects of the alcohol on the fetus/neonate last much longer. Ethanol can cause the neonate to be born intoxicated (if delivery takes place soon after treatment); it can also depress the central nervous and respiratory systems in the neonate causing respiratory distress. Its use therefore can no longer be recommended in the presence of safer, more effective alternatives.

Progesterone

Progesterone is a 'common sense' choice for a tocolytic since it is supposed to promote uterine quiescence. If used in prophylactic fashion, it might be able to bring about a reduction in preterm delivery rates and the incidence of low birth-weight infants. It is with this hope that it is used in certain Assisted Reproductive Technique (ART) programmes. By contrast, its efficacy in inhibiting active preterm labour is not proven (Keirse et al 1989). The effects of progesterone on myometrial cell physiology appear promising: it decreases myometrial oxytocin and α-adrenergic receptor concentrations and inhibits the appearance of intracellular gap junctions. However it was noticed long ago that even intravenous progesterone in doses up to 90 mg/hr was unable to inhibit uterine contractility in labour (Taubert and Haskins 1963). The use of progesterone is currently limited to prophylaxis rather than tocolysis.

Oxytocin analogues

It is known that there is an increase in myometrial oxytocin receptors in labour at term and that in preterm labour too oxytocin receptor concentration rises significantly (Fuchs et al 1982, Fuchs et al 1984). To use an analogue to competitively block these oxytocin receptors appears an attractive and logical approach to the inhibition of preterm labour (Akerlund et al 1987). Trials are presently in progress and their results will prove interesting.

Nitric oxide donors

Nitric oxide (NO) donors are not new: they have been used as vascular smooth muscle relaxants for a long time in cardiac conditions and nitroglycerine (GTN) is a classic example. There is gathering evidence that placental corticotrophin releasing hormone (CRH) acts as a promoter of human parturition. The regulation of placental CRH and NO metabolism has been demonstrated in placental villi and some work has shown that nitric oxide donors inhibit placental CRH secretion (Sun et al 1994). This hypothesis was tested in a small, uncontrolled, non-randomised trial on 13 patients at King's College Hospital (Lees et al 1994). The results appear promising with few side effects, but larger, properly conducted randomised controlled trials must be completed before the use of nitric oxide donors can be recommended for routine use as tocolytics.

A 10 mg nitroglycerine patch is applied over the uterine fundal region of the maternal abdomen. If tocolysis is not achieved in one hour another 10 mg patch can be applied, the maximum dose being 20 mg over 24 hours. The same dosage schedule can be followed for recurrence or maintenance.

Glucocorticoids to promote fetal lung maturity

This has become fairly well established since Liggins' work 20 years ago (Liggins and Howie 1972; Liggins et al 1977). They showed that the effects of the steroids were noted if delivery occurred after 24 hr of the first dose and within seven days. Controversy exists as to whether a second dose of steroids should be administered if the pregnancy is delayed beyond seven days. More recent studies confirm these beneficial effects of steroids on the fetus and even suggest some benefit from their use as early as 28 weeks (Avery et al 1986; Worthington et al 1983). The steroids appear to benefit other organ systems as well and decrease the incidence, apart from RDS, of necrotising enterocolitis, bronchopulmonary dysplasia and patent ductus arteriosus. Long-term follow up of the infants exposed in utero to antenatal corticosteroid therapy show no adverse effects upon growth, physical or mental development (MacArthur et al 1982; Collaborative group 1984).

Risks to the mother have been suggested repeatedly but these are small and under supervised circumstances avoidable. The majority of studies have not shown an increased propensity for the mother or fetus for infection. The steroids will aggravate the diabetogenic effects of concomitant β-mimetic tocolytic therapy but this can usually be kept in check. There is a theoretical risk of the steroid potentiating the possibility of pulmonary edema when used together with a tocolytic. All these risks must be weighed against the benefits accrued to the fetus from the glucocorticoid therapy.

There was some initial hope that thyrotropin releasing hormone (TRH) might act synergistically with glucocorticoids to enhance fetal lung maturity. Animal and in vitro studies suggested that glucocorticoids, thyroid hormone and prolactin act in concert to increase pulmonary phosphatidylcholine and improve fetal lung stability and distensibility (Ballard 1984). It was hoped that TRH which crosses the placenta and increases fetal thyroid hormone and prolactin might help improve fetal lung maturation. A recent study (ACTOBAT Study Group 1995) showed that this did not do so and that the significant maternal and perinatal risks presently inhibit any recommendation for widespread clinical use of the drug.

Prediction, early detection and prevention of preterm labour

In an attempt to achieve a real and dramatic reduction in the preterm delivery rate, there needs to be adequate primary prevention and effective secondary prevention. Many patients who present in preterm labour have already progressed to the point where inhibition is not possible. So the ability to predict patients who are at high risk of developing preterm labour, to educate them adequately, to recognise the early signs of the condition and the need to seek medical attention quickly and to modify their behaviour and lifestyle must all act synergistically to lower the incidence of preterm labour.

The three main lines of research in the prediction of preterm labour are risk-scoring systems, biochemical and biophysical methods. Risk-scoring systems based on history, in particular past reproductive history, and observed cervical changes have been developed. Though effective in predicting up to half the population that delivers preterm, they miss half and include many patients that never develop preterm labour (Papiernik 1977; Creasy et al 1980; Main et al 1987). The use of serum (or plasma) estradiol, progesterone and prostaglandin levels have not shown any promise so far (Block et al 1984; Mitchell et al 1978). Fetal fibronectin and CRH (*vide supra*) in maternal serum are now being actively investigated. Uterine activity monitoring with a portable home tocodynamometer was shown to be of some value in identifying women at high risk of preterm labour (Katz et al 1986). All these tests may prove helpful in patients already identified to be at high risk of preterm labour but unlikely to be of benefit as a screening tool in the general population (Lockwood and Dudenhausen 1993). Perhaps in time it will be a combination of historical, biochemical and biophysical factors put together that may be able to identify the woman at risk of preterm labour with reasonable sensitivity and specificity.

Early detection of preterm labour involves educating the women at risk in the symptoms that may portend early preterm labour: uterine contractions (frequently painless and which may be described as menstrual cramps), dull backache, pelvic pressure (these are constant symptoms) and a sudden increase in vaginal discharge or a pink-staining discharge. Changes in the cervix can be evaluated ultrasonographically or clinically (Smeltzer et al 1992) by a single or serial examination in the late second or early third trimester. Earlier concerns about examinations precipitating preterm labour, preterm prelabour rupture of the membranes or ascending infection have not been confirmed (Holbrook et al 1985). It appears that transvaginal ultrasonography appears superior to abdominal ultrasonography in evaluating cervical length and predicting the onset of preterm labour (Andersen et al 1990). Electronic monitoring of uterine activity by an ambulatory device allows an objective parameter that results in earlier detection of imminent preterm labour. Although not validated in randomised trials this has recently been included in various preterm birth prevention programmes.

Behaviour modification has been suggested and investigated but no particular method has been found to be universally effective. Perhaps the maximal advantage may be expected from the cessation of smoking, a proper diet and a reduction in psychological stress. The role of prophylactic bed rest and the avoidance of sexual intercourse in the third trimester has not yet been proven conclusively but may be recommended in women with a poor reproductive history. Cervical cerclage is not shown to be effective in reducing preterm delivery rates and should be reserved for patients with cervical incompetence (MRC/RCOG Working Party on Cervical Cerclage 1993). Looking for and treating cervical colonisation with Neisseria gonorrhoeae, Chlamydia trachomatis and group B streptococci and asymptomatic bacteriuria may be useful but is not proven to decrease the incidence of preterm labour.

The role of pharmacologic therapy in the prevention of preterm labour is as yet unclear. Since our present methods to identify 'high risk' patient are inadequate, the routine and liberal use of such therapy would expose a large number of patients to unnecessary risks. Prophylactic progesterone has been tried in the form of medroxyprogesterone (Ovlisen and Iverson 1963) and 17α-hydroxyprogesterone caproate (Johnson et al 1979). In a prospective double-blind study using 17α-hydroxyprogesterone caproate, Hauth et al (1983) were unable to demonstrate any beneficial effect in reducing preterm births. A decrease in the preterm birth rate was noted in a retrospective study using salbutamol at a dose and frequency that produced a mild maternal tachycardia (TambyRaja et al 1978) and this finding was confirmed in a few studies using terbutaline and ritodrine (Brown and Tejani 1980; Creasy et al 1980; O'Leary 1986). PGSIs and calcium channel blockers have not been evaluated for efficacy and safety in the prevention of preterm labour.

Finally, various birth prevention programmes have been initiated. They include ample education of patients at risk, increased awareness and surveillance by health care providers, patient detection of painless uterine contractions or ambulatory electronic measurements and prompt tocolysis if the diagnosis is established (Creasy 1983; Meis et al 1987). In France social support programmes which include financial support and liberal maternity leave policies have added impact to their preterm birth prevention programmes (Papiernik 1984). Such programmes may take years to be initiated in other countries and it may even then take up to 4 years before their impact becomes visible (Papiernik et al 1986).

Delivery

Ideally the delivery should take place in a centre equipped with adequate neonatal facilities to handle preterm infants. Occasionally this may mean temporary tocolysis to effect an in utero transfer. Having once decided that the labour is not to be inhibited, all tocolytics should be stopped. Preterm infants are extremely susceptible to hypoxia and intrapartum management should be geared to limit such insult (Martin et al 1974). A neonatologist should be present at delivery as most preterm babies will need some form of care and resuscitation. In all cases the mode of delivery and neonatal outcome should be discussed with the parents at the outset. These are discussed in the chapter dealing with neonatal resuscitation.

Analgesia and anesthesia

Parenteral sedatives and narcotics should be used cautiously as they have a depressant effect on the baby. Epidural analgesia is particularly useful in relaxing pelvic musculature and reducing resistance on the fetal head especially at the outlet. It also limits premature maternal expulsive efforts. General anesthesia may be used for caesarean section but an epidural may be preferable.

Route of delivery

So far there has been no evidence to support the need for caesarean section in the face of a vertex presentation. Indeed vaginal delivery may be of some benefit in expelling the amniotic fluid from the chest at delivery and facilitate lung expansion. The routes of delivery in breech and twin labours are controversial and if the labour progress is satisfactory in the first and second stage vaginal delivery can be anticipated.

Episiotomy and low (outlet) forceps

A generous episiotomy is certainly useful to reduce the length of the second stage and to decrease head compression and sudden decompression at the time of delivery. The place of the prophylactic forceps to reduce delivery trauma to the head has not been established (Schwartz et al 1983).

Postpartum care

The parturient and usually her partner undergo intensive emotional stress upon the delivery of a premature infant. She may experience shock, grief, denial, anger, guilt, anxiety and finally acceptance. During this difficult period she will need psychosocial support from the obstetrician, the neonatologist, nurses, a medical social worker and in some instances, a psychiatrist. She should be encouraged to visit the neonate in the nursery and to breast-feed in order to build mother-child bonding. Finally, all attempts should be made to try and identify the cause of the preterm labour and birth. At the postnatal visit she should be counselled regarding the possible risk of preterm labour in subsequent pregnancies. Abruption, fetal anomaly, PROM not due to infection and other similar causes are unlikely to operate in the next pregnancy and she should be reassured accordingly. If there are any preventable factors advice and care should be directed towards preventing a recurrence.

References

ACTOBAT Study Group 1995. Australian collaborative trial of antenatal thyrotropin-releasing hormone for prevention of neonatal respiratory disease. *Lancet* 345:877-882.

Adamsons K, Wallach RC 1984. Diazoxide and calcium antagonists in preterm labour. In: Fuchs F, Stubblefield PD, eds. Preterm Birth: Causes, Prevention and Management. New York: Macmillan, pp 249-263.

Andersen HF, Nugent CE, Wanty SD et al 1990. Prediction of risk for preterm delivery by ultrasonographic measurement of cervical length. *Am J Obstet Gynecol* 163:859.

Anderson ABM 1977. Pre-term labour: definition. In: Anderson ABM et al, eds. Proceedings of the Fifth Study Group of the Royal College of Obstetricians and Gynecologists. London: Royal College of Obstetricians and Gynecologists.

Andersson KE 1977. Inhibition of uterine activity by the calcium antagonist nifedipine. In: Anderson A, Beard R, Brudenell JM, Dunn PM, eds. Pre-term Labour. Proceedings of the Fifth Study Group of the Royal College of

Obstetricians and Gynecologists. London: Royal College of Obstetricians and Gynecologists, pp 101-114.

Arulkumaran S, Kitchener H, Balasingham S, Rauff M, Ratnam SS 1986. Myocardial strain associated with intravenous salbutamol therapy for preterm labour. *Sing J Obstet Gynecol* 17:54-58.

Avery ME, Aylward G, Creasy RK et al 1986. Update on prenatal steroids for prevention of respiratory distress. *Am J Obstet Gynecol* 155:2.

Bakketeig LS, Hoffman HJ 1981. Epidemiology of preterm birth: results from a longitudinal study of births in Norway. In: Elder MG, Hendricks CH, eds. Preterm Labour. London: Butterworths.

Ballard PL 1984. Combined hormonal treatment and lung maturation. *Seminars in Perinatology* 8:283.

Beard RW 1985. Fetal viability: an obstetric viewpoint. In: Beard RW, Sharp F, eds. Proceedings of the Thirteenth Study Group of the Royal College of Obstetricians and Gynecologists, London: RCOG.

Benedetti TJ 1983. Maternal complications of parenteral beta-sympathomimetic therapy for premature labour. *Am J Obstet Gynecol* 145:1.

Bieniarz J, Ibankovich A, Scommegna A 1974. Cardiac output during ritodrine treatment in premature labour. *Am J Obstet Gynecol* 118:910.

Block BSB, Liggins GC, Creasy RK 1984. Preterm delivery is not predicted by serial plasma estradiol or progesterone concentration measurements. *Am J Obstet Gynecol* 150:716.

Brazy JE, Pupkin MJ 1979. Effects of maternal isoxsuprine administration on preterm infants. *J Pediatr* 94:444.

Brown SM, Tejani N 1980. Terbutaline sulphate in the prevention of recurrence of premature labour. *Obstet Gynecol* 57:22.

Canadian preterm labour investigation group 1992. Treatment of preterm labour with a β-adrenergic agonist ritodrine. *New Engl J Med* 327:308-312.

Cano A, Tovar I, Parilla JJ, Abad L 1985. Metabolic disturbances during intravenous use of ritodrine: increased insulin levels and hypokalemia. *Obstet Gynecol* 65:356.

Cantor B, Tyler T, Nelson RM et al 1980. Oligohydramnios and transient neonatal anuria. A possible association with the maternal use of prostaglandin synthetase inhibitors. *J Reprod Med* 24:220.

Caritas SN, Lin LS, Toig G et al 1983. Pharmacodynamics of ritodrine in pregnant women during preterm labour. *Am J Obstet Gynecol* 147:752.

Caritas SN, Edelstone DI, Mueller-Heubach E 1979. Pharmacologic inhibition of preterm labour. *Am J Obstet Gynecol* 133:557-578.

Casey ML, MacDonald PC 1988. Biomolecular processes in the initiation of parturition: decidual activation. *Clin Obstet Gynecol* 31(3):533-552.

Castle BM, Turnbull AC 1983. The presence or absence of fetal breathing movements to predict the outcome of premature labour. *Lancet* 2:471.

Challis JRG, Brooks AN 1989. Maturation and activation of hypothalamic-pituitary-adrenal function in fetal sheep. *Endocrinology Review* 10:182-204.

Challis JRG, Olson DM 1988. Parturition. In: Knobil E, Neill J, eds. The Physiology of Reproduction. New York: Raven Press.

Chase HC 1977. Time trends in low birth weight in the United States 1950-1974. In: Reed DM, Stanley FJ, eds. The Epidemiology of Prematurity. Urban and Schwarzenberg, Baltimore, Maryland.

Collaborative Group on Antenatal Therapy 1984. Effects of antenatal dexamethasone administration in the infant. Long-term follow-up. *J Pediatr* 104:259.

Cotton DB, Gonik B, Dorman KF 1984. Cardiovascular alterations in severe pregnancy-induced hypertension: acute effects of intravenous magnesium sulphate. *Am J Obstet Gynecol* 148:162.

Creasy RK 1983. Prevention of preterm birth. *Birth Defects* 19:97.

Creasy RK 1989. Preterm labour and delivery. In: Creasy RK, Resnik R, eds. Maternal-Fetal Medicine: Principles and Practice. Philadelphia: WB Saunders.

Creasy RK, Golbus MS, Laros RK et al 1980. Oral ritodrine maintenance in the treatment of preterm labour. *Am J Obstet Gynecol* 137:212.

Creasy RK, Gummer BA, Liggins GC 1980. A system for predicting spontaneous preterm birth. *Obstet Gynecol* 55:692.

Cruikshank DP, Pitkin RM, Donnelly E, et al 1979. Effects of magnesium sulphate treatment on perinatal calcium metabolism. I. Maternal and fetal responses. *Am J Obstet Gynecol* 134:243.

Cruikshank DP, Pitkin RM, Donnelly E, et al 1981. Urinary magnesium, calcium and phosphate excretion during magnesium sulphate infusion. *Obstet Gynecol* 58:430.

Csaba IF, Sulyok E, Ertl T 1978. Clinical note: relationship of maternal treatment with indomethacin to persistence of fetal circulation syndrome. *J Pediatr* 92:484.

Dudley DKL, Hardie MJ 1985. Fetal and neonatal effects of indomethacin used as a tocolytic agent. *Am J Obstet Gynecol* 151:181.

Elliott JP 1984. Magnesium sulphate as a tocolytic agent. *Am J Obstet Gynecol* 147:277.

Elliott JP, O'Keefe DF, Greenberg P, et al 1979. Pulmonary edema associated with magnesium sulphate and betamethasone administration. *Obstet Gynecol* 134:717.

Epstein MF, Nichols E, Stubblefield PG 1979. Neonatal hypoglycaemia after beta-sympathomimetic tocolytic therapy. *J Pediatr* 94:440.

Ferguson JE, Hensleigh PA, Kredenster D 1984. Adjunctive use of magnesium sulphate with ritodrine for preterm labour tocolysis. *Am J Obstet Gynecol* 148:166-171.

Fredrick J, Anderson ABM 1976. Factors associated with spontaneous preterm birth. *Br J Obstet Gynecol* 83:342.

Freysz H, Willard D, Lehr A, Misser J 1977. A long-term evaluation of infants who receive a beta-mimetic drug while in utero. *J Perinat Med* 5:94.

Fuchs A-R, Fuchs F 1981. Ethanol for prevention of preterm birth. *Seminars in Perinatology* 5:236-251.

Fuchs AR, Fuchs F, Husslein P, Soloff MS, Fernstrom MJ 1982. Oxytocin receptors and human parturition: a dual role for oxytocin in the initiation of labour. *Science* 215:1396.

Garn SM, Bailey SM 1977. Genetics of maturation processes. In: Falkner F, Tanner JM, eds. Human growth. New York: Plenum Press.

Garn SM, Shaw HA, McCabe KD 1977. Effects of socioeconomic status and race on weight-defined and gestational prematurity in the United States. In: Reed DM, Stanley FJ, eds. The Epidemiology of Prematurity. Urban and Schwarzenberg, Baltimore, Maryland.

Garrioch DB 1978. The effect of indomethacin on spontaneous activity in the isolated human myometrium and on the response to oxytocin and prostaglandin. *Br J Obstet Gynecol* 85:47.

Gonik B, Creasy RK 1986. Preterm labour: its diagnosis and management. *Am J Obstet Gynecol* 154:3.

Goodlin RC 1969. Orgasm and premature labour. *Lancet* ii:646.

Goudie BM, Dossetor JFB 1979. Effect on the fetus of indomethacin given to suppress labour. *Lancet* 2:1187.

Green KW, Key TC, Coen R, Resnik RK 1983. The effects of maternally administered magnesium sulphate on the neonate. *Am J Obstet Gynecol* 146:29.

Greenhouse BS, Hook R, Hehre FW 1969. Aspiration pneumonia following intravenous administration of alcohol during labour. *JAMA* 210:2393-2395.

Hadders-Algra M, Touwen BCL, Huisjes HJ 1986. Long-term follow-up of children prenatally exposed to ritodrine. *Br J Obstet Gynecol* 93:156.

Hall DG, McGaughey HS, Corey EL, Thornton WN 1959. The effects of magnesium sulphate therapy on the duration of labour. *Am J Obstet Gynecol* 78:27-32.

Harbert GM, Cornell GW, Thornton WN 1969. Effect of toxemia therapy on uterine dynamics. *Am J Obstet Gynecol* 129:401.

Hardy JB, Mellitis ED 1977. Relationship of low birth weight to maternal characteristics of age, education and body size. In: Reed DM, Stanley FJ, eds. The Epidemiology of Prematurity. Urban and Schwarzenberg, Baltimore, Maryland.

Hatjis CG, Nelson LH, Meis PJ, Swain M 1984. Addition of magnesium sulphate improves the effectiveness of ritodrine in preventing premature delivery. *Am J Obstet Gynecol* 150:142.

Hauth JC, Gildtrap LC, Brekken AL, Hauth JM 1983. The effect of 17α-hydroxyprogesterone caproate on pregnancy outcome in an active-duty military population. *Am J Obstet Gynecol* 146:187.

Heinonen PK, Saarikoski S, Pystynen P 1982. Reproductive performance of women with uterine anomalies. *Acta Obstet Gynecol Scand* 61:157.

Herbst AL , Hubby MM, Blough RR et al 1980. A comparison of pregnancy experience in DES-exposed and DES-unexposed daughters. *J Reprod Med* 24:62.

Higby K, Xenakis EM, Pauerstein CJ 1993. Do tocolytic agents stop preterm labor? A critical and comprehensive review of efficacy and safety. *Am J Obstet Gynecol* 168:1247-56.

Holbrook RH, Lirette M, Creasy RK 1985. Weekly examination in the patient at high risk of preterm delivery. *Proceedings of the Society of Perinatal Obstetrics* 1:27.

Honnebier WJ, Swaab DF 1973 The influence of anencephaly upon intrauterine growth of fetus and placenta and upon gestation length. *J Obstet Gynecol Br Cwlth* 80:577.

Horowitz J, Creasy RK 1978. Allergic dermatitis associated with administration of isoxsupurine. *Am J Obstet Gynecol* 131:225.

Howie RN, Liggins GC 1977. Clinical trial of antepartum betamethasone therapy for prevention of respiratory distress in pre-term infants. In: Anderson ABM, Beard R, Brudenell JM, Dunn PM, eds. Pre-term labour. Proceedings of the Fifth Study Group of the Royal College of Obstetricians and Gynaecologists. London: RCOG, p 281.

Ingemarsson I, Arulkumaran S 1985. Beta agonists in obstetric practice. In: Malcolm Chiswick, ed. Recent Advances in Perinatal Medicine. London, UK: Churchill Livingstone, 2:39-58.

Ingemarsson I, Arulkumaran S, Kottegoda SR 1985. Complications of beta-mimetic therapy in preterm labour. *Aust NZ J Obstet Gynecol* 25:182-185.

Ingemarsson I 1976. Effect of terbutaline on premature labour. A double-blind placebo-controlled study. *Am J Obstet Gynecol* 125:520-524.

Itskovitz J, Abramovici H, Brandes JM 1980. Oligohydramnios, meconium and perinatal death concurrent with indomethacin treatment in human pregnancy. *J Reprod Med* 24:137.

Johnson JWC, Lee PA, Zachary AS et al 1979. High-risk prematurity--progestin treatment and steroid studies. *Obstet Gynecol* 54:512.

Kaltreider DF, Kohl S 1980. Epidemiology of preterm labour. *Clin Obstet Gynecol* 23:17.

Katz M, Robertson PA, Creasy RK 1981. Cardiovascular complications associated with terbutaline treatment for preterm labour. *Am J Obstet Gynecol* 139:605-608.

Katz M, Newman RB, Gill PJ 1986. Assessment of uterine activity in ambulatory patients at high risk of preterm labour. *Am J Obstet Gynecol* 154:44

Ke R, Vohra M, Casper R 1984. Prolonged inhibition of human myometrial contractility by intermittent isoproterenol. *Am J Obstet Gynecol* 149:841.

Keirse MJNC 1981. Potential hazards of prostaglandin synthetase inhibitors for the management of preterm labour. *J Drug Research* 6:915-919.

Keirse MJNC, Rush RW, Anderson AB, Turnbull AC 1978. Risk of preterm delivery or abortion. *Br J Obstet Gynecol* 85:81.

Keirse MJNC, Grant A, King JF 1989. Preterm labour. In: Chalmers I, Enkin M, Keirse MNJC, eds. Effective Care in Pregnancy and Childbirth. Vol 1. Oxford: Oxford University Press, pp 694-745.

Kincaid-Smith P 1968. Bacteriuria and urinary infection in pregnancy. *Clin Obstet Gynecol* 11:533.

Kirbinen P, Jouppila P 1978. Polyhydramnion. A clinical study. *Annales Chirurgiae et Gynaecologiae Senniae* 67:117.

Kirkpatrick C, Quenon M, Desir D 1980. Blood anions and electrolytes during ritodrine infusion in preterm labour. *Am J Obstet Gynecol* 138:523-527.

Kubli F. Discussion 1977. In: Anderson ABM, Beard R, Brudenell JM, Dunn PM, eds. Pre-term labour. Proceedings of the Fifth Study Group of the Royal College of Obstetricians and Gynaecologists. London: Royal College of Obstetricians and Gynaecologists, pp 218-220.

Lees C, Campbell S, Jauniaux E et al 1994. Arrest of preterm labour and prolongation of gestation with glyceryl trinitrate, a nitric oxide donor. *Lancet* 343:1272-1273.

Leopold D, McEvoy A, 1977. Salbutamol-induced ketoacidosis. *Br Med J* 2:1152.

Liggins GC, Fairclough RJ, Grieves SA, Forster CS, Knox BS 1977. Parturition in the sheep. In: The fetus and Birth. Ciba Foundation Symposium 47:5.

Liggins GC, Howie RN 1972. A controlled trial of ante-partum glucocorticoid treatment for prevention of respiratory distress syndrome in premature infants. *Pediatrics* 50:515-525.

Lipshitz J, English IC 1967. Hypermagnesemia in the newborn infant. *Pediatrics* 40:856.

Lipshitz J, Vinik AI 1978. The effects of hexoprenaline, a β_2-sympathomimetic drug, on maternal glucose, insulin, glucagon, and free fatty acid levels. *Am J Obstet Gynecol* 135:761.

Lockwood CJ, Dudenhausen JW 1993. New approaches to the prediction of preterm delivery. *J Perinat Med* 21:441-452.

Lundin-Schiller S, Mitchell MD 1990. Review: the role of prostaglandins in human parturition. *Prostaglandins Leukotrienes and Essential Fatty Acids* 39:1-10.

MacArthur BA, Howie R, Dezoete JA et al 1982. School progress and cognitive development of 6-year-old children whose mothers were treated with betamethasone. *Pediatrics* 70:99.

Main EK, Main DM, Gabbe SG 1987. Chronic oral terbutaline therapy is associated with maternal glucose intolerance. *Am J Obstet Gynecol* 157:664.

Mantell CD, Liggins GC 1970. The effect of ethanol on the myometrial response to oxytocin in women at term. *J Obstet Gynecol Br Cwlth* 77:976-981.

Martin CM, Siassi B, Hon EH 1974. Fetal heart rate patterns and neonatal death in low birth weight infants. *Obstet Gynecol* 44:503.

Martin RW, Gaddy DK, Martin JN, et al 1987. Tocolysis with oral magnesium. *Am J Obstet Gynecol* 156:433.

Meis PJ, Ernest JM, Moore ML et al 1987. Regional program for prevention of premature birth in northwestern North Carolina. *Am J Obstet Gynecol* 157:550.

Miller JM, Keane MWD, Horger EO III 1982. A comparison of magnesium sulphate and terbutaline for the arrest of preterm labour. *J Reprod Med* 27:348.

Mitchell MD, Flint AP, Bibby J et al 1978. Plasma concentration of prostaglandins during late human pregnancy: influence of normal and preterm labour. *J Clin Endocrin* 46:947.

Mitchell MD 1986. Pathways of arachidonic acid metabolism with specific application to the fetus and mother. *Seminars in Perinatology* 10:242-254.

Moise KJ, Huhta JC, Dawood S et al 1987. Indomethacin in the treatment of preterm labour: effects on the human fetal ductus arteriosus. Presented to the Society of Perinatal Obstetricians, Lake Vista, Florida.

Mordes D, Kreutner K, Metzger W, Colwell J 1982. Dangers of intravenous ritodrine in diabetic patients. *Am J Obstet Gynecol* 248:973.

MRC/ RCOG Working Party on Cervical Cerclage 1993. Final report of the Medical Research Council/ Royal College of Obstetricians and Gynecologists multicentre randomised trial of cervical cerclage. *Br J Obstet Gynecol* 100:516-523.

Neerhof M, MacGregor S, Retzity S, Sullivan T 1989. Cocaine abuse during pregnancy: peripartum prevalance and perinatal outcome. *Am J Obstet Gynecol* 161(3):633-638.

Niebyl JR, Witter FR 1986. Neonatal outcome after indomethacin treatment for preterm labour. *Am J Obstet Gynecol* 155:747.

Norton ME, Merrill J, Cooper BA, Kuller JA, Clyman RI 1993. Neonatal complications after the administration of indomethacin for preterm labour. *New Engl J Med* 329:1602-07.

O'Leary JA 1986. Prophylactic tocolysis of twins. *Am J Obstet Gynecol* 154:904.

Ott A, Hayes J, Polin J 1976. Severe lactic acidosis associated with intravenous alcohol for premature labour. *Obstet Gynecol* 48:362-364.

Ovlisen G, Iverson J 1963. Treatment of threatened premature labour with 6α-methyl-17α-acetoprogesterone. *Am J Obstet Gynecol* 79:172.

Papiernik E 1977. Discussion. In: Anderson ABM, Beard R, Brudenell JM, Dunn PM, eds. Pre-term labour. Proceedings of the Fifth Study Group of the Royal College of Obstetricians and Gynaecologists. London: Royal College of Obstetricians and Gynaecologists.

Papiernik E 1984. Proposals for a programmed prevention policy of preterm birth. *Clin Obstet Gynecol* 27:614.

Papiernik E, Bouyer J, Yaffe K et al 1986. Women's acceptance of a preterm birth prevention programme. *Am J Obstet Gynecol* 155:939.

Papiernik E, Kaminski M 1974. Multifactorial study of the risk of prematurity at 32 weeks of gestation: a study for the frequency of 30 predictive characteristics. *J Perinat Med* 2:30.

Parsons MT, Owens CA, Spellacy WN 1987. Thermic effects of tocolytic agents: decreased temperature with magnesium sulphate. *Obstet Gynecol* 69:88-90.

Petrie RH 1981. Tocolysis using magnesium sulphate. *Seminars in Perinatology* 5:266-273.

Philipsen T, Eriksen PS, Lynggard F 1981. Pulmonary edema following ritodrine-saline infusion in premature labour. *Obstet Gynecol* 58:304.

Post LC 1977. Pharmocokinetics of β-adrenergic agonists. In: Anderson PA, Beard R, Brudenell JM, Dunn PA, eds. Pre-term labour. Proceedings of the Fifth Study Group of the Royal College of Obstetricians and Gynaecologists. London: RCOG.

Powell TG, Pharoah POD, Cooke RWI 1986. Survival and morbidity in a geographically defined population of low birthweight infants. *Lancet* i:539-543.

Price HV, Cone BS, Keogh M 1971. Length of gestation in congenital adrenal hyperplasia. *J Obstet Gynecol Br Cwlth* 78:430.

Read MD, Wellby DE 1986. The use of a calcium antagonist (nifedipine) to suppress preterm labour. *Br J Obstet Gynecol* 93:933-937.

Reiss U, Atad J, Reuinstein I et al 1976. The effect of indomethacin in labour at term. *Int J Gynecol Obstet* 14:369.

Roberts G 1970. Unclassified antepartum hemorrhage: incidence and perinatal mortality in a community. *J Obstet Gynecol Br Cwlth* 77:492.

Roberts JS, McCracken JA, Gavagan JE, Soloff MS 1976. Oxytocin-stimulated release of prostaglandin F$_{2\alpha}$ from ovine endometrium in vitro: correlation with estrous cycle and oxytocin-receptor binding. *Endocrinology* 99:1107.

Robertson PA, Herron M, Katz M, Creasy RK 1981. Maternal morbidity associated with isoxsuprine and terbutaline tocolysis. *Eur J Obstet Gynecol Reprod Biol* 11:317.

Rush RW 1979. Incidence of preterm delivery in patients with previous preterm delivery and/ or abortion. *S Afr Med J* 56:1085.

Savarese MFR, Chang IW 1964. Incompetent cervical os. A collective review of the literature with a report of 30 new cases. *Obstet Gynecol Surv* 19:201.

Savory J, Monif G 1971. Serum calcium levels in cord sera of the progeny treated with magnesium sulphate for toxemia of pregnancy. *Am J Obstet Gynecol* 110:556.

Schreyer P, Caspi E, Ariely S, Herzianu I, User P, Gilboa Y, Zaidman JL 1979. Metabolic effects of intravenous ritodrine infusion during pregnancy. *Eur J Obstet Gynecol Reprod Biol* 9:97-103.

Schwartz DB, Miodovnik M, Lavin JP 1983. Neonatal outcome among low birthweight infants delivered spontaneously or by low forceps. *Obstet Gynecol* 62:283.

Schwartz S 1962. Prenatal care, prematurity and neonatal mortality. *Am J Obstet Gynecol* 83:591.

Skinner KA, Challis JA 1984. Changes in the synthesis and metabolism of prostaglandins by human fetal membranes and decidua in labour. *Am J Obstet Gynecol* 151:519.

Smeltzer J, Lewis J, Van Dorsten P, Cruikshank D 1992. Cervical dilation is the best predictor of risk for preterm birth. *Am J Obstet Gynecol* 166:364-366.

Steel JM, Parboosingh J 1977. Insulin requirements in pregnant diabetics with premature labour controlled by ritodrine. *Br Med J* 1:880.

Steer CM, Petrie RH 1977. A comparison of magnesium sulphate and alcohol for the prevention of premature labour. *Am J Obstet Gynecol* 129:1-4.

Stuart MJ, Gross SJ, Elrad H et al 1982. Effects of acetylsalicylic acid ingestion on maternal and neonatal homeostasis. *N Engl J Med* 307:909.

Sun K, Smith R, Robinson PJ 1994. Basal and KCl-stimulated corticotrophin-releasing hormone release from human placental syncytiotrophoblasts is inhibited by sodium nitroprusside. *J Clin Endocrin Metab* 79:519-524.

TambyRaja R, Atputhrajah V, Salmon Y 1978. Prevention of prematurity in twins. *Aust NZ J Obstet Gynecol* 18:179.

TambyRaja RL 1991. Current concepts in the management of preterm labour. In: Ratnam et al, eds. Contributions to Obstetrics and Gynecology, Volume 1. Singapore: Churchill Livingstone.

Taubert HD, Haskins HL 1963. Intravenous infusion of progesterone in human females: blood levels obtained and effect in labour. *Obstet Gynecol* 22:405-408.

Taylor PM, Hall BL 1979. Parent-infant bonding: problems and opportunities in a perinatal centre. *Seminars in Perinatology* 3:73.

Tchilinguirian NG, Najem R, Sullivan GB, Craparo FJ 1984. The use of ritodrine and magnesium sulphate in the arrest of premature labour. *Int J Obstet Gynecol* 22:117-123.

Thomas DJB, Dove AF, Alberti KGMM 1977a. Metabolic effects of salbutamol infusion during premature labour. *Br J Obstet Gynecol* 84:497.

Thomas DJB, Gill B, Brown P, Subbs WA 1977b. Salbutamol-induced diabetic keto-acidosis. *Br Med J* 2:1152.

Ulmsten U, Andersson KE, Wingerup L 1980. Treatment of premature labour with the calcium antagonist nifedipine. *Archives of Gynecology* 229:1-5.

Unbehaun V 1974. Effects of sympathomimetic tocolytic agents on the fetus. *J Perinat Med* 2:17.

US Department of Health and Human Services, Public Health Service, National Centre for Health Statistics: *Vital Statistics of the United States* 1980, Vol 1. Natality: Hyattsville 1984.

Van Kets H, Thiery M, Derom R, Van Egmond H, Baele G 1979. Perinatal hazards of chronic antenatal tocolysis with indomethacin. *Prostaglandins* 18:893-907.

Wagner NN, Butler JC, Sanders JP 1976. Prematurity and orgasmic coitus during pregnancy: data on a small sample. *Fertil Steril* 27:911.

Weber T, Obel E 1979. Pregnancy complications following conization of the uterine cervix. *Acta Obstet Gynecol Scand* 58:259.

Weitz CM, Ghodgaonkar RN, Dubin NH, Niebyl JR 1986. Prostaglandin F metabolite concentration as a prognostic value in preterm labour. *Obstet Gynecol* 67:496.

Wilkins IA, Goldberg JD, Phillips RN et al 1986. Long-term use of magnesium sulphate as a tocolytic agent. *Obstet Gynecol* 67(suppl):38.

World Health Organization 1969. Prevention of Perinatal Morbidity and Mortality. Public Health Papers 42, Geneva: WHO.

Ying YK, Tejani NA 1982. Angina pectoris as a complication of ritodrine hydrochloride therapy in premature labour. *Obstet Gynecol* 60:385.

Young DC, Toofanian A, Leveno KJ 1983. Potassium and glucose concentrations without treatment during ritodrine tocolysis. *Am J Obstet Gynecol* 145:105.

Yu VYH, Loke HL, Bajuk B, SzymonowiczW, Orgill AA, Astbury J 1986. Prognosis for infants born at 23 to 28 weeks gestation. *Br Med J* 293:1200-1203.

Yu VYH, Watkins A, Bajuk B 1984. Neonatal and postneonatal mortality in very low birthweight infants. *Archives of Disease in Childhood* 59:987-999.

Zuckerman H, Reiss U, Rubinstein I 1974. Inhibition of human premature labour by indomethacin. *Obstet Gynecol* 44:787-792.

17

Prolonged Pregnancy

S Arulkumaran
S Chua

The management of prolonged pregnancy is a subject of concern because of its known association with increased fetal morbidity and mortality (Clifford 1954, Nesbitt 1955, Evans et al 1963, Naeye 1978). Women worry when they have not delivered by the expected date of delivery (EDD) because they think post EDD is the same as prolonged pregnancy and because they have heard that prolonged pregnancy carries a risk to the fetus. Such anxiety should not arise if women are counselled on their first visit that they are most likely to deliver from between 38 to 42 weeks and not on the EDD and that prolonged pregnancy refers to gestations greater than 42 weeks. The anxiety increases even amongst doctors when a woman does not deliver by 41 weeks, because morbidity and mortality can occur between 41 and 42 weeks although it is more common beyond 42 weeks. Hence antenatal fetal wellbeing tests are instituted after 41 weeks (Guidetti et al 1989). It should be realised that the trials on induction versus conservative management in prolonged pregnancy were performed on a selected population where the fetus was thought to have 'minimal risk' (there being no situation called 'no risk') based on the fetal wellbeing tests at the end of 42 weeks. In those who are managed conservatively beyond 42 weeks, some develop signs suggestive of fetal compromise with the progress of time necessitating induction of labour. Centres vary in the availability of tests for fetal wellbeing and the ability to cope with the demand. The availability of appropriate medication for the successful induction of labour may also determine the timing of induction. Based on these factors it is difficult to have a uniform policy to manage prolonged pregnancy. The management has to be tailored to suit the facilities available in each centre. Any management policy should weigh the risk-benefit ratio of intervention versus nonintervention and should also take into consideration the patient's wishes after having given her the relevant information.

Prolonged pregnancy, postdated pregnancy, post-term, postdatism and post-maturity are terms used to denote a pregnancy which has gone beyond 42 weeks or 294 days from the first date of the last menstrual period (Gibb 1984). These terms are used with the idea of conveying a risk situation. But in practice it is useful to consolidate various views and adhere to one term. Prolonged pregnancy conveys the term most accurately and is defined by the International Federation of Gynecologists and Obstetricians (FIGO) as any pregnancy which exceeds 294 days from the first day of the last menstrual period (FIGO 1980). The term postdates and postdatism appear to convey different meanings to patients and doctors, some considering it a date which goes beyond the EDD. The term postdatism is best avoided in these situations, and the duration of pregnancy is stated as so many days post EDD, for example, 41 weeks and 4 days, unless it is more than 294 days when it can be labelled as prolonged pregnancy. The postmaturity syndrome refers to the description of a newborn who is coated with meconium, has dry peeling skin, overgrown nails, well developed creases on the palm and soles, an abundance of scalp hair, little vernix or lanugo hair, a scaphoid abdomen, minimal subcutaneous fat and an attentive apprehensive look (Clifford 1954). Though such a picture is associated with infants born after 42 weeks, they constitute only a small proportion. Infants with such features may be born even at 39 and 40 weeks and hence are not the norm or characteristic of prolonged pregnancy. Therefore the term prolonged pregnancy should be preferred to postmaturity for pregnancies beyond·42 weeks.

Incidence

The incidence of prolonged pregnancy varies from 3 to 10% or more depending on whether it is calculated in a prospective or retrospective manner. It will also vary depending on whether the calculation is based on the history and clinical examination alone or whether early ultrasound examination was utilised to calculate the gestation in the first half of pregnancy (Bierman et al 1965; Lindell 1956; Eik-Nes et al 1984; Ingemarsson and Heden 1989). The definition adapted and the factors considered in calculating the period of gestation will also influence the incidence. The calculation cannot be relied upon if the patient is not sure of her last menstrual period or if the period was immediately after the discontinuation of hormonal contraceptives or lactation. Allowance will have to be given if the cycles are long as it will influence the date of ovulation. The available literature suggests that about 20% of women could not remember their last menstrual period (LMP) and hence were unsure of their gestation (Hall et al 1985). One should be aware that perinatal mortality is increased in those with unknown dates (Dewhurst et al 1972) and some of these deaths may be due to unrecognised cases of prolonged pregnancy.

In centres where women book in the first trimester, and where a dating scan is done in the first half of the pregnancy the incidence of prolonged pregnancy is less than 5% (Eik-Nes et al 1984, Ingemarsson and Heden 1989). Places where the incidence of induction is high for various reasons will tend to reduce the true incidence of prolonged pregnancy (Lindell 1956; Chamberlain et al 1970).

Risks for the mother

Risks for the mother are that of operative delivery associated either with sponta-neous or induced labour. Induction of labour is performed as a routine by the 42nd week in some centres whilst in others it is done when poor fetal function tests prompt delivery. The incidence of operative delivery in prolonged pregnancy if the women are in spontaneous labour appears to be lower than induced labour in some series (Gibb et al 1982) whilst others have found no difference (Cardozo et al 1986); some have reported an increase in those managed conservatively with the help of antepartum testing (Dyson et al 1987). The risk of induction will depend on whether it was possible to successfully achieve vaginal delivery of a neonate in good condition within a reasonable time or whether the patient had a caesarean section for failed induction of labour. Other possibilities of morbidity like postpartum hemorrhage and infection will increase if labour is prolonged.

Two recent large multicentre randomised trials have returned conflicting results. Data from the National Institute of Child Health and Human Development Network of Maternal-Fetal Medicine Units (National Institute of Child Health and Human Development Network 1994) indicate that induction of labour in post-term pregnancies > 41 weeks is not associated with an increase in caesarean delivery rates. In 440 women with uncomplicated pregnancies at > 41 weeks, the caesarean delivery rate was 18% in the group managed expectantly and 23% and 18% respectively in the groups which had prostaglandin E_2 gel or placebo gel respectively 12 hours prior to induction of labour with oxytocin infusion. On the other hand, the Canadian multicentre study of 3,407 women with uncomplicated pregnancies of 41 weeks or more duration (Hannah et al 1992) showed a statistically significant decrease in caesarean section rates in the induction group (21.2%) as compared with the group who were managed conservatively with serial antenatal fetal monitoring while awaiting spontaneous labour (24.5%). It is worth noting that the higher caesarean section rate in the expectantly managed group was primarily due to a higher incidence of caesarean delivery for fetal distress in that group. The criteria for diagnosis of fetal distress in this trial was not controlled and the investigators have suggested that the differences in the rates of caesarean delivery may have been due to differences in the interpretation of fetal heart rate tracings.

A recent meta-analysis of 13 controlled trials where the intention to induce labour for prolonged pregnancy was compared with the intention to await spontaneous labour either indefinitely or until a specified date post-term (Crowley 1994) showed a small but statistically significant reduction in the likelihood of delivery by caesarean section when labour was induced at 41 weeks and 3 days. The risk of perinatal death was reduced in the induction group in spite of the decreased caesarean rate.

The success of induction depends on the parity and cervical score of the patient and the method of induction. The influence of the period of gestation on the outcome is dependent on the cervical score, the scores usually being better with increasing gestation.

In order to counsel the patient properly, the risk of caesarean section when labour is induced should be verified known according to parity, the cervical score and the method of induction. Table 1 summarises the risk of caesarean section (CS) for failed induction of labour related to parity and cervical score when labour was

Table 1: Caesarean Section rate for failed induction of labour according to parity and cervical score

Cervical Score	Para 0		Para 1 or more	
	n	%	n	%
0 – 3	27/59	(45.8)	2/26	(7.7)
4 – 6	30/292	(10.3)	10/257	(3.9)
– 10	3/208	(1.4)	2/215	(0.9)

induced for various indications by amniotomy and oxytocin infusion (Arulkumaran et al 1985a). For this study the cervix was assessed by giving a score of 0 to 2 for each of the cervical characteristics of position, consistency, length and dilatation of the cervix in addition to the station of the head in relation to ischial spines.

The CS rate in multiparae and nulliparae with a good score is not high. Nulliparae with a score of 3 or less had a CS rate of 65% for all indications and 45% for failed induction (Arulkumaran et al 1985a). In this study a diagnosis of failed induction was made when a CS was done for reasons other than fetal distress, cephalopelvic disproportion or failure to progress due to malposition. Those who had CS for failed induction did not show an improvement in cervical dilatation beyond 3 to 4 cm and did not enter the active phase of labour despite adequate use of oxytocin for a period of 10 – 12 hrs.

The incidence of failed induction in nulliparae with a poor cervical score can be reduced either by priming the cervix with prostaglandin or lamicel prior to the use of oxytocin and artificial rupture of the membranes (Tromans et al 1981; Sorensen et al 1985). Alternatively labour can be induced by prostaglandin vaginal pessaries or gel (Pearce et al 1979; Arulkumaran et al 1989a). Nulliparae with a poor cervical score of < 6 induced with oxytocin and artificial rupture of the membranes have significantly more CS when compared with those induced with two prostin E_2 vaginal pessaries (3 mg); each pessary being inserted four hours apart, followed if necessary by oxytocin and artificial rupture of the membranes 24 hours later (Table 2) (Kurup et al 1991). Yet the CS rates after prostaglandins are much higher compared with CS rates in nulliparae who were admitted in spontaneous labour (Arulkumaran et al 1985b).

Table 2:   Indication for caesarean section in nulliparae with a poor cervical score of < 6 according to treatment regimen

Treatment regimen	Oxytocin and Amniotomy		Prostaglandins	
	n = 230	%	n = 152	%
Fetal distress	27	(11.7)	13	(8.6)
CPD or malposition	10	(4.4)	8	(5.3)
Failed induction	55	(23.9)	14	(9.2)
Others	8	(3.5)	1	(0.7)
TOTAL	100	(43.5)[a]	36	(23.7)

[a] P < 0.001
CPD : cephalo-pelvic disproportion

The use of prostaglandin allows the postponement of induction if the woman does not become established in labour as the membranes are left intact. In prolonged pregnancy, because an appreciable number of women may be multiparous or nulliparous with a good cervical score, only a small number of nulliparae with a poor score will need prostaglandin. Hence the overall CS rate in induced labour may not be significantly higher compared with those managed conservatively. But the chances of needing CS based on different treatment regimens, parity and the cervical score should be of value in counselling the individual patient for induction or conservative management.

Risks for the baby

Descriptive and retrospective studies indicate that there is an increased risk of perinatal mortality after 42 weeks (Bakketeig and Bergsjo 1989). These deaths occur in the antepartum, intrapartum and the neonatal periods. The incidence of stillbirths before labour appears to contribute equally to that of intrapartum and neonatal deaths in prolonged pregnancy compared with the 37 to 42 weeks period when the antepartum deaths contribute about two-thirds of the perinatal deaths (Crowley 1989). However data from many of these older trials is confounded by uncertain dates, and variables like the presence of lethal congenital malformations, twin pregnancy, Rhesus disease, preeclampsia and antepartum hemorrhage, all of which may affect the perinatal mortality rates in both groups. The development and application of modern techniques of fetal monitoring have been associated with a reduction in perinatal risk in prolonged pregnancy. Thirteen studies performed between 1978 and 1987 in which antenatal surveillance was used for follow-up of the post-term pregnancy have shown that the risk of perinatal mortality was similar to that of pregnancies delivered at term (Dyson 1988). Because perinatal mortality in prolonged pregnancy is uncommon, and the prevalence of prolonged pregnancy in a well dated population is small, the numbers needed to show any change in perinatal mortality with either the induction of labour or fetal monitoring of the fetus while awaiting spontaneous labour would be very large. Meta-analysis of 13 randomised controlled trials (Crowley 1994) published from 1969 to 1992 to assess the outcome of a policy of induction of labour at 290 days gestation or greater have shown that perinatal mortality occurs at a rate of only 2.4 per thousand in normally formed babies in the control arm of these trials. Although none of the individual trials showed a statistically significant difference in perinatal mortality, meta-analysis of the 13 trials revealed a significant reduction in perinatal deaths (odds ratio 0.6; 95% confidence intervals 0.23 – 0.90) in the induction group compared with patients who had fetal monitoring while awaiting spontaneous labour.

There is also an increased morbidity in prolonged pregnancy due to a higher incidence of meconium stained amniotic fluid, hypoxia, shoulder dystocia and birth injuries with or without instrumental vaginal deliveries. Data from most individual trials is again non-conclusive. Meta-analysis (Crowley 1994) reveals that a policy of induction at 290+ days reduces meconium staining of amniotic fluid and appears to increase the incidence of neonatal jaundice, but the incidence of fetal heart rate abnormalities during labour and Apgar scores remain unchanged with either policy of management.

Management options

Pre-pregnancy counselling

The occurrence of prolonged pregnancy cannot be predicted. There is some evidence to suggest that primigravidae are likely to have a slightly higher incidence. Those who have had one previous prolonged pregnancy have a 30% chance and those who have had two prolonged pregnancies a 40% chance of another prolonged pregnancy (Bakketeig and Bergsjo 1989). There is conflicting evidence with regard to age related incidence. Since prolonged pregnancy is difficult to predict but is associated with an increased rate of obstetric interference and perinatal mortality, accurate knowledge of the last menstrual period is valuable in diagnosing the condition. To achieve this, one can educate women to keep an accurate note of their last menstrual period (LMP) and to seek early antenatal care during pre-pregnancy counselling. This will help to increase the number of women who will be certain of dates compared with the present situation where only 80% are able to remember their LMP (Hall and Carr-Hill 1985).

Antenatal management

Once the patient misses her period the earliest moment at which the pregnancy test becomes positive is important. If it is positive 5 weeks after her last menstrual period then it is worth taking note, as she is likely to be 5 weeks pregnant compared with a pregnancy test which is done at 7 weeks amenorrhoea when she could be 5, 6 or 7 weeks pregnant. It is equally important to perform a vaginal examination in the first trimester of pregnancy as the assessment of the uterine size in the majority of cases will give a good estimation of the period of gestation. Examination of the uterine size in the second trimester is not accurate for estimating the period of gestation.

An ultrasonic examination in the first or early second trimester is likely to give an accurate assessment of the dates within an error margin of one or two weeks. Ultrasonic examination in the late second trimester or third trimester is unlikely to give an accurate assessment of the dates. Assessment of dates by early ultrasound examination has reduced the incidence of prolonged pregnancy by half to two-thirds in many centres (Eik-Nes et al 1984; Ingemarsson and Heden 1989). Assessment of dates based on ultrasonic measurements, can now be made accurately for women who cannot remember their LMP or are uncertain of dates or have long or irregular cycles.

Once pregnancy proceeds beyond 41 weeks the risk to the fetus has to be carefully assessed. There is epidemiological evidence that women who had pregnancy complications like antepartum hemorrhage of unknown origin or a previous poor obstetric history of stillbirth or neonatal death are at increased risk of perinatal mortality (Butler and Bonham 1963). These women are better delivered by 40 weeks. There is a slightly increased incidence of hypertension when pregnancy advances in the late third trimester. In the majority of cases mild hypertension would have no major consequence on the mother or the fetus. But women with signs of placental insufficiency may have some adverse effects. These women have to be carefully assessed and are best delivered by induction around 40 weeks.

There are centres where pregnant women are not weighed in the clinics as there is no clear evidence to suggest that there is a decrease in perinatal morbidity or mortality in a population who had their weights taken. Sudden excessive weight gain might suggest the possible onset of hypertension whilst static weight or weight loss over a few weeks may indicate a possible compromise to the fetus, especially beyond 40 weeks. Static weight or weight loss at term was an indication for induction in many centres (Arulkumaran et al 1985a) but this has changed with the confidence in the newer methods of fetal surveillance. Reduction in amniotic fluid volume signifies possible fetal compromise but is difficult to quantify clinically especially in obese women. The use of ultrasound is helpful and will be discussed later.

Symphysial fundal height   Assessment of fetal size by the measurement of symphysial fundal height can be influenced by obesity, the amount of amniotic fluid, the level of presenting part, the fetal lie and abdominal wall tension. Although serial measurements are useful in following the progress of pregnancy, their value is limited in prolonged pregnancy; however they may help to identify an occasional case of growth retardation or a macrosomic baby which has been missed in the earlier examinations.

Tests of fetal wellbeing

The occurrence of prolonged pregnancy is unpredictable. Hence the mainstay of antenatal management lies first in the diagnosis of prolonged pregnancy. Once diagnosed the pregnancy can be terminated by induction of labour or managed conservatively till the spontaneous onset of labour. Whilst awaiting spontaneous onset of labour, fetal wellbeing should be monitored by available tests.

Biochemical methods   Few centres use biochemical methods to monitor fetal well being in current practice. For correct interpretation of the results the period of gestation should be known. Further, serial measurements are needed to make any meaningful conclusions because of the wide range of readings observed with these tests (Arulkumaran 1989). The tests need patients' blood or 24 hour collections of urine and a laboratory and trained personnel to perform the tests. The results obtained represent the fetal health for the previous few days and do not prognosticate it for the next few days. The results are usually not available till many hours after dispatching the test samples. In prolonged pregnancy the value of the test is limited as the patient might deliver before the results are known. Low oestriol values in an otherwise healthy fetus should suggest a rare condition of placental sulphatase deficiency (1 in 5,000 pregnancies). These women may have an autosomal recessive disorder of congenital ichthyosis (Harkness et al 1983).

Biophysical methods

Fetal movement chart   Fetal activity in the form of fetal movements has been found to be a reliable indicator of fetal health (Sadovsky et al 1974). One that has been commonly practised is the 'count to 10' fetal movement chart where 10 episodes of fetal activity are expected within a period of 12 hr (Pearson 1982). Many mothers feel 10 episodes of fetal movements within a few hours. Anxious mothers report less than optimal movements which might lead to unnecessary intervention. Mothers with less intelligence or those who are too busy may not seek attention or may come late with less than optimal or no fetal movements, leading to poor fetal outcome. For mothers who find it difficult to perceive fetal movements this method is not suitable. Although inexpensive, its value in monitoring the fetus in prolonged pregnancy has not been validated. A randomised study involving 68,000 women showed no benefit in providing the fetal movement chart as a routine compared with selective use when indicated (Grant et al 1989). Based on current data the fetal movement chart alone cannot be relied on in monitoring fetal health in prolonged pregnancy.

Maternal perception of sound provoked fetal movements   The fetus exhibits a flexion-extension type of limb movement or a startle reflex to a vibroacoustic stimulus, indicating an intact central nervous system and a somato motor sensory pathway (Gelman et al 1982; Divon et al 1985). Maternal perception of sound provoked fetal movement (mp SPFM) correlates well with the reactive nonstress test (NST) (Westgren et al 1987; Arulkumaran et al 1989b) and can be of value in centres where facilities are limited or non-existent to perform a NST. The correlation of the results of the NST to that of mp SPFM is given in Table 3.

Table 3: Correlation of the results of the NST to that of mp SPFM

mp SPFM	FM Present		FM absent		Total	
	(n = 1,009)	(%)	(n = 88)	(%)	(n = 1,097)	(%)
NST reactive	1,006	(99.7)	78	(88.6)	1,084	(98.8)
NST non-reactive	3	(00.3)	10	(11.4)	13	(1.2)

% is given within ( )

The sensitivity of the test was 92.8%, specificity 76.9%, positive predictive value 99.7% and negative predictive value 11.9%. When the mp SPFM is positive the chances that the NST will be reactive are high. The three cases who had positive mp SPFM but had a non reactive NST were cases under 33 weeks of gestation and were on multiple antihypertensive therapy (for severe preeclampsia) which is a factor known to decrease variability and accelerations (Montan et al 1984). There were 12.8% cases of prolonged pregnancy in the population studied and none had an adverse outcome. It may be possible to use mp SPFM to assess fetal wellbeing in prolonged pregnancy in centres where facilities for NST are not available or not possible to perform on a twice weekly basis due to technical reasons. However the reliability of mp SPFM in monitoring prolonged pregnancies without other forms of testing needs evaluation.

Nonstress test (NST)

A recording of the fetal heart rate (FHR) for a period of 20 to 30 min called the nonstress test (NST) has become one of the most popular methods of antenatal fetal surveillance including the surveillance of prolonged pregnancy (Cario 1984). Definitions of normal, suspicious and abnormal FHR patterns have been described by the FIGO (FIGO 1987). A normal reactive FHR trace is one with a baseline between 110 and 150 beats per min (bpm), a baseline variability of 10 – 25 bpm, no decelerations and two FHR accelerations of 15 beats or more above the baseline for > 15 sec in a 15 min window. In the absence of accelerations the trace should be continued for at least 40 min prior to labelling it as a nonreactive trace. The fetal acoustic stimulation test (FAST) where a vibroacoustic stimulus is used to elicit accelerations of the FHR is a useful way to reduce the number of nonreactive traces and to shorten the testing time (Smith et al 1985). The reliability of the NST to predict fetal wellbeing within a week of testing has been studied. The rate of false negative tests has been 7 per 1,000 cases when the results of 10,169 patients were analysed (Kubli et al 1977; Schifrin et al 1979; Keagan and Paul 1980; Flynn et al 1982). Some of the fetal demises within a week were associated with lethal malformations and others were cases with a reactive trace (with accelerations) which also had decelerations, indicating possible oligohydramnios (Barss et al 1985; Smith et al 1987; Garite et al 1979). Compromise to the fetus in prolonged pregnancy is generally due to oligohydramnios and will be discussed later. In a reactive trace with a good baseline variability isolated decelerations which are < 15 beats from the baseline rate lasting < 15 sec or < 30 sec following an acceleration do not signify fetal compromise. But if the trace is not reactive despite stimulating the fetus, or if it shows decelerations greater than the magnitude expressed, then it indicates possible compromise and should be an indication for termination of pregnancy.

Contraction stress test (CST) / Fetal acoustic stimulation test (FAST)

A good outcome has been reported with the contraction stress test utilised as a primary modality to assess fetal wellbeing in prolonged pregnancy (Freeman et al 1981). Though reliable, it is invasive, requires the patient to be restricted in bed and a short stay in hospital. The information obtained may be as good as that obtained by other noninvasive modalities of testing which are easier and convenient to perform on an outpatient basis. Its value may be important in a situation where a nonreactive nonstress test is encountered. But in current practice this problem has been resolved with the use of FAST. Not only does this produce a reactive trace but it also reduces the testing time (Smith et al 1985). It may not represent the stress of uterine contractions and thus does not reveal a situation of possible compromise in labour but it produces a reactive trace comparable to the NST and the perinatal outcome is similar whether the trace was reactive spontaneously or as a result of the FAST (Smith et al 1986). In fact, there is some evidence to suggest that the use of FAST in such situation is more discriminatory in selecting fetuses in good health (Trudinger and Boylan 1980).

Assessment of amniotic fluid volume

Fetal urine contributes significantly to the volume of amniotic fluid. Severe oligohydramnios is a common finding in bilateral renal agenesis. With diminished placental function, selective perfusion of the brain and heart and reduced perfusion of other systems including the kidneys take place. This leads to the reduction of fetal urine formation and thus the sequelae of oligohydramnios in severe intrauterine growth retardation. Fetal compromise that is due to gradual decline in placental function can therefore be monitored by assessing the amniotic fluid volume. In prolonged pregnancy the mechanism of fetal compromise appears to be cord compression (Leveno et al 1984) and evaluation of amniotic fluid volume has been found to be useful (Crowley 1980). Evaluation by palpation may be deceptive while an impression of the adequacy on ultrasound examination is more reliable.

Compared with the objective assessment of the vertical depth of the largest pool after excluding loops of the cord, addition of the vertical pockets (including the cord unless the entire pocket is filled with it) in the four quadrants of the uterus (the amniotic fluid index : AFI) correlates better with perinatal outcome (Moore 1990). In prolonged pregnancy, an amniotic fluid index < 5 cm or < 2 cm depth of the largest pocket is suggestive of reduced placental function. In these situations there is a possibility of fetal compromise antenatally or intrapartum due to cord compression. Delivery by induction and continuous electronic fetal monitoring during labour would be desirable. In prolonged pregnancy the decline in the AFI can be at a faster rate in some cases and it might be wise to determine the AFI twice weekly.

Biophysical profile   The biophysical profile consists of an ultrasound examination to evaluate fetal movements, fetal tone, fetal breathing movements, vertical depth of the largest amniotic fluid pocket and a nonstress test. Each of these parameters get a score of either 0 or 2 there being no intermediate score of 1. A score of 8 or 10 indicates a fetus in good condition and retesting can be done according to the high risk situation. In prolonged pregnancy it is best performed twice weekly. If the score is 6 then the score has to be reevaluated 4 to 6 hours later and a decision made based on the new score. A score of 4 or less is an indication for delivery (Manning et al 1980). Good perinatal outcomes have been reported with biophysical profile scoring in high risk pregnancies (Manning et al 1987) and as a primary modality of testing in prolonged pregnancy (Johnson et al 1986).

A modified biophysical profile where only the ultrasound parameters are evaluated (without NST) has been found to be equally reliable (Eden et al 1988). Due to the time and expertise needed to perform a biophysical profile, many centres perform a NST, if needed with FAST (when NST is not reactive) and an AFI. Excellent perinatal outcome has been reported with this approach in high risk pregnancies (Clark et al 1989). A simple plan for fetal surveillance is given in Fig 17.1 which should be carried out twice weekly in prolonged pregnancy. Indications for terminating the pregnancy are an AFI < 6, nonreactive NST despite FAST and retesting, decelerations > 15 beats lasting > 15 sec or > 30 sec if it followed an acceleration. There is a higher incidence of meconium stained amniotic fluid, caesarean section for fetal distress and babies with poor Apgar score when the pregnancy was terminated based on the above scheme compared with a control group of women with prolonged pregnancy but without features suggestive of the need for intervention (Rutherford et al 1987).

Doppler waveform studies   Doppler waveform studies have been used in high risk pregnancies to improve the predictive accuracy of other modalities of fetal assessment. The results of several small trials in prolonged pregnancy are conflicting. A doppler study of umbilical and uterine arteries has been shown to add little in itself to the follow-up of patients with prolonged pregnancies in predicting perinatal morbidity in terms of Apgar scores (Arabin et al 1994; Weiner et al 1993; Stokes et al 1991), although doppler flow measurement of the fetal descending thoracic aorta shows promise for identifying prolonged pregnancies at an increased risk of perinatal complications (Battaglia et al 1991).

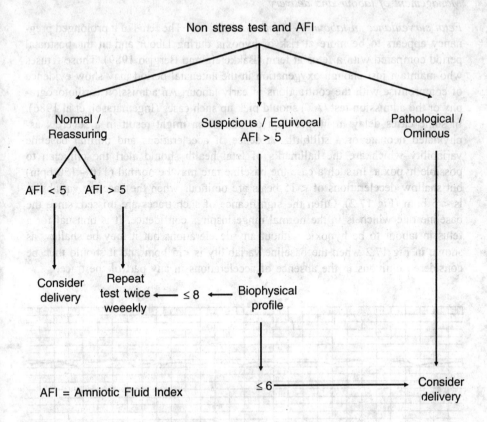

Fig 17.1 Suggestion for antenatal fetal monitoring of prolonged pregnancy

Counselling for induction of labour or conservative management

Obstetrics is a fine art built on facts gathered by scientific research. The same situation can be managed differently and will depend mainly on the skill of the obstetrician and the facilities available. When facilities are available to perform certain tests of fetal being the prolonged pregnancy can be managed conservatively. However the patient has to be told of the test results and counselled that she can wait a few more days till the onset of spontaneous labour. On the other hand an alternative way of managing by induction of labour should also be explained including the prospects of vaginal delivery based on her parity, cervical score and method of induction. She may select one of the options based on her knowledge, her social life and other personal considerations. A recent prospective study (Roberts and Young 1991) examined the attitude of 500 pregnant women at 37 weeks of gestation to a proposal of conservative management of prolonged pregnancy. Most women were unwilling to accept the conservative management of prolonged pregnancy, more so if they were undelivered at 41 weeks. The reasons for such an attitude varied from 'could not stand the thought of being pregnant for more than 42 weeks' to concern regarding fetal size or the feeling that 'there was no benefit in waiting'.

Management of labour and delivery

Fetal surveillance in labour — Admission test   The fetus of a prolonged pregnancy appears to be more at risk of hypoxia during labour and in the postnatal period compared with a fetus at term (Bakketeig and Bergjso 1989). Those fetuses who maintain just enough oxygenation in the antenatal period may show evidence of compromise with the contractions of early labour. An admission cardiotocography or the admission test (AT) should pick up such cases (Ingemarsson et al 1986). In some cases delay in intervention on admission might result in a severely asphyxiated neonate or a stillbirth. Absence of accelerations and normal baseline variability which are the hallmarks of fetal health should alert the clinician to possible hypoxia. In such a case the baseline rate may be normal (110 – 150 bpm) but shallow decelerations of < 15 beats are ominous when the baseline variability is < 5 bpm (Fig 17.2). Often the significance of such traces are missed, since the baseline rate which is in the normal range inspires confidence. It is unusual for a fetus in labour to be hypoxic without any decelerations but it may be shallow as shown in Fig 17.2 when the baseline variability is < 5 bpm and it should then be considered ominous in the absence of accelerations in any part of the trace.

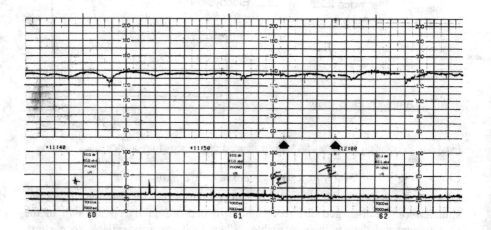

Fig 17.2 An admission test (AT) trace showing a normal baseline rate but reduced baseline variability (< 5 bpm) with shallow decelerations which are ominous in a non-reactive trace

In order to screen those at risk, it is useful to advise women after 41 weeks to come early when in labour and to have an AT on arrival. Precious time should not be wasted looking into other details of admission procedures prior to the AT. Electronic fetal monitoring at least for a brief period is mandatory to pick up subtle changes in the trace prior to those evident on intermittent auscultation. When there are no accelerations and the trace is suspicious, fetal acoustic stimulation can be employed to reduce the number of nonreactive traces (Ingemarsson et al 1988). This combined approach helps in selecting those who are already compromised or likely to be compromised in labour. An ominous trace (shown in Fig 17.2) in early labour in the presence of thick meconium stained amniotic fluid which is scanty in quantity warrants immediate delivery and procrastination to await further cervical dilatation to perform a fetal scalp blood sampling should be avoided. A suspicious or an abnormal admission test trace is an indication for continuous electronic fetal monitoring.

Continuous electronic fetal monitoring   Prolonged pregnancy is a high risk situation and continuous electronic fetal monitoring is ideal if equipment is available and the patient does not object. When there is limitation of equipment or the patient does not want continuous monitoring, a normal AT followed by meticulous intermittent auscultation may suffice in the presence of clear amniotic fluid. But a 20 – 30 min trace by electronic fetal monitoring every two to three hours should give more information and may be useful (Herbst and Ingemarsson 1994). Added risk factors like thick meconium stained fluid or no fluid at membrane rupture, induction or augmentation with oxytocin or prostaglandin, the use of epidural analgesia and suspected intrauterine infection following a prolonged period of membrane rupture demand the use of continuous monitoring as the fetal heart rate can become abnormal within a short time.

Colour and quantity of amniotic fluid   Meconium passage in utero may be a function of fetal maturity and the incidence of meconium stained fluid is higher in prolonged pregnancy. But fresh thick meconium staining with scanty fluid may indicate the possibility of intrapartum hypoxia (Miller et al 1975; Steer 1985; Wong et al 1985). Abnormal fetal heart rate patterns suggestive of hypoxia are more common with thick meconium stained fluid whilst the risk of thin or moderate meconium staining of the fluid appears to hold no greater risk than other high risk situations of pregnancy induced hypertension or diabetes in pregnancy (Meis et al 1978; Arulkumaran et al 1985c). The incidence of a low Apgar score is doubled with an abnormal FHR pattern in the presence of thick meconium compared with clear fluid. But there is no increase in the incidence of low Apgar scores in the presence of a normal trace whether the amniotic fluid was clear or meconium stained (Steer 1985). The umbilical cord arterial blood pH did not differ in the meconium stained or clear fluid group if the FHR pattern was normal. But the pH values were significantly lower in those with meconium compared with those with clear fluid if the FHR tracing was abnormal (Starks 1980).

Since there is a possibility of aggravating acidosis in the presence of meconium, hypotension with epidural anesthesia and hyperstimulation with oxytocics should be avoided and prompt action taken in the presence of an abnormal FHR pattern. Meconium aspiration leading to pneumonitis is the major threat with thick meconium, and there is some correlation between asphyxia and meconium aspiration (Bowes 1982). The meconium stained fluid in prolonged pregnancy tends to be more particulate with the presence of exfoliated skin, hair and vernix and this may block the airways causing more problems than nonparticulate meconium stained fluid found in pregnancies of earlier gestation. Post-term fetuses may be more prone to hypoxia due to reduced amniotic fluid volume, leading to a greater possibility of cord compression with uterine contractions (Leveno et al 1984). The appearance of meconium, the degree of staining based on the quantity of amniotic fluid and the FHR pattern have to be kept in mind in monitoring a patient with prolonged pregnancy.

Amnioinfusion in labour   Since the main problems appear to be due to oligo-hydramnios and cord compression, and since most problems occur in labour associated with the presence of meconium, it may be possible to use amnioinfusion of warm saline to reduce the possibility of fetal distress or meconium aspiration. A meta-analysis of recent published trials (Hofmeyr 1994) suggests that amnioinfusion in subjects with oligohydramnios decreases the occurrence of variable fetal heart rate decelerations. There was a significant reduction in caesarean section for 'fetal distress' as diagnosed by a cardiotocograph. Neonates in the amnioinfusion group had significantly better 1 and 5 minute Apgar scores and there were significantly less babies in the amnioinfusion group with cord arterial pH < 7.2. There was no effect of amnioinfusion on perinatal death in this series. In a meta-analysis of six recent trials (Hofmeyr 1994) to assess the effect of intrapartum amnioinfusion for meconium stained liquor in labour, treatment was associated with a marked reduction in caesarean section for fetal distress (3.7% vs 20.2%, odds ratio = 0.21; 95% confidence interval = 0.11=0.41). Meconium below the vocal cords and the incidence of the neonatal meconium aspiration syndrome was reduced in the amnioinfusion group.

Monitoring the progress of labour and care at delivery

There has been some debate about the progress of labour, some claiming an increase in dysfunctional labour whilst others find no such increase. The poor progress of labour might be either due to poor uterine contractions or some disproportion in the fetopelvic relationship. The fetuses attain the maximal weight gain by 270 days and the subsequent weight gain is not marked (Gruenwald 1967) although there is a higher proportion of heavy babies associated with prolonged pregnancy (Boyd et al 1983). There is also no evidence to suggest that the skull bones are significantly more ossified and that there is little moulding possibly leading to disproportion. It is reasonable to manage poor progress of labour in prolonged pregnancy as in term pregnancy.

In prolonged pregnancy increased perinatal morbidity and mortality have been attributed to birth trauma (Bakketeig and Bergjso 1989). This is best reduced by optimal monitoring of labour progress and intervention at the correct time. At the onset of labour birthweight should be estimated as around 2, 3, 4 or more kg. This estimation should be made early and not after 16 to 18 hr of labour at the time of CS or after traumatic instrumental vaginal delivery. A prolonged first stage, especially in the late first stage of labour when the cervix is loosely applied to the presenting part, followed by a prolonged second stage where there is marked caput and moulding and when there is difficulty in palpating the fetal ear, the possibility of difficult and traumatic instrumental vaginal delivery should be anticipated and avoided. The presence of meconium and/or an abnormal fetal heart rate pattern in addition would signify the possibility of hypoxia. Shoulder dystocia is always a possibility with abnormal labour patterns in prolonged pregnancy and each labour ward should be ready with a definitive plan of action. The delivery should be conducted in a stepwise fashion in the form of a drill: the 'shoulder dystocia drill' (Arulkumaran and Montan 1991).

Care of the neonate at and after delivery

Great care should be given to the neonate at delivery if the amniotic fluid is meconium stained. The oropharynx and nasopharynx should be sucked when the head is delivered, with the shoulder still in the maternal pelvis. Once the shoulder is delivered the oropharynx should be sucked before the nasopharynx to prevent the baby sneezing and aspirating the meconium. A pediatrician in attendance would be of help. A laryngoscope should be used to visualise the vocal cords and suck out any meconium. If meconium is present below the vocal cords a bronchial lavage might be useful (Carsons et al 1976). To prevent subsequent vomiting and aspiration of the stomach contents a gastric lavage should be undertaken to clear the thick particulate meconium from the stomach. The baby should be checked to exclude any birth injury. Hypoglycemia can be a problem in a large neonate and it may be useful to check the blood sugar and plan early feeding. Infants delivered after a prolonged pregnancy have been followed up for two years and no adverse mental or physical delay in milestones have been identified (Shime et al 1986).

Prolonged pregnancy cannot be predicted but when it is uncomplicated there is little risk to the fetus or the mother. Attempts to prevent prolonged pregnancy have taken the form of induction by medication or by the simple means of breast stimulation (Elliot and Flaherty 1984). These attempts are made because of the worry that prolonged pregnancy may be associated with fetal morbidity and mortality. Current biophysical methods of fetal health assessment are reliable and a combination of NST and AFI starting from the end of 41 weeks appears to be adequate. The testing when performed twice weekly is more reassuring. Women's wishes regarding induction or conservative management and the facilities for antepartum testing should be taken into consideration when the management is planned. Simple tests like the mp SPFM may be useful in centres with limited facilities for other forms of testing. The method of induction should be tailored according to the parity and cervical score to reduce caesarean section rates. When managed conservatively about 40 – 50% of nulliparae and multiparae deliver 4 – 5 days after 42 weeks (Ingemarsson and Heden 1989). Based on this knowledge and that of probable outcomes with different methods of induction it should be possible to counsel more mothers to adapt a conservative approach. An admission test, continuous cardiotocography and knowledge of the quantity and colour of the amniotic fluid are essential to provide optimal care to the fetus in labour. Amnioinfusion when warranted and the combined obstetric-pediatric approach to reduce the incidence of meconium aspiration should help to reduce the fetal morbidity and mortality associated with prolonged pregnancy to a minimum.

References

Arabin B, Becker R, Mohnhaupt A, Vollert W, Weitzel HK 1994. Prediction of fetal distress and poor outcome in prolonged pregnancy using Doppler ultrasound and fetal heart rate monitoring combined with stress tests (II). *Fetal Diagn Ther* 9:1-6.

Arulkumaran S, Gibb DMF, TambyRaja RL, Heng SH, Ratnam SS 1985a. Failed induction of labour. *Austr NZ J Obstet Gynaecol* 25:190-193.

Arulkumaran S, Gibb DMF, TambyRaja RL, Heng SH, Ratnam SS 1985b. Rising caesarean section rates in Singapore. *Sing J Obstet Gynecol* 16:6-15.

Arulkumaran S, Yeoh SC, Gibb DMF, Ingemarsson I, Ratnam SS 1985c. Obstetric outcome of meconium stained liquor in labour. *Sing Med J* 26: 523-526.

Arulkumaran S 1989. Antenatal monitoring of the high risk fetus. *Sing Med J* 30:202-204

Arulkumaran S, Adiakan G, Anandakumar C, Viegas OAC, Singh P, Ratnam SS 1989a. Comparative study of a two dose schedule of PGE 3 mg pessary and 1700 ug film for induction of labour in nulliparae with poor cervical score. *Prostaglandins Leukotrines and Essential Fatty Acids* 38:37-41.

Arulkumaran S, Anandakumar C, Wong YC, Ratnam SS 1989b. Evaluation of maternal perception of sound provoked fetal movements as a test of antenatal fetal health. *Obstet Gynecol* 73:182-186.

Arulkumaran S, Montan S,1991. The fetus at risk in labour - identification and management. In: Ratnam SS, Ng SC, Sen DK, Arulkumaran S, eds. Contributions to Obstetrics and Gynaecology, Vol I. Singapore: Churchill Livingstone, pp 179-190.

Bakketeig L, Bergsjo P,1989. Post-term pregnancy: magnitude of the problem. In: Chalmers I, Enkin M, Keirse MJNC, eds. Effective care in pregnancy and childbirth, Vol I. Oxford: Oxford University Press, pp 765-775.

Barss VA, Frigoletto FD, Diamond F 1985. Stillbirth after nonstress testing. *Obstet Gynecol* 65:541-544.

Battaglia C, Larocca E, Lanzani A, Coukas G, Genazzanni AR 1991. Doppler velocimetry in prolonged pregnancy. *Obstet Gynecol* 77:213-6.

Bierman J, Siegel E, French FE, Simonian K 1965. Analysis of the outcome of all pregnancies in a community Kauai pregnancy study. *Am J Obstet Gynecol* 91:37-45.

Bowes WA 1982. Steps to prevent meconium aspiration syndrome. *Contemp Obstet Gynecol* 19: 135-138.

Boyd ME, Usher RH, McLean FH 1983. Fetal macrosomia: prediction, risks, proposed management. *Obstet Gynecol* 61:715-722.

Butler NR, Bonham DG 1963. Perinatal mortality. The first report of the 1958 British perinatal mortality survey under the auspices of the National Birthday Trust Fund. Edinburgh and London: E & S Livingstone.

Cardozo L, Fysh J, Pearce JM 1986. Prolonged pregnancy: The management debate. *Br Med J* 293:1059-1063.

Cario GM 1984. Conservative management of prolonged pregnancy using fetal heart rate monitoring only: a prospective study. *Br J Obstet Gynecol* 91:23-30.

Carsons BS, Losey RW, Bowes WA, Simmons MA 1976. Combined obstetric and paediatric approach to prevent meconium aspiration syndrome. *Am J Obstet Gynecol* 126:712-715.

Chamberlain G, Philip E, Howlett B, Masters K 1970. British Births Vol 2: Obstetric care. London: Heinemann Medical Books, p 292.

Clark SL, Sabey P, Jolley K 1989. Nonstress testing with acoustic stimulation and amniotic fluid volume assessment: 5,973 tests without unexpected fetal death. *Am J Obstet Gynecol* 160:694-697.

Clifford SH 1954. Postmaturity with placental dysfunction. *J Pediatr* 44:1-13.

Crowley P 1980. Non quantitative estimation of amniotic fluid volume in suspected prolonged pregnancy. *J Perinat Med* 8: 249-251.

Crowley P 1989. Postterm pregnancy: induction or surveillance? In: Chalmers I, Enkin M, Keirse MJNC, eds. Effective care in pregnancy and childbirth, Vol I. Oxford: Oxford University Press, pp 776-791.

Crowley P, 5 May 1994. Elective induction of labour at 41 + weeks gestation. In: Enkin MW, Keirse MJNC, Renfrew MJ, Neilson JP, eds. Pregnancy and Childbirth Module. Cochrane Database of Systemic Reviews. Review No. 04144. Published through Cochrane Updates on Disk, Oxford: Update Software 1994, Disk Issue 1.

Dewhurst CJ, Beazley JM, Campbell S 1972. Assessment of fetal maturity and dysmaturity. *Am J Obstet Gynecol* 113:141.

Divon MY, Platt LD, Cautrell CJ, Smith CV, Yeh SY, Paul RH 1985. Evoked fetal startle response: A possible intrauterine neurological examination. *Am J Obstet Gynecol* 153:454-456.

Dyson DC, Miller PD, Armstrong MA 1987. Management of prolonged pregnancy - induction of labor versus antepartum fetal testing. *Am J Obstet Gynecol* 156:928-934.

Dyson DC 1988. Fetal surveillance vs labor induction at 42 weeks in postterm gestation. *J Reprod Med* 33:262-270.

Eden RD, Seifert LS, Kodack LD, Trofatter KF, Killam AP, Gall SA 1988. A modified biophysical profile for antenatal fetal surveillance. *Obstet Gynecol* 71:365-369.

Eik-Nes SH, Okland O, Aure JC, Ulstein M 1984. Ultrasound screening in pregnancy: A randomised controlled trial. i:1347.

Elliott JP and Flaherty JF 1984. The use of breast stimulation to prevent postdate pregnancy. *Am J Obstet Gynecol* 149: 628-632.

Evans TN, Koeff ST, Morley GW 1963. Fetal effects of prolonged iou pregnancy. *Am J Obstet Gynecol* 85:701-712.

FIGO News 1980. International classification of diseases: update. *Int J Gynecol Obstet* 17:634-640.

FIGO Subcommittee in Perinatal Medicine 1987. Guidelines for the use of fetal monitoring. *Int J Gynecol Obstet* 25:159-167.

Flynn AM, Kelly J, Mansfield H, Needham P, O'Connor M, Viegasá OAC 1982. A randomised controlled trial of non-stress antepartum cardiotocography. *Br J Obstet Gynecol* 89:427-433.

Freeman RK, Garite TJ, Modanlou H, Dorchester W, Rommal C, Devaney M 1981. Postdate pregnancy: Utilisation of contraction stress testing for primary fetal surveillance. *Am J Obstet Gynecol* 140:128-135.

Garite TJ, Linzey EM, Freeman RK et al 1979. Fetal heart rate patterns and fetal distress in fetuses with congenital anomalies. *Obstet Gynecol* 53:716-719.

Gelman SR, Wood S, Spellacy WN, Abrams RM 1982. Fetal movements in response to sound stimulation. *Am J Obstet Gynecol* 143:484-485.

Gibb DMF, Cardozo LD, Studd JWW, Cooper DJ 1982. Prolonged pregnancy, is induction of labour indicated? A prospective study. *Br J Obstet Gynecol* 89: 292-295.

Gibb D 1984. Prolonged pregnancy. In: Studd JWW, ed. The Management of Labour. Oxford, UK: Blackwell Scientific Publishers, pp 108-122.

Grant A, Elbourne D, Valentin L, Alexander S 1989. Routine formal fetal movement counting and risk of antepartum late death in normally formed singletons. *Lancet* Aug:345-349.

Gruenwald P 1967. Growth of human fetus. In: McLaren A, ed. Advances in reproductive physiology, Vol 2. London: Logos Press, pp 279-309.

Guidetti DA, Divon MY, Langer O 1989. Postdate fetal surveillance: Is 41 weeks too early? *Am J Obstet Gynecol* 161:91-93.

Hall MH, Carr-Hill RA, Fraser C, Campbell D, Samphier MI 1985. The extent and antecedents of uncertain gestation. *Br J Obstet Gynecol* 92:445-451.

Hall MH, Carr-Hill RA 1985. The significance of uncertain gestation for obstetric outcome. *Br J Obstet Gynecol* 92:452-460.

Hannah ME, Hannah WJ, Hellmann J, Hewson S, Milner R, Willan A and the Canadian Multicentre Post-term Pregnancy Trial Group 1992. Induction of labor as compared with serial antetnatal monitoring in post-term pregnancy - A Randomised Controlled Trial. *N Engl J Med* 326:1587-92.

Harkness RA, Taylor NF, Crawford MA, Rose FA 1983. Recognising placental steroid sulphatase deficiency. *Br Med J* 287:2.

Herbst A, Ingemarsson 1994. Intermittent versus continuous electronic monitoring in labour: randmised study. *Br J Obstet Gynecol* 101:663-668.

Hofmeyr GJ 1994a. Prophylactic vs therapeutic amnioinfusion for intrapartum oligo hydramnios. In: Enkin MW, Keirse MJNC, Renfrew MJ, Neilson JP, eds. Pregnancy and Childbirth Module. Cochrane Database of Systemic Reviews: Review No. 07642. Published through Cochrane Updates on Disk, Oxford: Update Software, Disk Issue 1.

Hofmeyr GJ 1994b. Amnioinfusion for meconium stained liquor in labour. In: Enkin MW, Keirse MJNC, Renfrew MJ, Neilson JP, eds. Pregnancy and Childbirth Module. Cochrane Database of Systemic Reviews: Review No. 05379. Published through Cochrane Updates on Disk, Oxford: Update Software, Disk Issue 1.

Ingemarsson I, Arulkumaran S, Ingemarsson E, TambyRaja RL, Ratnam SS 1986. Admission test: a screening test for fetal distress in labor. *Obstet Gynecol* 68:800-806.

Ingemarsson I, Arulkumaran S, Paul RH, Ingemarsson E, TambyRaja RL, Ratnam SS 1988. Fetal acoustic stimulation in early labor in patients screened with the admission test. *Am J Obstet Gynecol* 158:70-74.

Ingemarsson I, Heden L 1989. Cervical score and onset of spontaneous labor in prolonged pregnancy dated by second trimester ultrasonic scan. *Obstet Gynecol* 74:102-105.

Johnson JM, Hareman CR, Lange IR, Manning FA 1986. Biophysical profile scoring in the management of postterm pregnancy: An analysis of 307 patients. *Am J Obstet Gynecol* 154:269-273.

Keagan KA, Paul RH 1980. Antepartum fetal heart rate monitoring: non-stress test as a primary approach. *Am J Obstet Gynecol* 136: 75-80.

Kubli F, Boos R, Ruttgers H, Van Hagen SC, Vanselow H 1977. Antepartum fetal heart rate monitoring and ultrasound. In: Beard RW, Campbell S, eds. Obstetrics. RCOG Scientific Meeting, pp 28-47.

Kurup A, Chua S, Arulkumaran S, Tham KF, Tay D, Ratnam SS 1991. Induction of labour in nulliparas with poor cervical score: Oxytocin or prostaglandin vaginal pessaries? *Austr NZ J Obstet Gynecol* 31:223-226.

Leveno KJ, Quirk JG, Cunningham FG, Nelson SD, Santos Ramos R, Toofanian A, De Palma RT 1984. Prolonged pregnancy. I. Observations concerning the causes of fetal distress. *Am J Obstet Gynecol* 150:465-473.

Lindell A 1956. Prolonged pregnancy. *Acta Obstet Gynecol Scand* 35:136-163.

Manning FA, Platt LD, Sipos L 1980. Antepartum fetal evaluation: Development of a biophysical profile. *Am J Obstet Gynecol* 136:787-790.

Manning FA, Morrison I, Harman CR, Lange IR, Menticoglou S 1987. Fetal assessment based on fetal biophysical profile scoring: Experience in 19,221 referred high-risk pregnancies. *Am J Obstet Gynecol* 157:880-884.

McCarthy TG 1975. Relationship of a short period to conception. *Br J Obstet Gynaecol* 82:158

Meis PJ, Hall M, Marshall JR et al 1978. Meconium passage: a new classification for risk assessment during labor. *Am J Obstet Gynecol* 131:509-513.

Miller FC, Sacks DA, Yeh SY et al 1975. The significance of meconium during labor. *Am J Obstet Gynecol* 122:573-580.

Montan S, Solum T, Sjoberg NO 1984. Influence of beta-adrenoceptor blocker atenolol on antenatal cardiotocography. *Acta Obstet Gynecol Scand (Suppl)* 118:99-102.

Moore RT 1990. Superiority of the four- quadrant sum over the single-deepest pocket technique in ultrasonic identification of abnormal amniotic fluid volumes. *Am J Obstet Gynecol* 163: 762-767.

Naeye RL 1978. Causes of perinatal mortality excess in prolonged gestation. *Am J Epidemiol* 108:429.

Nesbitt REL Jnr 1955. Prolongation of pregnancy: A review. *Obstet Gynecol Surv* 10:311.

Pearce MF, Sheperd JH, Sims CD 1979. Prostaglandin E_2 pessaries for induction of labour. *Lancet* 1:572-575.

Pearson JF 1982. Monitoring high risk pregnancy. In: J Bonnar, ed. Recent advances in Obstet Gynecol, Vol 14; London: Churchill Livingstone, pp 3-34.

Roberts LJ, Young KR 1991. The management of prolonged pregnancy - an analysis of women's attitudes before and after term. *Br J Obstet Gynecol* 98:1102-1106.

Rutherford SE, Phelan JP, Smith CV, Jacobs N 1987. The four-quadrant assessment of amniotic fluid volume: An adjunct to antepartum fetal heart testing. *Obstet Gynecol* 70:353-356.

Sadovsky E, Yaffe H, Polishuk WZ 1974. Fetal movements in pregnancy and urinary oestriol in prediction of impending fetal death in utero. *Israel J of Med Sc* 10:1096-1099.

Schifrin BS, Foye G, Amato J, Kates R, Mackenna J 1979. Routine fetal heart rate monitoring in the antepartum period. *Obstet Gynecol* 54:21-25.

Shime J, Librach CL, Gare DJ, Cook CJ 1986. The influence of prolonged pregnancy on infant development at one and two years of age: A prospective study. *Am J Obstet Gynecol* 154:341-345.

Smith CV, Phelan JP, Paul RH, Broussard P 1985. Fetal acoustic stimulation testing: A retrospective experience with the fetal acoustic stimulation test. *Am J Obstet Gynecol* 153:567-568.

Smith CV, Phelan JP, Platt LD 1986. Fetal acoustic stimulation testing II: A randomised clinical comparison with the nonstress test. *Am J Obstet Gynecol* 155:131-134.

Smith CV, Nguyen HN, Kovacs B, McCart D, Phelan JP, Paul RH 1987. Fetal death following antepartum fetal heart rate testing: A review of 65 cases. *Obstet Gynecol* 70:18-20.

Sorensen SS, Brocks V, Lenstrup C 1985. Induction of labour and cervical ripening by intracervical prostaglandin E_2. *Obstet Gynecol* 65:110-114.

Starks GC 1980. Correlation of meconium stained amniotic fluid, early intrapartum fetal pH, and Apgar scores as predictors of perinatal outcome. *Obstet Gynecol* 56:604-609.

Steer PJ 1985. Fetal distress. In: Crawford J, ed. Risks of labour. Chichester: John Wiley and Sons, pp 11-31.

Stokes HJ, Roberts RV, Newnhan JP 1991. Doppler flow velocity waveform analysis in postdate pregnancies. *Aust NZ J Obstet Gynecol* 27-30.

The National Institute of Child Health and Human Development Network of Maternal Fetal Medicine Units 1994. A clinical of induction of labour versus expectant management in postterm pregnancy. *Am J Obstet Gynecol* 170:16-23.

Tromans PM, Beazley JM, Shenouda PI 1981. Comparative study of oestradiol and prostaglandin E_2 gel upon subsequent labour. *Br Med J* 282:679-681.

Trudinger BJ, Boylan P 1980. Antepartum fetal heart rate monitoring: Value of sound stimulation. *Obstet Gynecol* 55:265-268.

Weiner Z, Reichler A, Zlozover M, Mendelsom A, Thler I 1993. The value of Doppler ultrasonography in prolonged pregnancies. *Eur J Obstet Gynecol Reprod Biol* 48:93-97.

Westgren M, Almstrom H, Nyman M, Ulmsten U 1987. Maternal perception of sound provoked fetal movements as a measure of fetal wellbeing. *Br J Obstet Gynecol* 94:523-527.

Wong WS, Wong KS, Chang A 1985. Epidemiology of meconium staining of amniotic fluid in HongKong. *Austr NZ J Obstet Gynecol* 25:90-93.

18

Prolonged and Obstructed Labour

K. Bhasker Rao

Prolonged labour and obstructed labour are obstetric emergencies which are responsible for significant maternal and perinatal mortality and morbidity rates in developing countries. A proper understanding and management of the problem may contribute to reduction in the incidence of caesarean section for dystocia.

In over 80 per cent of nulliparous women, labour is complete within 12–14 hours of its onset (Stronge 1994). In multiparas, it is shorter in duration. The labour may be considered prolonged if a woman is not able to achieve a safe vaginal delivery within 18 hours of its onset. If it is delayed 24 hours or more, the risks to both the mother and child are undoubtedly higher. Hence the dictum, 'Do not allow the sun to set twice on a woman in labour'.

Etiology

In about 70 per cent of the cases of prolonged labour the delay is due to insufficient uterine contractions. In the remaining, the causes are cephalopelvic disproportion (CPD), malpresentations and malpositions such as the occipitoposterior (Stronge 1994; Arulkumaran and Chua 1994).

When labour is prolonged and further descent of the fetus in the birth canal is arrested, the delivery is impossible in the absence of any professional assistance and is called obstructed labour. This condition is more dangerous than prolonged labour and will be considered later in this chapter.

A partograph is a one-page documentation of the main events in labour graphically depicting the rate of cervical dilatation and descent of the presenting part against time. It also displays information on the frequency and intensity of uterine contractions, the colour of liquor, the degree of moulding and caput, maternal pulse, temperature as well as the fluids and drugs administered to the mother. Partography helps considerably in the prevention, early detection and proper management of prolonged labour. Normally, in the latent phase of labour, the cervical dilatation from 0 to 3 cm takes less than 8 hr. Subsequently, in the active phase of labour, the cervix dilates at the rate of 1 cm/hr reaching full dilatation (10 cm) in 7 hr. This observation has been confirmed in different ethnic groups in different countries (Philpott 1972; Studd 1973; Illancheran et al 1977). If the rate of dilatation is slower, it goes beyond the alert line in the partograph. The second stage of labour does not usually exceed one hour before the complete expulsion of the baby.

In a recent multicentric study covering over 35,000 parturients in Southeast Asia, partography was found useful in reducing the incidence of prolonged labour from 6.4% to 3.4 % (WHO 1994).

Types of prolonged labour

Prolongation of labour involves mostly the first stage of labour and sometimes the second stage and consists of the following types:

i.   Prolongation of the latent phase it may vary from 12–20 hr in nulliparas or 10–14 hr in multiparas.

ii.   In a prolonged active phase of labour or primary dysfunctional labour though the cervical dilatation reaches 3 cm normally, the subsequent dilatation is slower than i cm/hr. The same patient may at times show prolongation in the latent as well as active phases.

iii.   In secondary arrest of labour the cervix, after having dilated at the normal rate of 1cm/hr in the early active phase slows down prior to full dilatation. Besides arrest in the dilatation, there may be arrest or lack of progress in the descent of the presenting part.

iv.   In the case of delay in the second stage of labour: in this type, after full dilatation of the cervix, the delivery is not effected within one hour.

Prolonged latent phase

This varies greatly in duration as stated earlier. There are one or two painful uterine contractions in a 10-minute period, each contraction lasting for 20 sec. A patient admitted with a cervical dilatation of 1–2 cm may fail to reach the active phase of labour after 8 hr in a nullipara or 4–6 hr in a multipara. It is important to first find out whether the patient is actually in labour before arriving at this diagnosis. According to Stronge (1994) this is of critical importance. The criteria are:

i.   complete effacement of cervix, with dilatation of 1–3 cm

ii.   presence of 'show' — blood and mucus — with membranes present or liquor draining

iii.   painful uterine contractions of at least 2 in 10 min.

Management   If on reassessment, the patient is found not to be in labour, she is best left alone and transferred to the antenatal ward. In most instances, she may develop painful uterine contractions within 24–48 hr and deliver normally.

    If she is in labour and there is an associated CPD or malpresentation, caesarean section is indicated.

    In the absence of complications, the patient may need reassurance, hydration, nutrition and ambulation. Oxytocin augmentation at this stage, with the poor state of the cervix, is not useful. On the contrary it may increase the intrauterine pressure causing fetal anoxia and lead to unnecessary caesarean section or fetal death (Olah and Nielson 1994). The prolonged latent phase is therefore best managed conservatively.

Prolonged labour in the early active phase (primary dysfunctional labour)

If in a patient admitted in the active phase (cervix ≥ 3 cm dilatation), the labour progresses slowly with the nomogram showing a cervical dilatation slower than 1 cm/hr and crosses the alert line drawn at 1cm/hr, the main cause is inefficient uterine force. This is also the most common cause of prolonged labour. However genuine CPD, or that due to hydrocephalus, a large baby, malpresentations or a small pelvis have to be ruled out before oxytocin augmentation. After waiting for a grace period of 1–3 hr beyond the alert line if the progress is still slow, oxytocin augmentation should be considered.

The dose of oxytocin should not be too low and fail to stimulate the uterus adequately, or too high and cause hyperstimulation (with risk of uterine rupture) and fetal anoxia. Most centres prefer 2.5 U of oxytocin in 500 ml of normal saline and start at a rate of 10 drops a minute. It is advisable to commence with a dose of 2–6 mU/min of controlled oxytocin drip and increase the rate at half hourly intervals, monitoring the response with external tocography. With the dose not exceeding 8.0 mU/min and with 4 uterine contractions in 10 minutes, (each contraction lasting for 40 sec), labour progresses satisfactorily and 96% of cases deliver healthy infants vaginally (Arulkumaran 1991). For active management and better response to oxytocin in these cases, most physicians recommend amniotomy with a cervical dilatation of ≥ 3 cm. The duration of augmentation is normally about 4 hr. But if the uterine response is satisfactory with progressive descent of the presenting part oxytocin augmentation can be extended for 4 hours more, if necessary, so as to reduce the incidence of caesarean section. In many cases, failure of progress is due to failure on the part of the obstetrician to wait long enough.

Caesarean section is indicated in these cases when there is no satisfactory progress in cervical dilatation or descent of the presenting part or when the cardiotocography shows early or variable deceleration suggesting head compression due to CPD.

In cases of secondary arrest due to prolongation of the late first stage of labour after having had normal progress in the active phase earlier, if there is no CPD, oxytocin augmentation is indicated to promote the progress of labour and descent of the presenting part. If CPD is present, caesarean section should be performed.

Prolonged second stage of labour

Though the normal second stage lasts for an hour or less, it may be prolonged in those receiving epidural anesthesia (due to abolition of Ferguson's reflex), or in cases of malposition like the occipitoposterior due to slow descent and rotation. Some more time may be allowed for in these situations provided the mother and fetus are carefully monitored. In the absence of CPD, a uterine scar or multiparity, controlled oxytocin infusion may help if the contractions are not adequate (4 in 10 min each lasting > 40 sec). When labour progresses and the head descends, assisted vaginal delivery is undertaken. If there is no descent especially with evidence of maternal exhaustion or fetal distress, caesarean section is indicated after the least possible delay.

However if the head is adequately low in the pelvis when the patient is seen, forceps can be applied to deliver the child and steps taken to prevent PPH which may be associated with long labour.

The maternal consequences of prolonged labour are amnionitis (intrapartum sepsis), atonic postpartum hemorrhage, rupture of the uterus and later anemia and PID. In the fetus, anoxia, intracranial injury, pulmonary infection and later delayed milestones may be expected. Trauma and anoxia are leading causes of perinatal death in developing countries like India.

Prolonged labour is not always predictable. But good prenatal care (with early detection of CPD and malpresentations), monitoring with partography during labour and early reassessment when it crosses the alert line are valuable measures. As the commonest cause of the delay in the active phase is inefficient forces, amniotomy and augmentation with controlled oxytocin infusion drip are beneficial in most cases. When conservation fails, caesarean section is needed. Prophylactic broad spectrum antibiotics are necessary in all cases where the rupture of membranes to delivery interval is prolonged, for example, > 12 hours.

Obstructed labour

Obstructed labour results mostly from neglected obstetrics and is responsible for the majority of cases of rupture of the uterus and vesico-vaginal fistulae in developing countries.

In obstructed labour, the progress of labour is at a standstill with the presenting part jammed in the birth canal due to mechanical factors and without external assistance delivery is impossible. Its incidence is about 1–5% depending on the health care and transport facilities available (Dutta and Pal 1978; Gupta et al 1991; Kamala Jayaram 1993). Its exact incidence is difficult to estimate as some of these cases may be classified under complications like postpartum hemorrhage (PPH), ruptured uterus or puerperal sepsis. It contributes to about 10% of all maternal deaths in India.

Etiology

The leading causes of obstructed labour are
  i. cephalopelvic disproportion (contracted pelvis), a large baby
  ii. malpresentations (mostly, shoulder presentations) and malpositions, such as the occipito posterior

These two causes account for about 80 per cent of all cases of obstructed labour.
  iii. fetal anomalies such as hydrocephalus; also rarely, fetal ascites, conjoint twins
  iv. soft tissue lesions of the genital tract such as a scarred cervix following the Manchester operation; a prolapsed edematous cervix; a large cervical fibroid, other pelvic tumours, scarring due to genital mutilation and a 'Gishiri-cut' situation.
  v. vesical calculus complicating pregnancy (Sirohiwal et al 1994).

The risk factors are short statured nulliparas, unbooked women with bad obstetric history (BOH) and those residing far away from health facilities.

Pathology

About a third of women experiencing obstructed labour are nulliparas. In the presence of a malpresentation or CPD at the pelvic inlet nulliparas may rupture the bag of membranes prematurely and have prolonged labour with an edematous cervix resulting in a caput over the presenting part. Most of the liquor drains and intrapartum sepsis soon sets in. But rupture of the uterus is rare in a primigravida. If however she is a multipara, after the rupture of the membranes, the uterus acts strongly to overcome the obstruction. As labour progresses poorly, powerful uterine contractions with hardly any intervals of relaxation lead to fetal anoxia and death. The fetus is pushed down into the stretched out lower uterine segment with the presenting part jammed in the pelvis with a large caput. In cases of obstructed labour, the upper uterine segment is retracted and markedly thickened separating it from the abnormally stretched and thinned out lower segment forming the patho- logical retraction ring or Bandl's ring. In this state of threatened impending rupture of the uterus, the mother is usually exhausted, the baby moribund or dead and the uterus infected. Any further delay or intrauterine manipulation causes rupture of the already thinned out lower segment (mostly anteriorly) with escape of the fetus and placenta into the peritoneal cavity. If the rent extends to one of the uterine arteries, there will be intraperitoneal bleeding and hemorrhagic shock.

Depending on the cause and level of obstruction, the prolonged compression of the maternal soft parts by the jammed fetal head may cause ischaemic necrosis of bladder and vagina giving rise to vesico-vaginal fistula in the early puerperium irrespective of the mode of delivery. In some, it may also result in peroneal palsy.

Signs, symptoms and diagnosis

As the woman has been in labour for over 16–18 hours (and at least 4 hours after rupture of the membranes) she looks exhausted, dehydrated and is often infected with a rise in temperature and rapid pulse. Further examination very often shows the baby to be dead and reveals its presentation, position and the probable cause of obstruction. The level of Bandl's ring at or above the umbilicus with a tender stretched out lower segment suggests threatened rupture. The presence of the uterine outline confirms that the uterus has not yet ruptured. The fetal heart may be rapid, irregular or absent. Vaginal examination reveals an edematous vulva, a congested bruised vagina, a fully dilated cervix with marked moulding, large caput over the presenting part and offensive vaginal discharge. On catheterisation, the urine is often bloodstained. In about 10–15% of cases vaginal examination may show a neglected shoulder presentation.

The diagnosis is made from the history of prolonged labour after rupture of the membranes and from the abdominal and vaginal examination findings described earlier.

Prognosis   The maternal mortality is about 3–5% mainly due to hemorrhage and sepsis. Perinatal mortality is high as in most cases the fetus is dead prior to admission (Table 1). The important complications are hemorrhage, peritonitis, sep- tic shock, rupture of the uterus and later obstetric fistula (Rao 1992).

Management

Prophylaxis   Good prenatal care, early referrals of high risk cases and par- tographic monitoring of labour are useful preventive measures. Those who had operations on the cervix should be hospitalised near term and reassessed in early labour. In all cases of gross CPD and malpresentations where vaginal delivery is not possible caesarean section should be carried out.

Table 1:   Obstructed labour — Prognosis and management
(Except first row, figures in per cent)

	Dutta & Pal (1978)	Sahu & Sinha (1990)	Kamala Jayaram (1993)
No. of cases	307	298	126
Caesarean section	19.0	48.6	27.0
Embryotomy	51.8	27.5	8.0
Ruptured uterus	14.9	2.6	15.0
Maternal mortality	11.4	4.3	4.7
Perintal mortality rate	81.8	100.0	76.6

Curative   On admission, dehydration has to be corrected by administration of
1 – 1.5 L of IV fluids (normal saline, Ringer lactate) and sepsis should be combated
by parenteral broad spectrum antibiotics. Adequate quantities of blood should be
crossmatched to transfuse should the need arise due to rupture of the uterus, atonic
or traumatic PPH or septic shock. The rest of the management depends on the
condition of the fetus.

    a)   Fetus alive : If the head is unengaged or there is a malpresentation like
shoulder dystocia, immediate caesarean section should be performed. In
some countries, symphysiotomy is preferred in a borderline CPD as an
alternative to caesarean section.

In cases of obstruction by a pelvic tumour or a vesical calculus where
the head is unengaged, caesarean section is done. If it is a pedunculated
tumour it can then be removed. If a vesical calculus is the cause, after
the cystolithotomy careful repair of the bladder followed by drainage for
10 days is necessary.

In gross contracture of the pelvis when even after craniotomy, a vaginal
delivery is not possible, caesarean section is preferred.

If the fetal head has gone through the mid pelvic strait, forceps delivery
can be effected after a generous episiotomy.

    b)   Fetus dead: If the cervix is fully dilated, and the head is unengaged,
craniotomy is the treatment of choice. The axis traction forceps is applied
first to steady the head and craniotomy is done with the Oldham's or
Simpson's perforator. With further traction, the collapsed head can be
easily delivered vaginally.

In neglected shoulder presentation, internal podalic version is absolutely
contra-indicated. Decapitation is needed in such cases. With traction on the prolapsed hand, the neck can be reached easily and severed using the decapitating
hook and embryotomy scissors. Further traction on the prolapsed hand helps to
deliver the headless trunk and the head could be delivered by forceps or manually
by suprapubic pressure.

After any destructive operation the placenta should be removed manually and methyl ergometrine 0.2 mg IV given to prevent PPH. The uterus is then explored to ensure that there is no rupture of the uterus. The patient is watched for the next two to three hours for any septic shock and the bladder drained for seven days. If however the physician is not skilled in doing a decapitation, the alternative is a caesarean section. But the fetus in a neglected transverse lie cannot be delivered through a transverse lower segment incision; a midline vertical or an inverted T-shaped incision is required.

In hydrocephalus, the head is fixed by suprapubic pressure and perforation is done quite early in labour using a craniotomy forceps or sharp pointed scissors. There is no need for preliminary forceps application in these cases.

In obstructed labour, the embryotomy rate varies from 20–50% as these cases are brought in late. In some institutions in developing countries, the incidence of craniotomy is about 0.5% of all deliveries and 10–25% of obstructed labour may require this procedure (Table 1). Hence there is still a need to provide these skills to residents in some developing countries.

References

Arulkumaran S and Chua S 1994. Augmentation in labour. In: Ratnam SS, Sen DK et al, eds. Contributions to Obstetrics and Gynecology, Vol 3. New Delhi: BI Churchill Livingstone, pp 275-277.

Arulkumaran S 1991. Management of spontaneous labour. In: Ratnam SS, Rao KB, Arulkumaran S, eds. Obstetrics and Gynecology for Postgraduates. Madras: Orient Longman, pp 100-114.

Dutta DC and Pal SK 1978. Obstructed labour - A review of 307 cases. *J Obstet Gynecol India* 28: 55-58.

Gupta N, Vaid S and Acharya V 1991. Obstructed labour - A prospective clinical study of 70 cases. *J Obstet Gynecol India* 41: 52-55.

Illancheran A, Lim S M and Ratnam S S 1977. Nomograms of cervical dilatation in labour. *Sing J Obstet Gynecol* 8: 69-73.

Kamala Jayaram V 1993. Obstructed labour, an analysis of 126 cases. *J Obstet Gynecol India* 43: 60-63.

Olah KSJ, Nielson JP 1994. Failure to progress in the management of labour. *Br J Obstet Gynecol* 101: 1-3.

Rao KB 1992. Obstructed labour. In: Ratnam SS, Rao KB, Arulkumaran S, eds. Obstetrics and Gynecology for Postgraduates. Madras: Orient Longman, pp 127-133.

Sirohiwal D, Sangwan K, Sharma D et al 1994. Obstructed labour due to vesical calculus. *J Obstet Gynecol India* 44: 147-149.

Stronge JM 1994. Strategies for reducing the caesarean section rate. In: Popkin DR & Peddle LJ, eds. Women's Health Today. London: Parthenon Publishers, pp 55-58.

Studd J W W 1973. Partograms and Nomograms in the management of primigravid labour. *Br Med J* IV: 451-455.

WHO 1994. WHO Partograph in the management of labour, World Health Organisation, *Lancet* 343: 1399-1404.

19

Caesarean Deliveries — Changing Trends

K Bhasker Rao

It is of great importance to obstetricians to understand the evolution of caesarean section during the last hundred years not only in order to appreciate the alarming rise in its incidence during the last three decades but also to take suitable measures to bring it down to reasonable levels. The term 'caesarean' for the abdominal delivery of a child by cutting through the abdominal wall and the uterus was perhaps derived because of the 'Lex Caesarean' (Caesar's Laws), or most probably from the Latin word 'caedere' (to cut). Though there is a reference to postmortem caesareans in the *Susruta Samhita* (Rao 1952) and in the Talmud, it was not till the nineteenth century that the operation was done on the living with reasonable chances for the woman's survival. Kaufman (1995) describes eight caesarean sections performed in Edinburgh between 1737 and 1820 mainly for gross pelvic contraction caused by osteomalacia. In all these cases, the mothers died within 48 hours, and the child survived only in two. Fayrer (1870) describes in detail two caesarean sections done on two women in purdah for severe osteomalacia in early 1854 in Lucknow, India, in consultation with Dr Bonsfield. A longitudinal uterine incision was made in each case but the mothers died due to hemorrhage and sepsis within two days. The surgeon found at postmortem that the pelvis of both was so distorted that a finger could hardly be easily passed through it. Porros (1876) performed caesarean section with better results as the uterus was removed during the operation. It was only in 1882 that Max Sanger in Leipzig advocated the suturing of the uterus after delivering the child. This was the first major step towards reducing the risk of maternal deaths from hemorrhage, sepsis and rupture of the uterus during a subsequent pregnancy. The extraperitoneal operation described by Frank (1907) and Latzkos (1909) and revived 30 years later by Waters failed to gain popularity. But the transperitoneal lower segment operation with a vertical incision advocated by Kronig (1912) and later modified by Munro Kerr (1926) as a transverse lower segment operation proved much safer and has been universally accepted since then.

With the increasing safety following the introduction of modern anesthesia and blood transfusion, the operation which was primarily done as a last resort for severe contractions of the pelvis was liberalised to include other forms of dystocia, major degrees of placenta previa and severe eclampsia with a view to reduce maternal mortality. This was soon extended to cases of fetal distress, bad obstetric history (BOH) and as a safer alternative to difficult vaginal operative delivery so as to reduce perinatal mortality. With the introduction of modern technology in the labour wards and neonatology units, there was a further rise in the rate of caesarean deliveries performed to prevent potentially grave threats to fetal and neonatal life and wellbeing. Some obstetricians even opted for caesarean in VLBW babies to prevent 'possible intracranial trauma'. Besides, there have been numerous other obstetric, medical, social, ethical, economic and medicolegal factors which have added to the list of indications leading to alarmingly high rates of caesarean section all over the world.

Few countries have been reporting national caesarean section (CS) rates annually. From the figures published, we find that the CS rates which were hardly 1–2% in the early thirties in the USA, gradually increased to 4.5% in 1965. Thereafter, there has been an annual rise by 1% so as to reach a peak of 24.7% in 1988, resulting in one out of four deliveries in the USA being abdominal (Myers and Gleicher 1990). In Italy, the national data rose from 4.2% in 1980 to 14.5% in 1983 and 17.5% in 1987 (Signorelli et al 1991; Parazzini et al 1992). It must however be pointed out that the rising trends have not been uniform. They have been quite high in the USA and Canada; but the lowest rates have been reported in the Netherlands followed by Czechoslovakia, Norway and Hungary.

Table 1: Caesarean section rates per 100 deliveries
in selected countries (1970 – 1988)

Country	1970	1988
USA	5.5	24.7
Canada	5.7	19.5
Scotland	5.9	14.4
Australia	4.2	16.1
Hungary	2.2	10.2
Norway	2.2	9.4
CSFR	2.3	7.7
The Netherlands	2.1	6.5

(*Source:* Notzon et al 1987, Stephenson et al 1993)

Professional bodies were concerned at this enormous rise in the CS rates and appointed special committees to enquire into the causes of the sharply rising trends and suggest suitable measures to control these rates.

The epidemic of CS rates has not been limited to developed countries alone but has spread to developing countries too. The institutional rates in Women's Hospital, Madras, which were as low as 1–2% from 1930 to 1960, gradually rose to 3% in 1970, 10% in 1980 and peaked to 20% in 1992. The institutional rates in the Middle East (Kuwait, Saudi Arabia and Egypt) are about 10%. The rates for teaching hospitals in South and Southeast Asia are slightly higher ranging from 8.1% in Delhi to 21.1% in Trivandrum (Table 2). In a survey of 33 teaching institutions in India, the CS rates in 1993 varied from 8% to 36% (Rao 1994).

Table 2: Caesarean section rates in selected teaching hospitals
of South and Southeast Asia

Country	Per cent
Colombo (1992)	14.6
Karachi (1992)	16.3
Rawalpindi (1992)	15.1
Singapore (NUH) (1990)	12.3
Dacca (1990)	21.1
Bombay (W) (1992)	11.4
New Delhi (S.J.) (1993)	8.1
Madras (MH) (1993)	20.6
Calcutta (RGK) (1993)	21.6
Lucknow (1993)	20.6
Trivandrum (1993)	25.4

Probably the highest rates are reported from Brazil where they have gone up from 15% in 1974 to 31% in 1980 partly to enable some parous women to undergo sterilisation (Barros et al 1991).

Why are the CS rates on the increase?

1. Due to an increase in the number of repeat sections, as many obstetricians are reluctant to take risks in allowing subsequent trial of vaginal delivery.
2. Because with the use of continuous electronic fetal monitoring, more cases of fetal distress are 'detected'.
3. Because of increasing trends for caesarean section for uncomplicated breech presentations so as to reduce perinatal deaths.
4. Because of rising induction rates, with caesarean section for cases of failed induction.
5. Because obstetricians prefer caesarean to difficult vaginal delivery for pelvic arrests.
6. There are better 'chances of survival' of LBW and VLBW babies delivered by caesarean than delivered vaginally.
7. Because of better maternal and fetal prognosis in cases of antepartum hemorrhages (placenta previa or abruptio) with caesarean than by conservative vaginal delivery.
8. Caesarean section for severe PIH including eclampsia in primigravidae when urgent pregnancy terminations are needed or when there is no response to conservative therapy.
9. Because of the rising incidence or IUGR as made out by clinical and ultrasonologic methods.

10. To avoid malpractice suits for alleged neglect in vaginal delivery when the child has convulsions or cerebral palsy later. A physician with a history of malpractice claim is more likely to opt for caesarean due to defensive obstetrics.
11. Due to economic incentives because professional charges are higher for caesarean than for a successful vaginal delivery.
12. In some cases because of the lack of patience on the part of the patient or her physician. The physician factor in caesarean section was obvious from a study involving 11 physicians from a single institution where a caesarean rate varied from 19.1% to 42.3% depending on the physician's outlook and judgement (Goyert et al 1989).

Indications for caesarean section in modern obstetrics

Till 50 years ago, caesarean section was done primarily for pelvic dystocia (CPD, malpresentations like shoulder, mentoposterior, brow etc) and major degrees of placenta previa. In course of time, the list of indications has increased enormously contributing to a sharp rise not only in the total CS rates but also in the number of repeat sections.

Currently the important indications are previous caesareans, dystocia, fetal distress and breech presentations. From Table 3 it may be seen that in 1990 over two-thirds of the caesareans in the the USA were done because of previous caesarean section and dystocia. Compared to 1980, there has been an increase of 32–36% in these two indications in the course of 10 years. Similarly, in 1990 there has been a steep rise by 65% in the caesarean rates for fetal distress. For breech however the comparative rise has been less than 5%; and for 'others' there has been a fall by 18 per cent (Notzon et al, 1994). Similarly, in Madras, repeat sections and dystocia accounted for over 50% of caesareans in 1992, with a rise in the incidence of repeat sections and fetal distress and a decline for other indications.

Table 3: Indications for caesarean sections (All figures in per cent)

Indications	USA		Women's Hospital (Madras)	
	1980	1990	1970	1992
Repeat caesarean	31.9	37.5	19.2	33.4
Dystocia	28.4	30.0	23.4	19.4
Fetal distress	4.7	9.7	10.7	22.3
Malpresentation (Breech)	11.8	8.5	12.3	8.4
Others	22.5	13.5	34.4	16.5

(*Source:* Notzon et al 1994, Rao 1994)

Repeat caesarean section

It may be seen that previous caesarean section is a major indication in most centres, forming 15–45% of total caesarean sections. In selected South Asian teaching institutions, the repeat section rates were surprisingly high ranging from 18 – 40% of all caesareans. This leading cause for caesarean section can definitely be lowered by increasing the trial for vaginal delivery for patients with previous caesarean. By 1990, the vaginal births after caesarean (VBAC) were 19.5% in the USA (compared to hardly 3.0% in 1980), 52.9% in Sweden and as high as 56:2% in Norway (Notzon et al 1994).

VBAC is becoming more acceptable and quite safe. A meta-analysis of 31 studies of over 11,400 trials of labour following caesarean showed that VBAC was safe and that there was no difference in the rate of scar dehiscence whether a patient was given a chance to deliver vaginally or electively sectioned (Rosen et al 1991). In two recent series totalling 17,000 cases of VBAC from California, there was no rupture-related maternal death even though oxytocin augmentation was used whenever necessary (Miller et al 1994; Flamm et al 1994). The rupture of the scar with one previous caesarean section was 0.64% compared to 2.3% with two caesareans and 2.8% with three or more (Leung et al 1993). Therefore it is safe to allow a vaginal delivery after one caesarean section in the absence of CPD and malpresentation. Professional associations including American College of Obstetricians and Gynecologists have therefore recommended that women with previous lower segment transverse caesarean section should be counselled to undergo a trial of labour. It is hoped that most of the teaching institutions in developing countries too will give opportunities for previous caesarean cases to be delivered vaginally in large numbers. Currently the rates of VBACs are as disappointingly low at 20–40% in most of these centres.

Dystocia

The next important indication is dystocia which includes not only all difficult labour due to 'faults' in the passages but also in the 'forces'. Conservative management of dysfunctional labour with oxytocin augmentation, giving adequate time for cases of 'non-progress in labour' and availability of senior staff for consultation for emergencies contribute to reduction in caesareans for this indication. The midwife is mainly responsible for the management of delivery in some continental countries and to a large extent the very low caesarean rates in the Netherlands is due to the majority of deliveries in that country being conducted by midwives.

Fetal distress

The CS rates are high in institutions where continuous electronic fetal monitoring is carried out routinely. But in these institutions, with the rise in CS rates, the perinatal mortality rates (PNMR) have not declined (Klein et al 1993; MacDonald 1985). A prospective study of 35,000 women with selective and universal electronic fetal heart rate monitoring showed a higher rate of CS for the latter group, with similar rates of PNMR for the two groups (Leveno et al 1986). Perhaps more accurate diagnostic tools are needed for this condition, including fetal scalp blood sampling.

Breech presentations

Soni (1931) was the first to recommend CS for the reduction of perinatal mortality in breech presentations. For the last two decades, there has been a gradual increase in CS rates for breech presentations. In the Wadia hospital, Bombay, the CS rates for breech rose from 2.7% thirty years ago to 32% in 1987 (Nitwe et al 1987). In 1990, the CS rates for breech were 83% in USA and 60.8% in Norway (Notzon et al 1994). Though some advocate caesarean for preterm breech also, in the developing countries it has to be kept in mind that there is a resultant increase in maternal morbidity and risks of scar dehiscence in subsequent pregnancies (Viegas et al 1985). Caesarean section may be avoided by external cephalic version done between 32 and 36 weeks in uncomplicated breech and this is therefore advised in all cases where there are no contraindications for version. In a 11-year study of uncomplicated breech, Gordon (1994) recommended vaginal delivery in younger women with an adequate pelvis, an average sized baby and extended breech with no associated medical or obstetric complications. If however the baby is over 3.5 kg, and there is footling presentation, hyperextension of the head, associated IUGR, PIH, APH or diabetes, elective caesarean was suggested to be better. In all such cases, ultrasonography is advised to rule out congenital anomalies.

VLBW baby

Though it is claimed that intraventricular hemorrhage is a common neurological complication in preterm infants, prophylactic caesarean section as a routine is not recommended because of increased maternal morbidity and the findings that perinatal mortality rates are not appreciably reduced by an increasing CS rate in this group (Molloy et al 1989). Besides in the preterm vertex, caesarean section is controversial and technically difficult (Narayan and Taylor 1994).

Antepartum hemorrhages (APH)

In placenta previa, abdominal delivery is the route of choice as over 90% of cases are now delivered by caesarean compared to less than 30% four decades ago. This has resulted in the reduction of the maternal death rate to less than 1% and perinatal loss to below 30%. In abruptio placenta, the CS rate has gone up to over 50% compared to 3% twentyfive years ago (Bhatt 1989).

Induction of labour

The incidence of CS is about 2.5 times more in cases of failed induction compared to those who had spontaneous onset of labour (Arulkumaran et al 1986). With the availability of endocervical PGE_2 gel, the response to induction of labour has improved and the need for caesarean section is therefore less than before.

Other inductions

In twins, caesarean section may be preferred when both the fetuses (or the first one) have malpresentations. After the vaginal delivery of the first, if abdominal examination shows a malpresentation, external cephalic version can be done or the baby extracted after internal podalic version soon after the rupture of the second bag of membranes. The CS rate for twins varies from 18.5% in Calcutta (Kumar and Chakravarty 1989) to 45% in Sweden (Rydstrom et al 1990). Following IVF, the CS rates are obviously higher. In a collaborative study of over 2,300 such pregnancies the CS rate was 46.8% (Cohen et al 1988). Caesarean section is preferred in IUGR associated with PIH, BOH and diabetes to avoid the stress of labour for these infants (especially when biophysical profile on ultrasonography and nonstress test are not favourable).

Classical caesarean section is done rarely at present except for selected indications like (1) carcinoma of the cervix complicating pregnancy, (2) when the lower segment cannot be reached due to dense adhesions from previous surgery, (3) neglected shoulder presentation where the presenting part is jammed (even with a dead fetus when the obstetrician is not confident to do decapitation) and, rarely (4) in a myoma occupying the lower segment.

Prophylactic antibiotics for caesarean section

To lower the morbidity rates, prophylactic broad spectrum antibiotics have been advocated IV either an hour before surgery or during the operation, soon after clamping the cord. Though it is claimed to reduce the morbidity in these cases (Duff 1987), antibiotics are definitely indicated in all cases where membranes have been ruptured for over four hours and in those clinically diagnosed as having chorio-amnionitis. In such cases, it should be continued postoperatively till the patient becomes afebrile.

Have vaginal operative delivery rates decreased with rising CS rates?

The increasing CS rates seem to be associated with decreasing instrumental deliveries in a few countries. Mostly, the instrumental vaginal delivery rates have been stable, though CS rates have increased. It is claimed that oxytocin augmentation does not give rise to rising CS rates but does effect a slight increase in the vaginal operative delivery rates (Stephenson et al 1993). In some teaching centres in India, there has been a significant fall in the forceps delivery rate with rising CS rates probably due to the decrease in the number of midforceps or difficult vaginal operative deliveries (Rao 1994).

Is there any decrease in the maternal and perinatal mortality rates with rising CS rates?

A 12-country study concluded that a large proportion of interventions were unnecessary or marginally beneficial (Stephenson et al 1993). The increased CS rates contribute to increased morbidity due to anesthesia and surgery to both the mother and child, besides exposing the mother to risks in subsequent pregnancies and labour. There has not been any appreciable fall in the perinatal and maternal death rates attributable to the increased CS rates. Improved MCH care, better socio-economic conditions, and advances in perinatology have contributed to lowered perinatal mortality rates. O'Driscoll and Foley (1983) found that between 1965 and 1980, the CS rate was steady at around 4 per cent in Dublin but the PMR had declined from 42 per 1,000 to 16 per 1,000. There has also been no reduction in perinatal morbidity including that due to cerebral palsy with the increased CS rates. Besides, the incidence of cerebral palsy may not be related to intrapartum events (Illingworth 1985; Jonas and Dooley 1989).

Caesarean section no doubt carries a maternal mortality three to seven times higher than that associated with vaginal delivery (Miller 1988). The most important causes of maternal deaths following caesarean section are PPH and sepsis and rarely thromboembolism and anesthetic accidents (Rao and Saraswathy 1982). Prostaglandin $F_{2\alpha}$ is useful for the control of atonic PPH in caesarean cases (Hickl 1994).

How can the CS rates be reduced?

If the CS rates are alarmingly high and not beneficial to either the mother or the child, can these rates be reduced? Strategies to achieve this include :

1. Public and physician education.
2. Observing the guidelines and recommendations made by professional associations, especially in the management of previous CS so as to increase the VBAC rates.
3. Periodic institutional peer-review of CS cases.
4. A second consultation with no extra cost to the patient for elective caesareans.
5. Extra incentives for VBAC (King 1993).

The rising trends in CS rates should be checked by studies proving that there are equally good alternatives of managing obstetric problems. The decision to do a caesarean should be taken only when a safe vaginal delivery is no longer possible. Elective caesareans performed indiscriminately add not only to the rising CS rates but also to unnecessary morbidity rates and affect the woman's future reproductive performance. The lowering of CS rates is possible by reducing the primary CS rates especially for dystocia and also by increasing the VBAC rates. With physician education and increased motivation there has been a stabilisation of CS rates in several countries. A few countries like Sweden and many institutions have already shown an encouraging decline in caesarean section rates without in any way affecting the maternal and neonatal outcome.

Reference

Arulkumaran, S, Gibb, DMF, Heng, SH, Ratnam, SS 1985. Perinatal outcome of induction in labour. *Asia Oceania J Obstet Gynecol* 11:33-37.

Barros FC, Vaughan JP, Victoria CG et al 1991. Epidemic of caesarean sections in Brazil. *Lancet* 338: 161-169.

Bhatt RV 1989. Antepartum hemorrhages. In: Menon MKK, Devi PK, Rao KB, eds. Postgraduate Obstetrics and Gynecology, 4th edn. Madras: Orient Longman, pp 106-120.

Cohen J, Mayaux MJ, Guihard, Muscato, ML 1988. Over-view of pregnancy after IVF. *Ann NY Acad Sci* 541: 1-6.

Duff P 1987. Prophylactic antibiotics for caesarean delivery. *Am J Obstet Gynecol* 157: 794.

Fayrer 1870. Clinical surgery in India, London: Benjamin Pardon.

Flamm BL, Goings JR, Liu Y, Wolde-Tsadik G 1994. Elective repeat caesarean delivery versus trial of labour - a prospective multicentric study. *Obstet Gynecol* 83: 927-932.

Goyert GL, Bottoms SF, Treadwell MC et al 1989. Physician factor in caesarean section rates. *N Engl J Med* 320: 706-9

Gordon H. 1994. Appropriate role of caesarean section in modern obstetric practice - breech and multiple prenancies. In: Popkins DR and Peddle LJ, eds. Women's Health Today. London: Parthenon Publishers, pp 71-74.

Hickl EJ 1994. The safety of caesarean section. In: Popkin DR and Peddle LJ, eds. Women's Health Today. London: Parthenon Publishers, pp 65-70.

Illingworth RS 1985. A pediatrician asks - why is it called birth injury? *Br J Obstet Gynecol* 92: 122-130.

Jonas HS, Dooley SL 1989. The search for lower caesarean rate goes on. *JAMA* 262: 1512-1513.

Kaufman MH 1995. Caesarean operations performed in Edinburgh during 18th century. *Br J Obstet Gynecol* 102: 186-191.

King JF 1993. Obstetric interventions and the economic imperative. *Br J Obstet Gynecol* 100: 303-304.

Klein M, Lloyd L, Redman C, Bull M, Turnbull C 1993. A comparison of low risk pregnant woman booked for delivery in 2 systems of care. *Br J Obstet Gynecol* 90: 123-128.

Kumar B, Chakravarthy BK 1989. Caesarean section for twins. *J Obstet Gynecol India* 39: 212-214.

Leung AS, Leung EK, Paul RH 1993. Uterine rupture after previous caesarean delivery - maternal and fetal consequences. *Am J Obstet Gynecol* 169: 945-950.

Leveno KJ, Cunningham FG, Nelson S, Roark M et al 1986. A prospective comparison of selective and universal electronic fetal monitoring in 34,995 pregnancies. *N Engl J Med* 315: 615-619.

MacDonald DD, Grant A, Sheridan PM et al 1985. Dublin randomised control trials of intrapartum fetal heart monitoring. *Am J Obstet Gynecol* 152:524-539.

Miller JM 1988. Maternal and neonatal morbidity and mortality in caesarean section. *Obstet Gynecol Cl of N America* 15: 629.

Miller DA, Diaz FG, Paul RH 1994. Vaginal birth after caesarean - 10 year experience. *Obstet Gynecol* 84: 255-258.

Molloy MH, Rhoads GG, Schramm W, Land G 1989. Increasing caesarean section rates in VLBW infants. *JAMA* 262: 1475-1478.

Myers SA, Gleicher N 1990. 1988 US Caesarean section rate - good news or bad? *N Engl J Med* 323: 200.

Narayan H, Taylor DJ 1994. Role of caesarean section in delivery of a very preterm infant. *Br J Obstet Gynecol* 101: 936-938.

Nitwe MT, Motwani MN, Walvekar VR 1987. Changing trends in management of breech. *J Obstet Gynecol India* 9: 321-327.

Notzon FC, Plack PJ, Taffel SM 1987. Comparison of national caesarean section rates. *N Engl J Med* 316: 386-389.

Notzon FC, Cnattingius S, Bergsjo P et al 1994. Caesarean section delivery in 1980s: International comparison by indication. *Am J Obstet Gynecol* 170: 495-504.

O'Driscoll K, Foley M 1983. Correlation of decrease in perinatal mortality and increase in caesarean section rates. *Obstet Gynecol* 61: 1-5.

Parazzini F, Pirotta N, Veechia C et al 1992. Determinants of caesarean section rates in Italy. *Br J Obstet Gynecol* 99: 203-206.

Rao KB 1952. Obstetrics in Ancient India. *J Ind Med Assocn* 21: 210.

Rao KB 1994. Global aspects of a rising caesarean section rate. In: Popkin DR and Peddle LJ, eds. Women's Health Today. London: Parthenon Publishers, pp 65-70.

Rao KB, Saraswathi R 1982. Preventable factors in maternal mortality due to caesarean section. Paper presented at World Congress Obst and Gynecol (FIGO), San Francisco, Sept. 1982.

Rosen MG, Dickinson JC, Westhoff CL 1991. Vaginal birth after caesarean - A meta-analysis of morbidity and mortality. *Obstet Gynecol* 77: 465-470.

Rydstrom H, Ingemarsson I. Ohrlander S 1990. Lack of correlation between high caesarean rates and prognosis for LBW babies in twins. *Br J Obstet Gynecol* 97: 229-233.

Signorelli C, Elliott P, Cattarruzza MS et al 1991. Trends in caesarean section in Italy, an examination of national data 1980-85. *Int J Epidemiol* 20: 712-6.

Soni M R 1931. Breech presentations. *Br Med J* i: 547-548.

Stephenson PA, Bakoula C, Hemminki E et al 1993. Patterns of use of obstetric interventions in 12 countries. *Pediatr Perinat Epidemiol* 7: 45-54,

Viegas OAC, Ingemarsson I, Sim LP et al 1985. Collaborative study on preterm breech. Vaginal vs Caesarean. *Asia Oceania J Obstet Gynecol* 11: 349-355.

20

Management of Women with Previous Caesarean Section Scar

S Chua
S Arulkumaran
R Haththotuwa

Concern expressed over the rapid rise in caesarean section (CS) rates in many industrialised countries in the 1970s and early 1980s appear to have given way to stabilisation of CS rates in the late 1980s and 1990s (Table 1) (Notzon et al 1994). However there remains a great diversity in the levels of national CS rates and in the pace and extent of change from country to country.

Table 1: National CS rates 1980 – 1990

	1980	*1985*	*1990*
Norway	8.4	11.6	12.8
Scotland	11.7	13.0	14.2
Sweden	11.0	11.5	10.7
United States	16.9	22.7	23.6

Source: Notzon et al 1994

The population of women with previous CS scar are at high risk of a repeat CS, and previous CS is a major indication for CS in many countries. Repeat CS is the commonest indication for CS (Bolaji and Meehan 1993) and accounts for as high as 30% of the increase in CS rates in the United States (NIH 1981). Indeed, it has been reported that 99% of women with a previous CS were delivered by repeat CS in American hospitals in 1974 (Saldana et al 1979). The contribution of this indication to the overall CS rate varies. In a recent review of CS trends in the industrialised countries (Notzon et al 1994), the contribution of previous CS to the overall CS was two times as high in the United States as in Scotland and Sweden. Underlying the national differences in the contribution of previous CS were strong differences in the attitudes to vaginal delivery after CS in the different countries (Table 2). If overall CS rates are to be stabilised, the different management policies for a woman with a previous CS needs to be assessed critically.

In 1918, Craigin introduced the concept of 'once a CS always a CS' (Craigin 1916), when referring to a classical uterine incision. Since then anesthesia, blood transfusion facilities, and antibiotics have improved, and a classical caesarean section, which is associated with a higher incidence of scar rupture, is rarely

Table 2:   Rates of vaginal delivery after CS, 1980 – 1990

	1980	1985	1990
Norway	56.9	53.8	56.2
Scotland	38.7	56.3	50.0
Sweden	40.7	47.4	52.9
United States	3.0	7.0	19.5

Source: Notzon et al 1994

performed. Maternal mortality associated with CS can be ten times that of a woman delivered vaginally (Ritchie 1986). In one study, there was a 27-fold increase in maternal mortality with CS as compared with vaginal delivery and one-third of deaths occurred in cases of repeat CS (Evrard and Gold 1977). Maternal morbidity after CS is also increased compared with vaginal delivery. Yet many obstetricians prefer to deliver women with previous CS by a repeat CS even though the incidence of scar rupture is as low as 0.3–1.7% (Lavin et al 1982; Nielsen et al 1989; Flamm et al 1990). Data shows (Gibbs 1980; Clark 1988) that loss of integrity of a transverse low segment incision (window or dehiscence referring to intact visceral peritoneum, frank rupture) occurred as frequently in women without labour as in those allowed a trial of labour. Many series have shown that the rupture of a transverse low-segment incision does not carry an increased fetal risk if appropriately managed. Maternal mortality from rupture of a previous CS scar is very uncommon in modern obstetrics.

Reluctance to give a trial is because of the difficulty in assessing the integrity of the uterine scar and the fear of scar rupture late in pregnancy or in labour. This fear is understandable as the diagnosis of scar rupture is retrospective and cannot be predicted prospectively. However review of the literature on vaginal birth after a previous CS has shown that rupture of a prior lower segment uterine incision is often incomplete whereas spontaneous or traumatic rupture of an unscarred uterus is often complete and may be catastrophic. Bloodless dehiscence is the commonest form of loss of integrity of the lower segment CS scar, and has few clinical signs and usually does not cause significant morbidity and mortality. It is more often than not diagnosed at the time of abdominal delivery for some other indication such as failure to progress, or after vaginal delivery (Arulkumaran et al 1992).

Most series in which rupture in scarred and unscarred uteri were differentiated show a striking difference in fetal mortality in the two groups (Muller et al 1961; Schrinsky and Benson 1978; Golan et al 1980). Golan et al (1980) noted that the fetal mortality was 74% with rupture in the group with unscarred uteri and 22% in the group with a previous uterine scar. Maternal mortality was also strikingly different between the two groups of women; there were nine maternal deaths in the series (9.7%), all occurring in the women with unscarred uteri (nine of 61 or 14.7%). Likewise, Muller et al (1961) noted in a review of a series of uterine ruptures that high maternal mortality rates associated with rupture of the uterus occurs with spontaneous and traumatic ruptures and not in ruptures of post CS scars.

Uterine activity in labour in women with a previous caesarean scar

The scar is breached with stretching of the uterine scar due to uterine contractions. The stronger the contractions and the more the contractions necessary to achieve delivery (that is, the more the uterine activity necessary to achieve vaginal delivery), the greater the chance of scar rupture.

Uterine activity during spontaneous labour after a previous lower segment CS has been documented (Arulkumaran et al 1989). The uterine activity of women with a previous CS done electively or in the latent phase of labour, who have had no previous vaginal delivery has been compared with a control group of nulliparae and multiparae. Similarly the uterine activity in spontaneous normal labour in those who had a previous CS done in the active phase of labour, but who had no vaginal delivery and women with previous CS who also had a vaginal delivery prior to or after that event were compared with the uterine activity of nulliparae and multi-parae. The results show that a first pregnancy that progressed to the active phase of the first stage of labour needs less uterine activity in a subsequent labour which is more similar to that of multiparae than nulliparae. A multiparae who had a previous CS and a normal vaginal delivery prior to or after the CS had uterine activity similar to that of a multipara with no previous CS. An intact scar did not influence uterine activity if the patient had had a previous vaginal delivery.

The same study also showed that there is a steep rise of uterine activity in the late first and second stages of labour. This increase in uterine pressure for a prolonged period of time may not be advisable in the presence of a uterine scar, and supports the practice of well-timed prophylactic forceps in the second stage of labour described by many authors (Birnbaum 1956; Douglas et al 1963; Meehan et al 1972).

In selected women a properly conducted trial of labour after previous caesarean delivery constitutes the best and safest form of obstetric management. Reported success rates of vaginal delivery after previous CS varies from 38–93% (Lawrence 1953; Meehan et al 1972; Saldana et al 1979). These women must be carefully selected, based on a review of the events leading to the CS in the previous pregnancy, as well as factors affecting the feasibility of a trial of labour in this pregnancy.

Type of scar

Most authors exclude women with classic CS from trials of labour. Among women with previous classical CS scars, the incidence of uterine rupture is increased two- to tenfold (Wilson 1951; Muller et al 1961; Lavin et al 1982); maternal and perinatal mortality is five to ten times (Dewhurst 1957; Muller et al 1961) when compared with patients with a previous lower segment CS. The clinical picture is also less serious after a ruptured lower segment scar compared with the classical CS scar. In Dewhurst's (1957) series, two-thirds of the women with a classical rupture collapsed and required transfusion and urgent treatment compared with less than one-tenth of cases after a lower segment scar rupture. In this review, there were five maternal deaths after 100 ruptured classical scars and no deaths with 55 ruptured lower segment CS scars. In all reports, the complete rupture occurred more frequently in classical CS scars and the incomplete in the lower segment CS scars. In a review of 33 cases of complete uterine rupture at trial of labour after previous CS (Muller et al 1961), classical CS scars were responsible for 30 ruptures. Twenty-four infant deaths occurred after complete rupture of a classical CS scar with none in women with a lower segment CS scar. Women with inverted T incisions, extensive lateral tears and perforations of the fundus are better excluded from trials of labour. However women with unknown scars have been shown to be able to undergo trial of labour without an increase in maternal or fetal complications (Beall et al 1984). Those with lower segment transverse CS scars are the most suitable for a trial of labour (Nielsen et al 1989).

Post-operative convalescence

Evidence of uterine wound infection following a previous CS as suggested by high swinging temperature, features of peritonitis, acute uterine tenderness and purulent vaginal discharge, may suggest the possibility of scar weakness (Holland 1921). In many countries repeat CS is performed in women with a history of uterine wound infection. However this practice is supported by very little objective evidence of the relationship between morbidity at the time of primary CS and an increased predisposition to uterine rupture in a trial of labour in a subsequent pregnancy (Case et al 1971; Lavin et al 1982). Wilson (1951) found that 50% of cases of uterine rupture after previous CS had a morbid course after the primary CS, but the morbidity among women who did not experience uterine rupture was not stated. Microscopic examination of scars at laparotomy revealed that complete myometrial regeneration or fibrosis after a previous CS was not related to the presence of puerperal infection in the previous CS; indeed some women with a history of infection appeared to demonstrate a 'tougher' scar than those with an uncomplicated puerperium. In the series by Case et al (1971), 99 women with a history of genital tract infection after primary CS had the state of their scars noted at subsequent CS. Only three women had evidence of scar dehiscence/rupture. The rest of the scars were presumably intact. In another series (Morewood et al 1973), 33 women with proven genital tract infection after their first CS were considered for trial of labour. No uterine ruptures were noted in this group. A history of abdominal wound infection will not exclude the patient from having trial of labour in a subsequent pregnancy.

Number of previous incisions

Trial of vaginal birth after one previous lower segment CS has, in carefully selected women, become an accepted option with a success rate of 38–93% (Lawrence 1953; Meehan et al 1972; Saldana et al 1979). Trial of labour in women with more than one previous CS remains controversial. There appears to be no unanimity on this point, and the question of whether uterine scar rupture is influenced by the number of previous CS scars remains unanswered.

Several authors suggest that multiple scars rule out the possibility of vaginal delivery because the risk of uterine dehiscence or rupture increases the greater the number of previous uterine incisions (Tahilramaney et al 1984; Pedowitz and Schwartz 1987). Others believe that the number of previous CS should bear little significance on the outcome in a subsequent pregnancy when deciding on a trial of labour (Meier and Porreco 1982; Porreco and Meier 1983; Tahilramaney et al 1984; Phelan et al 1987; Chattopadhyay et al 1994). In a recent trial of planned vaginal delivery after two previous CS (Chattopadhyay et al 1994), the rates of vaginal delivery, scar dehiscence, uterine rupture and associated complications among 115 women with two previous sections who underwent trial of labour were compared with 1,006 women with two previous CS who did not have a trial of labour. 103 (89%) of the women who had a trial of labour were delivered vaginally. Prostaglandin was used for induction of labour in 37 (32%) women and augmentation of labour with oxytocin was required in 32 (28%) in the trial of labour group. One scar dehiscence (0.8%) was detected among the 115 women who had a trial of labour after two previous CS compared with seven (0.7%) among 1,006 women with two previous CS scheduled for elective CS over the same period of time. The woman who developed scar dehiscence during trial of labour had secondary arrest of labour, and the dehiscence was detected and repaired at CS. She subsequently went on to have two uncomplicated CS. Caesarean hysterectomy was performed on one patient (0.8%) in the trial of labour group because of atonic postpartum hemorrhage at CS for secondary arrest in labour. Fifteeen (1.4%) hysterectomies were performed in women scheduled for elective repeat section, eight for atonic postpartum hemorrhage and seven for placenta accreta. There was one maternal death among the women scheduled for elective repeat section. The authors concluded that a trial of labour in selected women with two previous CS appears to be a reasonable option.

Indication for previous CS

In considering trial of labour in women with a previous CS, the indication for the previous CS has traditionally been a significant factor. Analysis of combined data from several previous reports (Lavin et al 1982) suggests that women with previous CS for CPD compared with CS for other non-recurrent indications have a poorer prognosis for subsequent vaginal delivery, although a substantial number of these women can be expected to deliver vaginally.

Discussion about recurrent vs non-recurrent indications for CS is abundant and some studies specifically exclude women with previous CS done for cephalopelvic disproportion from trial of labour because of fear of scar rupture but others include them (Morewood et al 1973; Saldana et al 1979; Seitchik and Rao 1982; Benedetti et al 1982; Clark et al 1984; Tahilramaney et al 1984; Chua et al 1989; Miller and Leader 1992). An analysis of the obstetric outcome in 305 women with a previous lower segment CS scar (Chua et al 1989) showed that women with CS done for recurrent indications like CPD and no progress of labour had a vaginal delivery rate of 63.3% and a CS rate of 36.7% whilst the women with CS done for nonrecurrent indications had a vaginal delivery rate of 73.4% and a CS rate of 26.6%. These differences were statistically not significant. There was no maternal or fetal mortality in either group. It was concluded that with careful selection and appropriate management, women who had a previous CS for CPD/failure to progress can be given a trial of labour safely. Blanket exclusion of women from a trial of labour after a previous LSCS for CPD or failure to progress is not justified. In some of these women failure to progress in the previous labour could be due to malposition (relative cephalopelvic disproportion). In a subsequent pregnancy if the fetus presents in the normal position with adequate uterine activity vaginal delivery may be achieved safely (Morewood et al 1973; Seitchik and Rao 1982; Chua et al 1989; Miller and Leader 1992).

Exclusion of fetopelvic disproportion

Passage   The adequacy of the pelvis relative to fetal size can be assesssed clinically although in some instances, X-ray pelvimetry may be preferred (Gibbs 1980; Lavin et al 1982; Nielsen et al 1985) because it is thought to be less subjective. The reliability of routine antepartum X-ray pelvimetry for deciding between trial of labour or elective CS in women with previous CS has recently been challenged (Thubisi et al 1993). Indeed routine X-ray pelvimetry in women with a previous CS may increase the elective CS rate without assuring vaginal delivery in women considered for a trial of labour (Wilson 1951; Thubisi et al 1993).

Passenger   The fetal size should be estimated considering the period of amenorrhoea, the size of the patient, the size of the fetal head, clinical experience and knowledge of fetal weight at different gestations. The role of ultrasound for estimating fetal weight is contentious. Even in women with macrosomic babies larger than in previous pregnancies a trial of labour may be given, if labour is progressing well without any evidence of fetal distress or poor progress (Phelan et al 1984).

Facilities available for trial of labour

To conduct a trial of labour, blood transfusion facilities, anesthetic and pediatric facilities, continuous fetal monitoring and an operating theatre should be ideally available when required.

Scar rupture can present with clinical symptoms and signs of bleeding per vaginum, scar tenderness, continuous pain in the lower uterine segment, increased maternal pulse rate or abnormal fetal heart rate pattern. Acute fetal bradycardia of < 80 beats/min may indicate scar dehiscence and such bradycardia lasting > 10 min from whatever cause is likely to be associated with severe acidosis and hence needs immediate delivery ideally within 10–15 minutes of decision making (Ingemarsson et al 1985). Hence facilities should be available to perform a caesarean section within 15 minutes and the decision termed as 'immediate' rather than 'emergency' CS to indicate the urgency to the anesthetist and the operating theatre staff.

Counselling   The woman and her partner should be properly counselled regarding the benifits and risks of the trial of labour and how the trial will be performed.

Use of oxytocin

Clinicians are reluctant to use oxytocin to augment labour in women with a previous CS scar because of the fear of complete uterine rupture or partial rupture referred to as dehiscence. Hence a trial of labour may be abandoned prematurely in women with inadequate uterine contractions. However recent studies do not show an increased risk of rupture, or any change in maternal or perinatal outcome with the judicious use of oxytocin (Horenstein et al 1984; Clark 1988; Flamm et al 1987;

Horenstein and Phelan 1985; Arulkumaran et al 1989; Chua et al 1989; Flamm et al 1990).

Uterine activity profiles in women with a CS scar and abnormal labour have been described (Arulkumaran et al 1989). In 63 women with one previous CS who did not progress in labour due to poor uterine activity but with no clinical evidence of cephalopelvic disproportion, labour was augmented using syntocinon. Following augmentation, 78% delivered vaginally and 22% needed CS. The study showed that there was no difference in the frequency or amplitude of uterine contractions and uterine activity integral, between the vaginal delivery group and the caesarean section group prior to augmentation. After augmentation, the frequency, amplitude and uterine activity were significantly but similarly elevated in the two groups. The median uterine activity in these two groups were higher than in the women with previous CS who had normal progress of labour without oxytocic augmentation and vaginal delivery. The women who delivered vaginally dilated at a rate of 1.5 cm/hr whilst the women who finally had a CS dilated only at the rate of 0.3 cm/hr. All CS were for CPD and the mean birthweight of babies born by CS (3,598 g) was significantly heavier than that of babies born vaginally (3,230 g). Those with heavier babies had CPD and failed to progress despite adequate uterine activity for a sufficient length of time. Satisfactory cervical dilatation in the presence of optimum uterine activity for the next few hours after augmentation is an important factor in predicting the mode of delivery.

In a previous study, the same authors studied the characteristics and outcome of labour in 1,158 nulliparae and 1,360 multiparae who had no previous CS scar. Of these, 220 nulliparae and 99 multiparae had dysfunctional first stage of labour (Arulkumaran et al 1987). The majority, that is 65.5% of nulliparae and 83.3% of multiparae with dysfunctional labour responded with satisfactory progress within the first 4 hr of augmentation. The CS rate was low (1.3%) in this group who had satisfactory progress and the neonatal outcome was good. In nulliparae who did not show satisfactory progress in the first 3–4 hr with oxytocic augmentation the CS rate was 49% despite a 15 hr labour. In multiparae the CS rate in those who did not respond satisfactorily to augmentation was 66% despite 14 hr of labour.

Women with previous CS and dysfunctional labour can be subjected to judicious oxytocic augmentation. The rate of progress during the first 3–4 hr after augmentation appears to indicate the likely outcome and hence should help in the decision of whether to continue oxytocin. Scar rupture appears to be associated with prolonged infusion of oxytocin for 6 hr despite poor progress of labour (Arulkumaran et al 1992). Despite reports of scar dehiscence with the use of oxytocin, the benefits outweigh the risks, provided the patient is monitored appropriately.

Symptoms and signs of scar rupture

Many studies have shown that the classical symptoms and signs described with scar rupture like scar pain or tenderness, bleeding per vaginum, maternal tachycardia and hypotension are poor indicators of a rupture. They may be evident in various combinations, and may occur late, after a severe degree of rupture (Arulkumaran et al 1992; Leung et al 1993). Fetal distress manifested by prolonged, late or variable decelerations, acute bradycardia or prolonged variable deceleration with a rise in the baseline rate within a short time is not an uncommon finding with scar rupture (Leung et al 1993).

Beckley et al (1991) analysed ten cases of scar rupture in labour in a subsequent pregnancy after a previous lower segment CS. All the women were monitored with continuous electronic fetal heart rate recording and intrauterine pressure measurements. In four cases, recordings showed a marked fall in uterine activity because of clipping off of pressure peaks and these features occurred before fetal heart rate changes were identified. In another report of nine cases of scar rupture (Arulkumaran et al 1992), three cases showed abrupt reduction of uterine activity and one showed fetal bradycardia.

These findings suggest that continuous fetal heart rate monitoring and, where available, intrauterine pressure measurement may provide early signs of scar rupture, compared with other clinical symptoms and signs which may develop later with further loss of scar integrity (Arulkumaran et al 1992).

Monitoring of labour

Internal tocography is preferred to external tocography because sudden reduction of uterine pressure may be an early sign of scar rupture. Loosening of the belt or change in position of the woman may account for reduction in uterine activity when external tocography is used (Arulkumaran et al 1992). However intrauterine pressure monitoring should not be a substitute, nor an overriding factor in the overall clinical appraisal of the woman during a trial of labour. It should not in itself be regarded as a 'safeguard' against scar rupture, and the decision to continue labour, especially when augmentation of labour with oxytocin is necessary, should be based on the assesment of the progress of labour.

Epidural anesthesia

The place of epidural anesthesia in women with a previous CS remains unresolved. Epidural anesthesia is not used by some because of the fear that it may mask the clinical features of abdominal pain and tenderness when uterine rupture occurs (Gibbs 1977), and also because epidural anesthesia may result in sympathetic blockade or paralysis, which might delay the diagnosis of uterine rupture and even prevent adequate response to hemorrahge in the event of a catastrophic rupture. However it has been shown that pain and uterine tenderness are unreliable symptoms in predicting scar rupture (Case et al 1971; Arulkumaran et al 1992) and epidural anesthesia is unlikely to mask the visceral pain due to scar rupture. In a review of 20 caesarean sections done because of severe lower abdominal pain and tenderness thought to be indicative of scar rupture, a rupture was found only in 5% of the women (Case et al 1976). Regional anesthesia is relatively safe but the number of women with a prior CS in whom this technique has been used is small and future studies are warranted.

Postpartum examination of the uterine scar

Although some authors have recommended transcervical postpartum palpation of the uterine scar (Lawrence 1953; Case et al 1976; Merril and Gibbs 1977), there is a risk of inducing scar dehiscence at the time of examination and it is uncomfortable for the patient. Even if a small tear is detected the management is unlikely to change in the absence of bleeding. Palpation of the scar should be undertaken under general anesthesia if there is continuous bleeding in the third stage which may be due to a dehisced scar.

Vaginal ultrasound and magnetic resonance imaging have been used in the antenatal period to give accurate and objective information about the thickness and continuity of the lower uterine segment scar after previous CS. Their use has not been properly validated in clinical practice.

Medicolegal aspects

Clinicians are also reluctant to give a trial of labour because of the fear of medico-legal consequences in cases of scar rupture. It is important to (a) carefully select the women for a trial of labour; (b) explain clearly to both the woman and her husband the conduct of the trial of labour, its benefits and risks, and document the discussion; (c) conduct the labour in a fully equipped centre, preferably with continuous electronic fetal heart rate monitoring and where facilities permit intrauterine pressure monitoring; (d) have facilities and training for emergency intervention when required; and (e) to act promptly when the situation demands. Such attention to details in practice is safe and will not be considered medicallly negligent.

In properly selected cases, vaginal delivery is the best and safest form of obstetric management. The incidence of scar rupture in women with a previous lower segment CS scar is low and maternal and fetal morbidity are not severe when such trials of labour are appropriately managed. An overwhelming majority of consultants (97%) in the United Kingdom are in general agreement (Roberts et al 1994) with the recommendations of the Canadian policy statement that a trial of labour after a previous CS is recommended for women who meet the following criteria : one low transverse incision caesarean section, a singleton vertex presentation and no absolute indication for caesarean section in the present pregnancy (Panel and Planning Committee 1986). The National Institute of Health (NIH 1981) has also produced similar guidelines, although consultants in the United States are less aggressive in pursuing a vaginal delivery than their colleagues across the Atlantic. Based on the discussion in this chapter, attention to details should help many women with previous CS to deliver safely with minimal morbidity and/or mortality.

References

Arulkumaran S, Gibb DMF, TambyRaja RL, Heng SH, Ratnam SS 1985. Rising caesarean section rates in Singapore. *Sing J Obstet Gynecol* 16:1: 5-14.

Arulkumaran S, Koh CH, Ingemarsson I, Ratnam SS 1987. Augmentation of labour - mode of delivery related to cervimetric progress. *Aust NZ J Obstet Gynecol* 27: 304-8.

Arulkumaran S, Gibb DMF, Ingemarsson I, Kitchener HC, Ratnam SS 1989. Uterine activity during spontaneous labour after previous lower-segment caesarean section. *Br J Obstet Gynecol* 96:933-938.

Arulkumaran S, Imgemarsson I, Ratnam SS 1989. Oxytocin augmentation in dysfunctional labour after previous caesarean section. *Br J Obstet Gynecol* 96:939-941.

Arulkumaran S, Chua S, Ratnam SS 1992. Symptoms and signs with scar rupture - value of uterine activity measurements. *Aust NZ J Obstet Gynecol* 32(3):208-212.

Beall Marie, Eglinton Garry S, Clark Steven L, Phelan Jeffrey P 1984. Vaginal delivery after caesarean section in women with unknown types of uterine scar. *J Reprod Med*, 29:1:31-35.

Benedetti TJ, Platt LD, Druzin M 1982. Vaginal delivery after previous caesarean section for a non-recurrent cause. *Am J Obstet Gynecol* 112:358.

Birnbaum S 1956. Post caesarean obstetrics management of subsequent pregnancy *Obstet Gynecol* 7:611.

Bolaji II, Meehan FP 1993. Post CS Delivery. *Eur J Obstet Gynecol* 51:181-192.

Beckley S, Gee H, Newton JR 1991. Scar rupture in labour after previous lower uterine segment caesarean section: the role of uterine activity measurement. *Br J Obstet Gynecol* 98:265-269.

Caesarean childbirth: report of the NICHD Task force on caesarean childbirth Bethesda Maryland : National Institutes of Health 1981, DHHS publication no NIH 351-74

Case B, Corcoran R, Jeffcoate N, Randle GH 1971. Caesarean section and its place in modern obstetric practice. *J Obstet Gynaecol Br Cwlth* 78:203.

Chalmers I 1985. Trends and variations in the use of caesarean section. In: Clineh J, Mathews T, eds. Perinatal Medicine. Lancaster: MTP Press, pp 145-149

Chattopadhyay SK, Sherbeeni MM, Anokute CC 1994. Planned vaginal delivery after 2 previous caesarean sections. *Br J Obstet Gynecol* 101:498-500.

Chua S, Arulkumaran S, Piara Singh, Ratnam SS 1989. Trial of labour after previous caesarean section : Obstetric outcome. *Aust NZ J Obstet Gynecol* 29:12-17.

Clark Steven L, Eglinton Gary S, Beall Mary, Phelan Jeffrey P 1984. Effect of indication for previous caesarean section on subsequent delivery outcome in patients undergoing a trial of labor. *J Reprod Med* 29:1:22-25.

Clark SL 1988. Rupture of scarred uterus. In *Obstet Gynecol Clin N Am* 15:737-744.

Craigin EB 1916. Conservatism in Obstetrics *NY Med J* 104:1.

Crawford J S 1976. Letter. *Lancet* 1:1304.

Demianczuk Nestor N, Hunter David JS, Taylor D Wayne 1982. Trial of labor after previous caesarean section: Prognostic indicators of outcome. *Am J Obstet Gynecol* 142:640-2

Dewhurst CL 1957. The ruptured caesarean section scar. *J Obstet Gynaecol Br Cwlth* 64:113-8.

Douglas R, Birnbaum S, MacDonald F 1963. Pregnancy and labour following caesarean section. *Am J Obstet Gynecol* 986-961.

Evrard J, Gold E 1977. Caesarean section and maternal mortality in Rhode Island; incidence and risk factors 1965-1975. *Obstet Gynecol* 50:594.

Flamm B, Goings J, Fulbright N-J et al 1987. Oxytocin during labour after previous CS. Results of a multicentre study. *Obstet Gynecol* 70:709-712.

Flamm BL, Naoman LA, Thomas SJ, Fallon D, Yoshida MM 1990. Vaginal birth after caesarean delivery : results of a 5 year multicenter collaborative study. *Obstet Gynecol*, 76:750-753.

Francome C, Savage W 1993. CS in Britain and the United States. *Soc Sci Med* 37:1199-1218.

Gibbs C 1980. Planned vaginal delivery following caesarean section. *Clin Obstet Gynecol* 23:507-515.

Golan A, Sandbank O, Rubin A 1980. Rupture of the pregnant uterus. *Obstet Gynecol* 56:549-559.

Hebisch G, Kerkinen P, Haldemann R, Pakkoo E, Hiech A, Huch R 1994. Comparative study of lower uterine segment after caesarean section using ultrasound and magnetic resonance tomography. (German trans). *Ultraschall Med* 15(3): 112-6.

Holland E 1921. Uterine scar rupture. *J Obstet Gynaecol Br Cwlth* 28:475-87.

Horenstein Janet M, Eglinton S Garry, Thilramaney Mona P, Boucher Marc, Phelan Jeffrey P 1984. Oxcytocin use during a trial of labor in patients with previous caesarean section. *J Reprod Med* 29:1:26-30.

Horenstein JM, Phelan JP 1985. Previous CS - Risks and benefits of oxytocin usage in trial of labour. *Am J Obstet Gynecol* 151:564-9.

Ingmarsson I, Arulkumaran S, Ratnam SS 1985. Bolus injection of terbutaline in labor. Effect on fetal pH in cases with prolonged bradycardia. *Am J Obstet Gynecol* 153:859-865.

Lawerence R 1953. Vaginal delivery after caesarean section. *J Obstet Gynecol Br Emp* 60:237.

Lavin JP, Stephens RS, Miodovnik M, Barden TP 1982. Vaginal delivery in patients with a prior caesarean section. *Obstet Gynecol* 59:135-47.

Leung AS, Leung EK, Paul RH 1993. Uterine rupture after previous caesarean delivery: Maternal and fetal consequences. *Am J Obstet Gynecol* 169:945-50.

Meehan F, Moolgaoker A, Stallworthy J 1972. Vaginal delivery under coudal analgaesia after caesarean section and other major uterine surgery, *Br Med J* 2:740.

Meier PR, Porreco RP 1982. Trial of labor following caesarean section : A two year experience. *Am J Obstet Gynecol* 144:671-678.

Merrill B, Gibbs C 1977. Planned vaginal delivery following caesarean section. *Obstet Gynecol*, 52:50.

Miller M, Leader R 1992. Vaginal delvery after caesarean section. *Aust NZ J Obstet Gynecol* 32:213-216.

Molloy B, Shell O, Duignan NB, Deluy 1987. Caesarean section: review of 2,176 consecutive cases. *Br Med J* 294:1645-1647.

Morewood GA, O'Sullivan MJ, McConney J 1973. Vaginal delivery after caesarean section. *Obstet Gynecol* 42:589-95.

Muller PF, Heise W, Grahanm W 1961. Repeat caesarean section. *Am J Obstet Gynecol* 867-876.

Nielsen TF, Hokegard K-H, Moldin PG 1985. X-ray pelvimetry and trial of labor after previous cesarean section. *Acta Obstet Gynecol Scand* 64:485-90.

Nielsen TF, Ljungblad Ulf, Hagberg H 1989. Rupture and dehiscence of caesarean section scar during pregnancy and delivery. *Am J Obstet Gynecol* 160:569-73

NIH Consensus Development Task Force 1981. NIH Consensus Development Task Force statement on cesarean childbirth. *Am J Obstet Gynecol* 139:902-9.

Notzon FC, Cnattingius S, Bergsjo P, Cole S, Taffel S, Irgens L, Daltveit AK 1994. Caesarean section delivery in the 1980s: International comparison by indication. *Am J Obstet Gynaecol* 170:495-504.

O'Driscoll K, Foley M 1983. Correlation of decrease in perinatal mortality and increase in caesarean section rates. *Obstet Gynecol* 61:1.

Panel and Planning Committee of the National Consensus Conference on aspects of caesarean birth 1986. Indications for caesarean section: final statements of the panels of the National Consensus Conference on aspects of caesarean birth. *Can Med Assoc J* 134:1348-52.

Pedowitz B, Schwartz RM 1987. The true incidence of silent rupture of caesarean section scar. A prospective analysis of 403 cases. *Am J Obstet Gynecol* 74:1071-1081.

Phelan JP, Eglinton GS, Horenstein JM, Clark SL, Yeoh SY 1984. Previous caesarean birth. Trial of labor in women with macrosomic infants. *J Reprod Med* 29:36-44

Phelan JP, Clark SL, Diaz F, Paul RH 1987. Vaginal birth after caesarean section *Am J Obstet Gynecol* 157:1510-1515.

Porreco RP, Meier PR 1983. Trial of labour in patients with multiple caesarean section. *J Reprod Med* 28:770-772.

Ritchie JWK 1986. Obstetric operations and procedures. In: Dewhurst's Textbook of Obstetrics and Gynaecology for Postgraduates 4th ed. Blackwell Scientific Publications, pp 428-441.

Riva H, Teich J 1961. Vaginal delivery after caesarean section. *Am J Obstet Gynecol* 81:501.

Roberts LJ, Beardsworth SA, Trew G 1994. Labour following caesarean section : current practice in the United Kingdom. *Br J Obstet Gynecol* 101:153-5.

Saldana L, Schulman H, Reuss L 1979. Management of pregnancy after caesarean section. *Am J Obstet Gynecol*, 135:555.

Salzmann B 1964. Rupture of lower segment caesarean section scars. *Obstet Gynecol*, 23:460.

Schrinsky DL, Benson RL 1978. Rupture of the pregnant uterus. A Review. *Obstet Gynecol Surv* 33:217.

Seitchik J, Rao VRR 1982. Caesarean delivery in nulliparous women for failed oxytocin augmented labour. Route of delivery in subsequent pregnancy. *Am J Obstet Gynecol* 143:393.

Steer PJ, Carter ML, Beard RW 1984. Normal levels of active contraction area in spontaneous labour. *Br J Obstet Gynecol* 91:211-219.

Tahilramaney Mona P, Boucher Marc, Eglinton Garry S 1984. Beall Marie, Phelan Jeffrey P. Previous caesarean section and trial of labor; factors related to uterine dehiscence. *J Reprod Med* 29:1:17-21.

Thubisi M, Ebrahim A, Moodug J, Shweni PM 1993. Vaginal delivery after previous CS. Is pelvimetry necessary? *Br J Obstet Gynecol* 100:421-424.

Wilson A 1951. *Am J Obstet Gynecol* 62:1225-1233.

21

Rupture of the Uterus

K Bhasker Rao

Rupture of the uterus is one of the gravest emergencies in obstetrics. The hospital incidence of rupture of the uterus in developing countries varies from 1 in 100 to 1 in 500 deliveries (Table 1). Most of these cases are brought in late from outside the hospital.

Etiopathology

In India, spontaneous rupture of the uterus is the commonest (68.1%), followed by scar dehiscence (21.4%) and traumatic (10.5%) (Dhar 1989).

The contributory causes of spontaneous rupture are the same as those for obstructed labour: CPD, malpresentations and hydrocephalus. Rarely, there is a history of previous curettage or manual removal of the placenta. Oxytocin augmentation of labour should always be done under supervision with a controlled IV drip and tocographic monitoring to avoid hyperstimulation and rupture. Traumatic rupture is often due to intrauterine manipulations in late labour or extraction through an incompletely dilated cervix. Rarely, it may follow destructive operations.

The commonest site of complete rupture is the anterior lower uterine segment, and often occurs as as a transverse rent. In about 15%, it may be incomplete involving the lateral wall and with a broad ligament hematoma. Rarely the rupture is at the uterovaginal fornix (colporrhexis). The rupture may extend to the bladder in 5–10% of cases (Rao 1992).

Clinical picture

In a typical case, there is evidence of hemorrhagic shock. Examination shows the abdomen to be tender and shows loss of uterine contour. Fetal parts are felt superficially and the fetal heart is absent. On vaginal examination, there is evidence of obstructed labour with a large caput over the presenting part or if the presenting part has receded, there is some vaginal bleeding.

However in early cases of rupture of the uterus the general condition may be surprisingly good. In rupture of the lateral wall, the diagnosis may be missed as the fetus is still in utero but maternal tachycardia, absent fetal heart sounds and vaginal bleeding with a markedly tender lower abdomen should arouse a suspicion.

Prognosis

The maternal mortality in rupture of the uterus is about 5–15% (Table 1) depending on the cause and site of rupture, the interval between rupture and surgery, availability of adequate blood, associated sepsis and the type of operation done. It is worse in traumatic and incomplete varieties due to delayed diagnosis.

Table 1:   Rupture of the Uterus in labour in developing countries — incidence
and prognosis

Country, Author and Year	No. of cases	Inci- dence	MMR (%)	PMR (%)
Srinagar, India (Dhar 1989)	152	1:490	9.0	82.0
Baroda, India (Mody et al 1991)	73	1:234	4.1	42.5
Nigeria (Harrison 1985)	203	1:112	8.4	—
Nigeria (Ezem et al 1983)	123	1:148	14.6	82.9
Turkey (Kafkas and Taner 1990)	41	1:96	7.3	83.0

MMR — Maternal Mortality Rate;   PMR — Perinatal Mortality Rate

Treatment

Good prenatal and intranatal care prevents obstructed labour and uterine rupture.
Traumatic rupture can be eliminated by avoiding intrauterine manipulations in late
labour and by not extracting the fetus through an incompletely dilated cervix. The
scar dehiscence is rare (less than 1%) in labour following lower segment caesarean
section and can be suspected early by clinical and cardiotocographic monitoring.

Once a diagnosis of rupture of the uterus is made (or even suspected) no
attempt should be made at vaginal delivery. Immediate steps should be taken to
resuscitate the patient with IV fluids and blood transfusion followed by a laparotomy. After removal of fetus, placenta, blood and clots the uterine rent is identified.
If it is a clean-cut rent in the lower segment, repair with sterilisation is carried out.
If the mother has no living child, sterilisation may be deferred so that in next
pregnancy elective caesarean with sterilisation can be done. A quick subtotal hysterectomy may be preferred in cases where the rent is irregular, friable and in
lateral tears or if the uterus is infected. In colporrhexis, total hysterectomy may be
easier to perform. If the bladder is involved in the rupture, it is carefully closed
in two layers and continuously drained for 12 days.

Postoperatively all cases of rupture of the uterus following obstructed labour
will require broad spectrum antibiotics to control infection, and bladder drainage
to prevent obstetric fistula.

References

Dhar G 1989. Rupture of the uterus. In: Rao KB, ed. Postgraduate Obstetrics and Gynecology, 4th edn. Madras: Orient Longman, pp192-197.

Ezem BV, Otabum JA, Barnes B 1983. Rupture of the pregnant uterus. *Asia Oceania J Obstet Gynecol* 9: 163-167.

Harrison K A 1985. Mode of delivery with noteson rupture uterus and vesicovaginal fistula. *Br J Obstet Gynecol* 95 (Suppl 6); 41-71.

Kafkas S, Taner C E 1990. Rupture uterus. *Int J Gynecol Obstet* 34: 41-44.

Mody, H R, Pagi, S I, Gohil, J T, Patel B C 1991. Rupture uterus, 5 years review. *J Obstet Gynecol India* 41: 56-58.

22

Management of Eclampsia

S Arulkumaran
S S Ratnam

Hypertension occurs in 6 to 8% of women, making it the most common high risk complication in pregnancy. A great part of the resources in the antenatal clinics are spent in the identification and surveillance of suspected and established cases of hypertension in pregnancy. Hypertensive disease contributes significantly to intrauterine growth retardation and iatrogenic prematurity leading to fetal, neonatal and infant deaths. Preeclampsia and eclampsia are also major contributors to maternal deaths both in developing countries and developed countries like Sweden (Hogberg 1986), England and Wales (HMSO 1989), and the USA (Kaunitz et al 1985). Despite such statistics there are centres where no maternal deaths have been attributed to eclampsia or its associated complications over the last two decades due to good antenatal screening, early and appropriate treatment of hypertension and good management of severe preeclampsia and impending eclampsia. In most institutions such cases are managed in the labour ward which has better facilities for intensive care, and because of the intent of early delivery.

Maternal mortality and morbidity due to eclampsia can be brought to a minimum by
  a. predicting and preventing or reducing the incidence of preeclampsia
  b. aggressively managing all the cases of severe preeclampsia and impending eclampsia
  c. appropriate management of eclampsia and the ensuing complications.

Table 1:   Risk factors in eclampsia and their identification

A. Risk Factors	B. Tests available	C. Drugs
history of hypertension renal disease SLE past history of pregnancy induced hypertension strong family history of hypertension diabetes multiple pregnancy in current pregnancy	roll over test angiotensin sensitivity studies uterine arcuate arterial blood flow velocity waveform by 20 to 24 weeks angiotensin II receptors in platelets in early pregnancy absence of the drop in blood pressure in the second trimester of pregnancy.	low dose aspirin as little as 75 mg per day magnesium and calcium supplementation reported to be effective.

Averting eclampsia

It is possible to avert eclampsia by prophylactic treatment of the susceptible groups based on the known risk factors either from the history, present obstetric condition or by screening the low risk population through various tests to identify those who are likely to develop hypertension and by treating them (Montan and Arulkumaran 1994). These are summarised in Table 1.

Control of severe preeclampsia/impending eclampsia

Control of severe preeclampsia and impending eclampsia can abort an attack of eclampsia and hinges essentially on the appropriate and adequate use of anticonvulsant and antihypertensive therapy.

Symptoms and signs of impending eclampsia

Identifying symptoms and signs of impending eclampsia will be present in nearly 80 per cent of those at risk and are shown in work done by Sibai et al (1981), given below:

SYMPTOMS	PATIENTS IN WHOM PRESENT (%)
Headache	83
Hyper-reflexia	80
Proteinuria	80
Edema	60
Clonus	46
Visual signs	45
Epigastric pain	20

Management

Management of eclampsia can be considered under the following four subsections:
  a. general management
  b. drugs for control of convulsions (including appropriate antidotes)
  c. antihypertensive therapy
  d. specific obstetric management, for example, delivery of the fetus

Facilities necessary for proper management   Although ideally any of the rooms in the labour ward should be suitable and equipped to manage a patient with eclampsia, it is expensive to have all the necessary equipment in every room. When the funds are limited at least one room should have such facilities. The room should not have bright lights that might dazzle the eyes of the patient but should be adequately lit so that cyanosis, which may be the earliest sign of cardiac failure in these patients is not missed. Undue sound stimulation that may precipitate an eclamptic fit should be avoided. The patient is ideally nursed in a bed with facilities to tilt the head down. Suction apparatus should be handy by the bed side to suck out secretions which otherwise might lead to aspiration and its consequences. The patient might develop respiratory arrest with the anticonvulsant therapy, or develop problems with breathing due to laryngeal edema and heavy sedation, or develop status eclampticus with repeated convulsions despite maximal anticonvulsive therapy. In these circumstances the only lifesaving measure is endotracheal intubation and ventilation. Facilities should be available to carry out the procedure or at least to initiate it when the emergency arises and then to transfer the patient to an intensive care bed. In severely ill patients continuous arterial pressure monitoring and ECG monitoring facilities will be useful.

Preventing asphyxia and injury as a first step   The mouth should be kept open by a soft gag. This prevents injury to the tongue by the teeth, and helps to remove dentures and false teeth. The secretions can be sucked out effectively and a suitable airway can be placed to prevent the tongue from falling back and obstructing the oropharynx. Patients should be nursed in the left lateral position with the head low to reduce the risk of aspirating secretions. Along with these general measures, specific anticonvulsive and antihypertensive therapy should be commenced to control the convulsions, to prevent recurrence and to avoid complications of the severe hypertensive process.

Anticonvulsive therapy

Magnesium sulphate   Magnesium sulphate has been a popular drug for many decades. The dosage proposed by Pritchard (1975) has stood the test of time. The immediate dose consists of 4 g intravenously as a 20 ml 20% solution administered over 3–5 mins, followed by 10 g as 10 ml of 50% solution given deep intramuscularly into each buttock. The follow up dose is 5 g as 5 ml of 50% solution every 4 hr alternately in each buttock. Care must be taken not to administer this intermittent dose if knee jerks are absent or if the respiratory rate is less than 16 per min or the urine output less than 25 ml per hr. Lower volumes can be given to Asian women with lesser body and gluteal mass.

Magnesium sulphate can also be administered totally as an intravenous regime as described by Zuspan (1966). The priming dose is as in the earlier regime of 3–4 g (20 ml of 20% solution administered over 3 to 5 min), followed by an infusion of 1 g every hr. The umbilical cord magnesium levels are higher with the infusion regime (Lipsitz 1971) but are not high enough to cause problems to the neonate.

Magnesium sulphate is an effective cerebral depressant and hence reduces neuromuscular irritability. The blood levels needed for depression of various functions vary, and the patellar reflex is abolished long before the drug can cause respiratory depression. Based on this principle it is best to test the patellar reflex before each intramuscular injection, and to test the reflex every hour when the patient is on an intravenous regime. Since the mode of excretion of the drug is via the kidneys, a urinary output of greater than 25 ml per hr should be maintained when the patient is on therapy. If the urinary output is poor, the blood levels of magnesium have to be checked, the dosage adjusted accordingly and the problem of early renal failure corrected. In case of overdosage with magnesium, 10 ml of 10% calcium gluconate should be given intravenously over a period of 3 min as an antidote.

Table 2 gives the effects associated with various serum magnesium levels to illustrate the margin of safety with this drug.

Table 2:   Effects associated with various serum magnesium levels

Effect	Serum Level mEq/Litre
anticonvulsant prophylaxis	4 – 6
EKG changes	5 – 10
loss of deep tendon reflexes	10
respiratory paralysis	15
general anesthesia	15
cardiac arrest	> 25

Magnesium sulphate and the newborn   Magnesium sulphate crosses the placenta freely but there is little evidence of toxicity to the newborn, provided maternal safe limits are observed.

The safety and efficacy of intravenous magnesium sulphate therapy has been well documented (Sibai et al 1981) (Table 3).

Table 3:   Efficacy of magnesium sulphate therapy in eclampsia

	n	%
treated	1870	
seizures	11	0.6
seizures morbidity	1	0.05
treatment morbidity	0	0

Benzodiazepines   The use of lytic cocktail constituting multiple drug regimes has become historical after the introduction of benzodiazepines in the 1960s by Lean et al (1968). To control convulsions 100 mg of chlordiazepoxide or 10 to 40 mg of diazepam was used intravenously. The subsequent maintenance was by titrating 100 mg chlordiazepoxide in 500 cc 5% dextrose saline. Of 90 eclamptics admitted during the study period, there were three deaths, two of whom died on admission due to cerebral hemorrhage. The perinatal mortality was 11%, and all babies weighing more than 1,360 g survived.

Diazepam

Immediate therapy   For women with eclampsia and impending eclampsia, 10 mg diazepam is given intravenously over 1 to 2 min. The dose is repeated every 5 min if necessary till the patient is well sedated and can be aroused only with difficulty. The total dose used with the confidence that no respiratory depression would occur was 40 mg for any one episode.

Maintenance therapy with diazepam   Although chlordiazepoxide 100 mg in 500 cc of saline titrated to achieve the desired state of sedation was the mainstay of treatment, the non-availability of chlordiazepoxide and the familiarity of diazepam has made maintenance with a diazepam infusion an acceptable regime. A total of 40 mg of diazepam in 500 cc saline can be titrated to keep the patient well

sedated and drowsy but arousable. To prevent recurrent convulsions the maintenance regime is continued for 24 hours after the last convulsion or after delivery
whichever was the last event. For the next 24 hours 20 mg diazepam in 500 cc
saline can be titrated to prevent withdrawal effects or recurrence of symptoms like
restlessness and convulsions (Arulkumaran and Ratnam 1985).

Complications

The dose of diazepam required to prevent convulsions can sedate the patient heavily
and at times cause depression of the central nervous system especially that of
respiration. The cough reflex may also be suppressed leading to the risk of aspiration and pneumonia. Nursing the patient in the 'recovery' position should minimise this risk. Complications can be avoided by not injecting the bolus dose of
the drug too rapidly (can cause apnoea) and by avoiding build up of the drug by
cumulative doses or prolonged therapy when the drug is not needed. Accidental
overdose by a repeated large bolus dose or too rapid infusion while titrating should
be kept in mind.

Respiratory depression   If respiratory depression evidenced by irregular or la-
boured breathing is encountered or if cyanosis is noted, the infusion should be
stopped. Attention should be given to maintaining a clear airway, and if necessary
oxygen should be administered by a mask.

Nursing the patient in the recovery position will help to avoid the tongue
falling back and obstructing breathing. If the respiration does not normalise 5 to
10 min after this therapy and especially if cyanosis is present, after excluding cardiac
failure an antidote for diazepam should be administered.

Respiratory arrest   If respiratory arrest occurs during treatment with diazepam,
the infusion should be stopped and the patient intubated and ventilated. Positive
pressure ventilation should continue till spontaneous regular respiration resumes.
The process can be enhanced by giving the antidote specific for diazepam.

Flumazenil as a specific antidote for diazepam   Flumazenil 0.2 mg in 2 ml
solution should be given intravenously over 15 sec (Chua and Arulkumaran 1995).
If the desired level of consciousness is not obtained in 45 sec, a further 0.2 mg
dose can be given every 60 sec up to a maximum total dose of 1 mg, that is,
5 doses over a period of 5 min. If the desired effect is still not obtained or if
resedation occurs after recovery then flumazenil can be repeated in 20 min, up to
another dose of 1 mg but at 0.2 mg increments every minute. The total dose of
this drug that can be administered with safety is 3 mg for any one hour. Since the
antidote itself will have some effect on the drugs used by the pediatrician and the
anesthetist, they should be warned.

Diazepam/Phenytoin regime

Diazepam can be used in bolus doses of 5 mg till convulsions stop and the therapy
then maintained by using phenytoin. A loading dose of 1 mg/kg phenytoin should
be given followed by 5 mg/kg two hours later. Oral phenytoin, 200 mg, can be
given 12 hours later and the dosage continued every 12 hours for a period of 48
hours after delivery to prevent recurrence of convulsions. This regime has less

sedative effect compared with the diazepam maintenance regime. However the efficacy of this regime has to be tested in large trials.

Benzodiazepines have stood the test of time as a useful agent in the management of impending eclampsia and eclampsia. In our institution, we had 26,173 deliveries over the last seven years (1986 – 1992). The incidence of hypertensive disease during this period was 5.9% and the incidence of eclampsia was 0.05% (n=13), almost all these cases were unbooked. There were no maternal deaths or morbidity related to eclampsia (Ratnam and Arulkumaran 1995).

In an attempt to answer the question which of the three anticonvulsants (magnesium sulphate, diazepam or phenytoin) was useful in the management of eclampsia, a large multicentric randomised trial of 1,680 cases was recently undertaken by the Eclampsia Trial Collaborative Group (1995). It was found that women allocated to magnesium sulphate had 56% lower risk of recurrent convulsions than those allocated to diazepam; and women in the magnesium sulphate group had a 67% lower risk of recurrent convulsions than those allocated to the phenytoin. No significant difference in the maternal or perinatal mortality or morbidity was seen in the three different groups. The study concluded that 'there is now compelling evidence in favour of magnesium sulphate rather than diazepam or phenytoin in the treatment of eclampsia'.

Maternal mortality and eclampsia

Although eclampsia is a dramatic event to the onlooker, maternal mortality is essentially due to a cerebrovascular accident and other cerebral lesions. This is illustrated by Tables 4 and 5.

Antihypertensives

Because of the great risk of cerebrovascular accidents antihypertensive therapy is the mainstay in reducing maternal mortality. The vasoconstriction of severe preeclampsia does not respond well to methyldopa, clonidine, debrisoquine or guanethidine, which are effective in mild to moderate preeclampsia. Hydralazine, diazoxide and its derivatives which paralyse the arterial smooth muscle by direct action are more appropriate.

Hydralazine   Immediate reduction of blood pressure is desired if the systolic blood pressure is > 170 mmHg and the diastolic blood pressure > 110 mmHg. Hydralazine can be given as 2 mg intravenous bolus injections or as 5 mg intramuscular injections and repeated every 15–30 min. For maintenance therapy 100 mg hydralazine in 500 cc saline can be titrated to get the desired effect. Usually the drip is titrated by escalating the drip rate by 10 drops (0.1 mg/min) every 5 min till the diastolic blood pressure is < 110 mmHg and the systolic blood pressure is < 170 mmHg. The patient should be monitored carefully with an intensive care chart which records the blood pressure, pulse rate, respiratory rate and the fluid input and output. Some patients are hypersensitive to hydralazine and may act dramatically by a sudden steep drop in blood pressure. This can affect the fetus if it is growth retarded and recording of the fetal heart rate will indirectly give a forewarning of when the blood pressure falls drastically. If the desired control of blood pressure is not seen within a short time, intermittent bolus doses of the drug

Table 4:   Maternal mortality in the UK (1985–1987)

	n	%
pulmonary embolism	29	20.9
hypertensive disorders	27	19.4
ectopic pregnancy	16	11.5
antepartum and postpartum hemorrhage	10	7.2
amniotic fluid embolism	9	6.5

Table 5:   Causes of maternal deaths from hypertensive disease
(England and Wales, 1973–84: UK 1985–87)

Cause of death	1973-75		1976-78		1979-81		1982-84		1985-87	
	n	%	n	%	n	%	n	%	n	%
Cerebral hemorrhage	17	44	17	59	9	25	13	52	11	41
Other CNS pathology	6	15	4	14	8	22	8	32	11	41
Hepatic pathology	4		1		8		1		1	
Pulmonary pathology	1		1		2		3		12	

(Source : DHSS 1979, 1982, 1986 and DHA 1989, 1991)

can be used in addition to the titration. Once the blood pressure is controlled and stable for over 4 hr, the infusion rate can be reduced gradually at a rate of 10 drops every 30 min and finally the infusion tailed off.

Other preferred drugs used for hypertensive emergencies are given in Table 6. It gives the onset of action, the time taken for maximal action and the duration of action. The dosage, the interval between doses and the mechanism of action is also given.

Labetalol   Labetalol has also been tried out in these situations in recent times. A dose of 200 mg labetalol can reduce the blood pressure by 10 to 20 mmHg in 60 min. A further dose of 200 mg labetalol can be given when required. The drug can also be given intravenously as a slow 50 mg dose, followed by 300 mg in 60 ml (5 mg/ml) by syringe pump. The titration can be started at 12 ml per hour and increased up to 48 ml per hour till the desired effect is achieved.

Obstetric management of eclampsia

There is always a debate about the obstetric management in a patient with eclampsia: whether to conserve the pregnancy or to terminate it and, if the pregnancy is to be terminated, whether should it be by induction or by caesarean section. In addition the hydration and nutrition of the patient have to be carefully balanced

Table 6:   Different drugs used in the treatment of hypertensive emergencies

| Drug | Time | | | Dosage | | | Mechan-ism of action |
	Onset	Maxi-mum	Dura-tion	IM	IV	Interval between doses	
Hydralazine	10–20 min	20–40 min	3–8 hr	10–50 mg	5–25 mg	3–6 hr	Direct dilatation of arterioles
Diazoxide	1–2 min	2–3 min	4–12 hr	—	50–300 mg	3–10 hr	Direct dilatation of arterioles
Sodium nitroprusside	1/2–2 min	1–2 min	3–5 min	—	IV solution 0.01 g/L Infusion rate 0.2–0.8 mg/min	----	Direct dilatation of arterioles and veins
Trimethaphan camsylate	1–2 min	2–5 min	10 min	—	IV solution 2 g/L Infusion rate 1–15 mg/min	----	Ganglionic blockade

during the time of crisis. The answers to these can be derived by looking at Tables 7 and 8 which illustrate the maternal and perinatal mortality in relation to the first convulsion to delivery interval.

Delivery and resolution of the PE process

Based on Tables 7 and 8 there is no doubt that earlier the delivery is undertaken, the better it is for the mother and the fetus. The delivery will also result in the resolution of the PE process and hence is of great advantage to the mother. This may not however be optimal for the fetus, depending on its maturity and whether it has already been compromised by the process of preeclampsia. If the fetus is older than 34 weeks and is mature and alive, then caesarean section gives it the best chance if the patient is not in labour and if the contemplated induction delivery interval is going to be long. If the fetus is immature or dead, the feasibility of

Table 7: Convulsion–delivery interval and matenal mortality in eclampsia

First convulsion to delivery (hr)	Maternal mortality (%)
0 -- 2	7
2 – 4	13
4 – 8	19
8 – 12	22
12 – 18	25
18 -- 24	32
> 24	42
887 cases	17

(*Source* : Menon 1961)

Table 8: Convulsion–delivery interval and perinatal mortality in eclampsia

First convulsion to delivery (hr)	Perinatal mortality (%)
< 6	14
6 -- 12	19
12 -- 24	62
> 24	53
88 cases	33

(*Source* : Lopez–Llera 1967)

induction and vaginal delivery should be sought; however if the induction fails, early resort to caesarean section will help to arrest the preeclamptic process.

Eclampsia and its associated complications

Severe preeclampsia and eclampsia are known to be associated with a number of complications. Most of them are due to the hypertensive process and may occur even without eclampsia. But the management becomes difficult when eclampsia occurs at the same time. The known complications are listed below:

a. fatal cerebaral hemorrhage
b. left ventricular failure
c. status eclampticus
d. respiratory failure
e. aspiration with convulsions
f. rupture of the liver
g. abruptio placentae
h. renal impairment
i. DIVC/HELLP syndrome
j. hyperpyrexia

The limited space here permits only discussion of the management of some of these complications.

Abruptio placentae

Due to heavy sedation or coma, the pain of abruption and the sign of tenderness elicited at the time of examination might be masked. Additional signs should be sighted, like uterine irritability, disappearance of the fetal heart rate, bleeding per vaginum and restlessness of the patient. Tense uterus, hypotension and decreased urinary output are some of the other signs that may be observed. Pre-eclamptic patients do not tolerate hypotension well and it is important to replace the blood volume quickly, preferably with blood, failing which, with colloids. If the blood pressure has to be corrected with crystalloids it takes about four times the volume transfused compared with the colloids. Central venous pressure monitoring is useful in preventing overtransfusion and causing cardiac-failure. The problem of disseminated intravascular coagulation can be avoided by expediting the delivery. DIVC should be anticipated and managed if it sets in.

Artificial rupture of the membranes releases the tension within the uterus thereby reducing the chance of extrinsic tissue thromboplastin being forced into the maternal circulation from within the uterus. Frank bleeding seen without clots, or the failure of the blood to clot by the bedside would be late signs. If the problem of bleeding is to be tackled early laboratory tests are useful. Although it is known that the fibrin degradation products in DIVC inhibits clotting and gives rise to bleeding, and fibrinogen is not advised in a patient with DIVC (adding fuel to the fire), more often than not the patient bleeds due to the consumption of the essential clotting factors including fibrinogen, leaving behind blood in the circulation which does not have sufficient factors to clot. This phenomenon where the clotting factors are below the critical levels is also referred to as the 'washout phenomenon'. Appropriate therapy in these situations can be instituted by having a hemotherapy chart (Arulkumaran and Ratnam 1988). The hemotherapy chart records the Hb, platelets, fibrinogen level, pt, ptt, and fibrinogen degradation products. A typical chart from a patient is given below. The blood can be observed to clot as long as the fibrinogen level was over 1 g. The moment it droped below that level the blood was not clotting. This can also be attributed to the raised fibrin degradation product level (> 320 mg/L). However replacement with fresh frozen plasma and cryoprecipitate elevated the fibrinogen and other clotting factor levels and the blood started clotting despite the raised levels of fibrin degradation products.

Cardiac failure

Cardiac failure is at times missed when it is associated with eclampsia. This is because of the difficulty in recognising the signs of cyanosis, breathlessness and difficulty in breathing due to cardiac failure from symptoms and signs due to the eclamptic process itself or that caused by the drugs used to control convulsions. The cyanosis should not be missed and nursing these patients in semi-darkness should be avoided. The pulmonary edema might be due to unrelieved hypertension. The eclamptic process and the exhaustion that follows and the poor fluid and electrolyte balance can contribute to the cardiac failure. Govan (1966) described specific myocardiac lesions in these patients in cardiac failure, but to what degree it is contributory is debatable. Therapy is by propping up the patient properly. The convulsions must be controlled and 40–60 mg frusemide given as a diuretic at 2–4 hourly intervals. The value of digoxin in these patients is debated. Oxygen inhalation by mask or nasal tube will help.

Renal failure

Renal failure should be diagnosed when there is oliguria of < 20 ml per hour. Increasing azotemia would be another sign. Renal failure can be due to a pre-renal

HEMOTHERAPY CHART
24.04.86

Time	Hb (gms/dl)	Plate-lets (10⁹/ml)	PT	PTT (sec)	Throm-bin time (sec)	Fibri-nogen (g/L)	FDP (mg/L)	Hemo-therapy
12.20	13.2	305	1.0	33	14	2.75	> 32	—
14.00	12.2	250	1.0	37	14	2.00	80–110	5 units of blood
16.10	10.1	209	1.2	40	14	1.53	160–320	—
18.45	9.2	127	1.6	52	23	0.85	> 320	—
				Blood not clotting				15 packs cryoprecip-itate +4 packs group specific fresh frozen plasma

25.04.86

Time	Hb	Platelets	PT	PTT	Thrombin	Fibrinogen	FDP	Hemotherapy
00.45	9.5	70	1.4	40	20	1.1	> 320	5 units of blood
				Bed side clotting 4 min				
01.45	Delivered a fresh stillbirth — no fresh bleeding. 2.5 L of clots and old blood evacuated from uterus							
02.00	9.0	70	1.4	40	20	0.93	40–80	—

cause if the patient had an abruption and hypotension. Alternatively, patients can develop renal failure due to acute tubular necrosis or massive cortical necrosis. Management consists of a challenge by intravenous frusemide 60 to 80 mg followed by osmotic diuresis with mannitol once diuresis has commenced. In most situations the process of delivery itself can reverse the process of renal shutdown. Once the diuresis starts, it can cause rapid changes in fluid and electrolyte balance and this has to be checked by repeated estimation of electrolytes. It is easy to overload these patients with fluids and central venous pressure monitoring is handy to avoid such problems. Hypokalemia and acidosis have to be thought of if there is rapid diuresis. Frequent acid base and potassium level determinations are important both at the oliguric and diuretic phase. Dialysis has to be resorted to, if the renal failure persists or if there is grossly disordered electrolyte balance.

Hyperpyrexia

Hyperpyrexia or a marked rise in body temperature without any evidence of infection is a known complication of eclampsia. This is thought to be due to anoxic changes in the temperature regulating centre in the midbrain. If the temperature rises to more than 41°C it could be a considerable strain on the heart and if the temperature persists it may result in irreversible brain damage. The incidence is small and cases that have recovered are too sporadic to define the detail or the extent of damage. Frequent temperature recordings should be taken and cooling of the patients undertaken if the temperature rises beyond 39°C in order to avoid any deleterious effects. Blankets kept in refrigerators or deep freeze or ice caps need to be used to reduce the temperature.

Recent advances in therapy

Unfortunately most of the hypertensive calamities happen in the villages or where the patient had no access to proper antenatal care or in the absence of medical personnel in the labour ward. Modern drugs which are effective antihypertensives and anticonvulsants and which can be administered sublingually or rectally by paramedical personnel allow prompt action. Sublingual nifedipine for hypertensive crisis and rectal diazepam to prevent convulsions are increasingly used in clinical practice especially when there is difficulty in establishing an intravenous line immediately.

Nifedipine　　　Sublingual nifedipine starts acting within 1 to 5 min and the peak plasma concentration is achieved in 20 to 30 min. If the same capsule is swallowed the peak action takes 60 min. So in an eclamptic patient, the capsule can be pierced and the fluid squeezed under the tongue for rapid onset of action. The usual dosage is 10 mg every 15 min as required and a maximum of 180 mg can be used per day. Generally 10 to 20 mg is adequate to control the blood pressure in a hypertensive crisis. Its effectiveness is due to its powerful vasodilator action. Reflex tachycardia may develop with a 20 mg dose but the effect is short lasting. Once the blood pressure is decreased and stable at a certain level, it is maintained for at least two hours. This makes it ideal for its use in the field, as no parenteral form of administration is needed and once the blood pressure is stable, the patient can be referred to a nearby centre with facilities to manage convulsions should they occur, and the pregnancy may be terminated should such an event becomes necessary. The drug is also suitable in a modern setting as it can be easily repeated and continued orally after delivery of the baby.

　　　The nifedipine capsule is best stored between 15 to 25°C, as the gelatin capsule might melt at higher temperatures. Currently the capsule is available in blister packages which is more temperature tolerant than loose capsules. The keeping quality beyond 25°C is not known and hence it is kept in a cool place. It has to be protected from light. The drug is metabolised in the liver and excreted in the urine in 3–4 hours. The known side effects of the drug are flushing, palpitations, hypotension, dizziness, syncope and headaches.

Anticonvulsant - stesolid or diazepam rectal tube　　　Diazepam is available as a rectal tube. When administered rectally it is rapidly and completely absorbed with the peak concentration attained within 10 min. It is preferable to store the drug below 15°C but it tends to have a shelf life of up to one year when stored at temperatures just above 25°C. The elimination half-life of this drug is biphasic, with an initial half-life of 7–10 hours, followed by a second half-life of 2–6 days. Usually extensive metabolism occurs to active metabolites with less than 25% of the drug excreted unchanged in the urine. So the drug can be used safely unless there is severe liver derangement. Due to the long duration of action, once the desired effect of sedation is reached the patient can be transferred to a centre with more facilities if treatment was undertaken in a peripheral centre. The drug is attractive because syringes and trained personnel to administer it are not necessary, and it is possible to obtain a rapid onset of action.

Total paralysis and intermittent ventilation

Total paralysis and intermittent ventilation are lifesaving in certain situations. These are listed below:

- If the patient gets repeated convulsions despite maximal anticonvulsive therapy, that is status eclampticus.
- When the patient is restless despite maximum doses of sedation.
- When the sedative dose cannot be increased any further because of possible respiratory depression as shown by cyanosis.
- When there is difficulty in breathing with sedation due to laryngeal edema pre-operatively or after intubation and surgery.
- Paralysis can be achieved by d-tubocurarine. The patient is intubated and ventilated. This should be done by an anesthetic colleague and preferably in the intensive care unit. Care should be taken not to extubate in a hurry in an edematous patient; should there be obstruction to breathing due to laryngeal edema, it may be difficult to re-intubate.

The secret of the successful management of eclampsia lies in using a familiar drug regime both for cases of impending eclampsia and eclampsia. To avoid maternal mortality associated with cerebrovascular accidents hypertension has to be treated early and aggressively, preferably with peripheral vasodilating drugs. The only definitive way to resolve the crisis and to reduce the mortality is by terminating the pregnancy. At times there should be no hesitation to intervene operatively. Anticipation and management of complications should help to reduce maternal morbidity. It is essential to manage these patients with an anesthetist and help should be requested if it is felt that paralysing and ventilating the patient for 24 to 48 hours might save her life.

References

Arulkumaran S, Ratnam SS 1985. Eclampsia - Prevention and Management. *J Paed Obstet Gynaecol* Jan/Feb 7-13.

Arulkumaran S, Ratnam SS 1988. Caesarean sections in the management of severe hypertensive disorders in pregnancy and eclampsia. *Sing J Obstet Gynecol* 9:61-66.

Chua S, Arulkumaran S 1995. Eclampsia - No room for complacency. *Sing Med J.* In press

Department of Health and Social Services 1979. Report on confidential enquiries into maternal deaths in England and Wales 1973-1975,

London: HMSO, pp 21-29.

Department of Health and Social Services 1982. Report on confidential enquiries into maternal deaths in England and Wales 1976-1978, London: HMSO, pp 19-25.

Department of Health and Social Services 1986. Report on confidential enquiries into maternal deaths in England and Wales 1979-1981, London: HMSO, pp 13-21.

Department of Health and Social Services 1989 Report. on confidential enquiries into maternal deaths in England and Wales 1982-1984, London: HMSO, pp 10-19

Department of Health, Welsh Office, Scottish Home and Health Department and Social Services, Northern Ireland 1991 Report on confidential enquiries into maternal deaths in the United Kingdom 1985-1987, London: HMSO, pp 17-27

The Eclampsia Trial Collaborative Group 1995. Which anticonvulsant for women with eclampsia? Evidence from the Collaborative Eclampsia Trial. *Lancet* 345:1455-63

Govan ADT 1966. Myocardial lesions in fetal eclampsia. *Scottish Med J* 11:187-191.

Hogberg U 1986. Maternal deaths in Sweden 1971-1980. *Acta Obstet Gynecol Scand* 65:161-167.

Kaunitz AM, Hughes JM, Grimes DA et al 1985. Causes of maternal mortality in the United States. *Obstet Gynecol* 65:605-612.

Lean TH, Ratnam SS, Sivasamboo R 1968. The use of benzodiazepines in the management of eclampsia. *J Obstet Gynecol Br Cwlth* 75:856-859.

Lipsitz PJ 1971. The clinical and biochemical effects of excess magnesium in the newborn. *Paediatrics* 47:501-504.

Lopez-Llara M 1967. Eclampsia 1963-1966. *J Obstet Gynecol Br Cwlth* 74:379-383.

Menon MKK 1961. The evolution in the treatment of eclampsia. *J Obstet Gynecol Br Cwlth* 68:417-421.

Montan S, Arulkumaran S 1994. Prediction and prevention of pre-eclampsia. In: Ratnam SS, Sen DK, Ng SC and Arulkumaran S (eds) Contributions to Obstetrics and Gynaecology, Vol 3, Singapore: Churchill Livingstone, pp 195-210.

Pritchard JA 1975. Standardised treatment of 154 consecutive cases of eclampsia. *Am J Obstet Gynecol* 123:543-548.

Ratnam SS, Arulkumaran S 1995. Prise en charge de la crise d'eclampsie. *Gynecologie Internationale.* In press.

Sibai BM, McCubbin JH, Anderson GD, Lipshitz J, Diets PV 1981 Eclampsia I. Observations from 67 recent cases. *Obstet Gynecol* 58:609-613.

Zuspan FP 1966. Treatment of severe pre-eclampsia and eclampsia. *Clin Obstet Gynecol* 9:954-959.

23

Neonatal Resuscitation and the Management of Immediate Neonatal Problems

Roy Joseph

Modern obstetric care results in the acquisition of much knowledge of the disease states that a particular baby is likely to be predisposed to, not just in the moments after birth but also in the neonatal period and beyond infancy. Thus the task at birth is no longer confined to resuscitating and facilitating a smooth and uncomplicated transition into extrauterine existence. The additional task is to initiate in the healthy newborn appropriate, cost effective, physical and investigative evaluation for disease states that the child may be at risk for and the establishment of healthy communication between parent and physician. These steps are the foundation of the subsequent management of the anticipated disease. The majority of the world's babies are born in situations where a pediatrician is not readily available. It becomes imperative that the delivery team be aware of their primary and extended tasks and be competent in accomplishing them (Joseph 1990).

Conceptually, the tasks are resuscitation, management of the high risk newborn and management of the healthy newborn. While fulfilling these tasks, there must be a constant awareness that the atmosphere at the point of delivery is always slightly charged, with parents being unusually perceptive and sensitive. Thus care needs to be taken to ensure that the actions and speech of the attending staff are never found wanting nor capable of leading to misunderstanding.

Resuscitation

The transition from the fetal to the neonatal state is a hazardous point in the life of the human fetus and is accomplished without any assistance by a majority of babies. A small number need assistance which if not provided promptly and appropriately will result in an increased morbidity and mortality in the neonatal period and, more importantly in life-long neurological deficits.

The neonate who is in need of assistance at birth is usually labelled as being asphyxiated. It is now known that not every baby who needs assistance with transition is biochemically asphyxiated, that is hypoxic, hypercarbic and acidotic. The diagnostic label asphyxia should therefore be used cautiously.

Incidence

Observation at the National University Hospital over a five-year period starting in 1990, indicated that in general about ten per cent of babies needed assistance at birth. Only about one per cent however needed assistance in the form of ventilatory and or circulatory support. The incidence of those needing assistance at birth varies with the nature of the obstetric population and may be much higher in situations where there is minimal antenatal and intrapartum care.

Anticipation

Anoxia, drug effect, prematurity, anomalies, trauma and infection are the primary conditions leading to a difficult transition and consequent asphyxia. A variety of well-known clinical diseases predispose the fetus to one of the above pathological states.

Advances in antenatal care have enabled the identification of the compromised fetus well before its birth in the majority of pregnancies. However a significant number, estimated to be about 30%, are still not identifiable until after birth, even in centres with the most sophisticated antenatal and intrapartum fetal monitoring (Ho 1988). The occurrence of inadequate resuscitation as a result of lack of pre-paredness, incompetent personnel or equipment failure, all of which are usually avoidable, is unacceptable. The prevention of such occurrences call for a high degree of readiness.

Personnel　　The compromised fetus necessitates the presence at delivery of a person trained in resuscitation. Since a pediatrician cannot always be available, it is mandatory that the obstetric attendant be capable of initiating and maintaining the resuscitative procedures. Particularly in the less developed countries, this person is likely to be not a doctor but a nurse; the value of training and empowering non-physician birth-attendants to resuscitate cannot be underestimated. A second person is also necessary to provide assistance. These two persons should ideally have no responsibility other than caring for the baby.

Equipment　　The following must be available on site: a resuscitation table with attached sources of light and warmth and a stop clock; suction bulbs, a pump (50–100 cm H_2O) and catheters (size Fg 4, 6 and 8); oxygen and air supply with reducing valves, flow meter and blender; face masks of different sizes; a resuscitation bag with pressure blow off at 30 cm H_2O and pressure measuring device, connectors for the face mask and endotracheal tube; laryngoscopes with Miller blades size 0 and 1 ; endotracheal tubes, size 2.5–3.5; sterile towels, scissors and cord clamps; antiseptic cleaning solution and alcohol swabs; adhesive tapes precut to appropriate lengths; a stethoscope with an infant endpiece, sets for intravenous administration, an umbilical catheterisation set, syringes (2, 5 and 10 ml) and blood specimen containers.

Drugs　　The few drugs that are needed are adrenaline, sodium bicarbonate, volume expanders, naloxone and dopamine. Non-essential drugs and drugs meant for the mother should not be stored with the drugs used in resuscitation. Sodium bicarbonate and adrenaline are usually supplied in strengths that are higher than those required and must therefore be appropriately diluted with water before use. Likewise there are two strengths of naloxone. There is no evidence for the use of either atropine or calcium during the resuscitation of newborns.

Assessment　　Errors in resuscitation often arise from inadequate assessment of the baby's condition. Evaluation is usually accomplished by the Apgar scoring system. Immediate and repeated scoring provides a rapid but dependable measurement of physiological status and a guide to selecting resuscitation measures. Most term infants will have scores of 8 or more at and beyond one minute. Extremely premature infants though not asphyxiated may have low scores which nevertheless indicate their need for assistance (Simmons 1978).

Besides scoring the baby, assessment should also include a rapid estimation of the gestational age and weight, and the recognition of major congenital anomalies and extensive soft tissue injuries of the head. The history of the mother's major medical and obstetric problems should ideally have been ascertained before the baby's birth. All these put together enables the resuscitator to have a proper perspective of the pathophysiological changes in operation and the manner in which the baby is going to respond to resuscitative measures.

Resuscitative procedures as guided by the Apgar scores

Apgar 8–10   Healthy infant, pink, active, responsive, vigorously crying with a rapid heart rate. The first step is to prevent heat loss by placing the infant under a heated radiant warmer, quickly drying the infant of amniotic fluid and removing all wet towels. The baby should be positioned on the back with the neck in the neutral position. Brief low pressure suction of the mouth and nose should follow. A reassessment must be made in five minutes. When the vital signs become stable, the stomach can be aspirated.

Apgar 6–7   Slightly cyanotic, moving with decreased tone, shallow or periodic breathing, with a heart rate > 100/min. The baby should be wiped dry, kept warm and suction applied; she should be stimulated by gentle slapping of the sole, flicking of the heel and or rubbing of the back. Oxygen should be administered through a mask held just above the face. If the baby improves, the oxygen should be continued until the baby becomes pink and vigorous and then removed; a reassessment should be done to confirm that Apgar scores are maintained. If the baby does not improve, treatment is as described in the situations that follow.

Apgar 3–5   cyanotic, poor tone, weak respiratory efforts and slowing heart rate < 100/min. The baby is wiped dry, kept warm, given suction and ventilated with 100% oxygen through a mask, using pressure adequate to move the chest. Careful ventilation through the mask will be sufficient in all but a very small number; success in this procedure is dependent on the size of the mask, its application, the attainment of a good seal and creation of a positive pressure that is sufficient to create a visible expansion of the chest. The concentration of oxygen delivered is about 40% if the bag does not have a reservoir.

Effective ventilation will result within a minute in, rising and stable heart rates, abolition of cyanosis and maintenance of other vital signs. The chest should be auscultated and equal air entry should be ensured. If the baby improves, ventilation must be continued until respiration becomes regular and the heart rate is stable and > 100/min. If the baby does not improve, the chest does not move or the air entry is unequal or poor, treatment is as in the next group.

Apgar 0–2.   Asphyxia likely: deeply cyanotic or pale, limp, apnoeic or gasping and heart rate slow or absent. The baby should be wiped dry and kept warm, brief suction is done of the upper airway. Laryngoscopy should be performed, the trachea aspirated and the baby intubated and ventilated with 100% oxygen at 40–60 breaths/min using an inspiratory pressure sufficient to move the upper chest wall. Cardiac massage should be performed if the heart rate is < 60/min or between 60 and 80 and not increasing.

For effective cardiac massage, the back should have a firm support, the sternum be compressed to a depth of 0.5–0.75 inch and interposed with ventilation in a 3:1 ratio, that is, at a ventilating rate of 30 breaths and chest compression rate of 90/min, the compressing force is applied at the lower end of the sternum about a finger breadth above the xiphoid. The force is to be applied vertically either with the thumbs, one placed above the other or placed side by side or by two fingers.

The majority of babies will improve within 1–2 minutes, showing initially a rise in heart rate followed by the disappearance of pallor or cyanosis and restoration of tone, respiration and responses. If the response is prompt and strong and sustained with spontaneous breathing efforts, then extubation can be tried; if the baby responds by crying as the tube is withdrawn, the timing is right. The child may however continue to need oxygen and must be observed carefully over the next few minutes to decide on the type of assistance that must be provided during transfer to the special care nursery.

Special situations

Meconium passage before birth   The majority of babies who are meconium stained are neither hypoxic during labour nor do they have meconium in their lower airway. Inappropriate management based on rigid protocols often produces more harm than good. At the same time, failure to clear especially the lower airway of particulate meconium will result in morbidity if not mortality. The anxiety associated with the prevention of meconium aspiration syndrome should not cause the resuscitating team to forget that preexisting hypoxia will need equal if not more attention in the newborn period.

As the risk of aspirating meconium into the trachea and bronchi is high, the nose and mouth must be cleared before the chest is delivered. This is followed by immediate laryngoscopic visualisation of the pharynx and glottis for meconium; and if detected, it is reasonable to assume that there is meconium distal to the cords. Three procedures are available for this task of removing particulate and viscous meconium. They are : insertion of an endotracheal tube, connecting a meconium aspirator to it, followed by application of a negative pressure through it as it is withdrawn; next is the insertion of a thick suction catheter (about 10Fr) into the trachea followed by application of suction as it is rotated during withdrawal; lastly the application of suction through a suction catheter in the endotracheal tube. This last method is less capable of withdrawing meconium but is the safest from the point of maintenance of access to the airway; also the risk of laryngospasm and trauma from repeated intubation is least in this method. The possibility of damage to the tracheal epithelium and the drastic reduction of the functional residual capacity that takes place in all three techniques must be remembered. I have found it best to use the third technique, but do not hesitate to move up the list. Inexperienced persons should use the third method. The technique of meconium clearance from the trachea is nowhere as important as avoidance of prolonged fetal hypoxia, timely delivery and early aspiration of meconium from the pharynx.

Endotracheal suction need not be performed in meconium stained babies who are vigorous and pink.

When coexisting hypoxia and acidosis are almost certain, deliberate attempts must be made by IPPV to correct the chemical disturbance after the airway has been cleared. The temptation is again to ventilate hard and fast (? directly related to the degree of anxiety experienced by the resuscitator) in the hope of a quick correction of hypoxia and acidosis. The danger is over-ventilation of expanded alveoli, creation of lobar or segmental emphysema and or pneumothorax when there are ball valve-like obstructions from meconium plugs in the bronchi; this will result in compression of the blood vessels and raising of pulmonary vascular resistance, culminating in the worsening of a ventilation perfusion mismatch and of pulmonary hypertension. Both these will perpetuate hypoxia and acidosis, the very disturbance that the intervention aimed to correct.

What is necessary is gentle ventilation with a generous (especially in term infants) concentration of oxygen and just sufficient pressures to produce a visible chest expansion and vigilant inspection and auscultation to detect unequal expansion and/or aeration, the first sign of pneumothorax or emphysema. Not to be forgotten is the often continued need for oxygen in the first hours, even when ventilatory support is not needed or cyanosis is not apparent.

Persistent apnoea   Most babies will begin to breathe within a short time of resuscitation; a small number however remain apnoeic, make weak or infrequent spontaneous breathing efforts, but have healthy heart rates, colour and perfusion. Though this could be due to asphyxia, it can also be due to opiates or other CNS depressant agents, hypovolemia, central nervous system abnormality or no apparent cause. Intravenous naloxone 100 ug/kg should be given at this stage through the umbilical vein if there is a history of recent (within 4 hours) maternal opiate sedation. Naloxone comes in two preparations, the readily available adult preparation containing 1.0 mg/ml; a 3 kg infant will require 0.3 ml. The other preparation has a concentration of 0.25 mg/ml; the required amount is therefore 0.25 ml/kg.

Cyanosis   It is not at all uncommon to come across a neonate who remains cyanosed in spite of what is considered to be good respiratory effort, heart beat and vitality. The immediate reaction is to either consider the possibility of a cyanotic heart condition or a pulmonary complication like aspiration. Statistically the likely diagnosis is a persistence of the transitional circulation; this is characterised by the continued flow of venous blood across the foramen ovale and the ductus arteriosus into the systemic circulation.

The majority of such states will spontaneously revert provided the baby is not compromised by hypothermia secondary to exposure, or airway obstruction caused by reflex vocal cord spasm which is induced by repeated pharyngeal irritation by a suction catheter or laryngoscope blade. The transition may be facilitated by the gentle administration of oxygen through a mask.

In the absence of a falling heart rate the desperate desire to do something must be resisted. Once the normal pattern of circulation is attained the baby should have a subsequent uneventful transition. However the babies should be nursed in a special care nursery as they are more likely to respond to hypothermia, hypoxia and acidosis with reversal to the transitional circulation.

Respiratory distress   It will reveal itself with two or more of the following symptoms: tachypnoea, retractions, cyanosis and grunting. The baby may be hypoxic but not cyanosed; warm humidified oxygen should be promptly administered and if not associated with stable vital signs, treatment must be intensified by ventilation either with a mask or through the endotracheal tube.

Hypotonia   Severe neuromuscular diseases arising from congenital brain abnormalities or infections, antepartum hypoxic states, spinal cord injury and congenital myopathy are characterised by a good colour, heart rate and perfusion, but profound hypotonia that does not improve with ventilatory support. It is very often mistaken for an acute asphyxial state. Closer examination will reveal changes in muscle bulk brought on by wasting and positional deformities of the extremities. Such babies are also at high risk of becoming asphyxiated after birth if their respiratory inadequacy is unrecognised. Treatment unfortunately centres on the asphyxia and attention is diverted from the underlying neuromuscular disease state. Although the fatal outcome may not be changed by awareness of the disease, opportunities for determining the etiology and recurrence risks may be lost by lack of awareness and worse still, obstetrical management of labour may be blamed.

Hypovolemia   These babies will present initially with a low Apgar score and with resuscitation they will show pallor, tachycardia, poor pulse and slow capillary filling, and collapsed umbilical cord vessels. There may or may not be a preceding history of vaginal bleeding in labour or bloodstained liquor. Transfusion with 10–20ml/kg of synthetic plasma protein solution or Group O negative blood will be immediately needed. If either of the preceding two are not immediately available, a crystalloid solution should be used.

A similar clinical presentation of poor peripheral perfusion may be seen when there is poor myocardial contractility especially after prolonged hypoxia and acidosis. The liver and umbilical vessels will tend to be engorged in this case; treatment would then be the administration of a dopamine infusion.

Bradycardia   Though rare, bradycardia may be due to an arrhythmia rather than to asphyxia. If so, other bodily functions will be seen to be adequate unless the bradycardia is so profound (< 60/min) as to diminish cardiac output.

Diaphragmatic hernia   This is often easily recognisable by the triad of severe respiratory distress, mediastinal shift and a scaphoid abdomen; survival is inversely related to the degree of hypoplasia of the contralateral lung and not by the rapidity with which the hernia is reduced; ventilation by mask is contraindicated; there should be prompt intubation followed by careful ventilation using the lowest inspiratory pressure possible that will result in expansion of the contralateral chest. Correction of cyanosis will be slow and should not be countered with higher inspiratory pressures, or repeated intubations arising from fears of a misplaced endotracheal tube. The thrust of management is to lower the raised pulmonary vascular pressures and minimise damage to the remaining healthy lung.

Hydrops   The prognosis of hydropic babies is not uniformly fatal; often the hydropic state is secondary to self-limiting or treatable conditions like acute infections particularly syphilis, parvo virus infection, chronic anemia of immune origin or secondary to chronic fetomaternal hemorrhage or placental vascular abnormalities. These babies have a good prognosis with proper resuscitation and continued intensive care for about a week.

The babies require ventilatory support, raising of hematocrit by isovolumetric partial exchange transfusion, restoration of blood volume by fresh frozen plasma containing high molecular weight proteins (albumin is contraindicated as it may aggravate existing ascites or pleural effusion), removal of pleural and ascitic fluid to facilitate ventilation, frusemide for pulmonary edema and dopamine to improve peripheral perfusion and cardiac contractility. Cannulation of the umbilical vein and measurement of the central venous pressure will facilitate management.

Dwarf   The handling of dwarfs calls for much experience. From a management point of view, they come in two groups: those that are lethal (associated with thoracic and pulmonary hypoplasia) and those that are not. Though it is rare for the lethal variety not to be sick from birth, it is not uncommon for the non-lethal variety (for example, those with achondroplasia) to need assistance at birth. This places the resuscitator in a dilemma. The preferred approach is to resuscitate all unless a firm diagnosis of a lethal variety (achondrogenesis or thantophoric dwarf) has been made antenatally and the lethal nature conveyed to the parents who in turn have had time to accept the diagnosis and prognosis. In the absence of documentary evidence of all of the above it is prudent to resuscitate, transfer to the nursery and only after evaluation by specialists and obtaining the parents' consent should ventilatory efforts be stopped.

Dysmorphic baby   The management of a dysmorphic neonate calls for a similar approach to that of a dwarf. The important difference is that though the prognosis for normal neurological function may be extremely poor, the cardiorespiratory function may not be always affected, that is, they are less likely to be lethal. This creates a problem as to the extent to which basic or special care should be given and a decision will have to be made. There is no right or wrong way to proceed. Different approaches arising from multiple social factors, the doctor-family relationship and the local medicolegal climate are practised. What is important to realise is that what may work with one family cannot be prescribed for all babies even if the pathology is the same.

Particular care must be taken when the nature of abnormalities are in the realm of cosmetic inadequacies, for example, facial clefts or reduction deformities of the limbs rather than severe functional limitations. The temptation to give up is high and must be resisted.

Suspected lethal abnormality   Advances in surgical techniques, medical support, and facilities for safe transport even over long distances have all been of help to affected infants and have drastically reduced the number of abnormalities that are considered to be lethal. Hydrocephalus, Down's syndrome with surgical complications, diaphragmatic hernia, oesophageal atresia, exomphalos and exstrophy of the bladder are highly amenable to treatment. Anencephaly, encepahlocoel, hypoplastic left heart syndrome, pulmonary hypoplasia and lymphangiectasia, bilateral renal agenesis and E and D trisomies are among the abnormalities considered to be lethal even in highly developed societies. The list is significantly longer in localities where intensive care is less developed and transport inappropriate. Babies suspected to have chromosomal abnormalities because of multiple abnormalities and who are dying should have their blood sampled in the delivery room for chromosomal analysis. Obstetricians, physicians and surgeons should in agreement draw up a list of abnormalities that are lethal in their practice. This will ensure that parents are provided with prompt, clear and consistent advice on the nature and prognosis of their child's abnormalities.

Absent heart beat at birth   Resuscitation must be immediate as a few may respond and survive. It has been found that all neonates who had no spontaneous heart beat at 10 minutes or by 30 minutes remained apnoeic either died or survived with very severe disability (Jain et al 1991). Hence resuscitation can be stopped at 30 minutes. In some instances it may be prudent not to stop but to treat vigorously for about 24–48 hours during which time investigations and consultations that confirm the poor prognosis can be obtained and parents counselled prior to the withdrawal of intensive care.

Failure of resuscitative efforts

Three groups of conditions may present with difficulty or failure of resuscitative efforts. The first group comprises oesophageal intubation, bronchial intubation, a blocked endotracheal tube, insufficient airway pressure, inappropriate gas, pneumothorax and hypovolemia which are all readily diagnosable with a systematic approach and which when corrected will result in rapid improvement.

The second group are those with diaphragmatic hernia, bilateral pleural effusion, congenital pneumonia, massive aspiration and pulmonary hemorrhage. These conditions are sometimes difficult to diagnose and always difficult to resuscitate, but with perseverance they can be salvaged.

The third group with pulmonary hypoplasia or severe prolonged hypoxia are usually not salvageable.

Medications   These are indicated if the heart rate is < 80/min in spite of 30 seconds of ventilation and cardiac massage. Vascular access is obtained by catheterising the umbilical vein.

Cardiac contractility is improved by giving adrenaline rapidly 1:10,000 in a dose of about 0.1–0.3 ml/kg. The drug, after diluting 1:1 with normal saline, can also be given intratracheally; after five minutes the dose can be repeated. The drug may be repeated intravenously if there is no response to intratracheal instillation.

At this stage, the possibility of hypovolemia is to be considered and corrected by rapidly infusing over ten minutes, about 10 ml/kg of a volume expander, the order of preference being : Group O negative whole blood compatible with the mother's blood, 5% albumin solution, normal saline or Ringer lactate. Another 10 ml/kg can be given if partial improvement is noted.

Little or no improvement raises the possibility of metabolic acidosis. This is corrected by administering sodium bicarbonate in a dose of about 2 mmol/kg, (4 ml/kg of a 4.2% solution) at a rate of about 1 mmol/kg/min. Effective ventilation must precede and accompany sodium bicarbonate administration. Risks of intra-ventricular hemorrhage in prematures can be minimised by using the recommended concentration and rates.

If the heart rate recovers but there is poor peripheral perfusion with a thready pulse and continued evidence of shock, Dopamine infusion is begun at 5 mcg/kg/min. If at least intermittent respiratory efforts are not present within 30 minutes then resuscitative procedures should not be continued.

Practical hints

Prolonged oropharyngeal suction can cause reflex bradycardia, vocal cord spasm and apnoea. The neck must not be kept in a hyperextended position during venti-lation or intubation. For effective ventilation a complete seal must be ensured be-tween the mask and the face. A size 2.5 endotracheal tube needs to be used only when the baby is below 1 kg. Air entry and breath sounds may be deceptively normal with oesophageal intubation. Bronchial intubation occurs very easily. Drugs should not be injected intramuscularly as the poor blood supply to the muscles that accompanies hypoxic states will prevent them from reaching the systemic circula-tion. Direct injection into the umbilical vein is also to be avoided as the chances of extravasation or mistaken entry into the umbilical artery are high. The compli-cations from intracardiac injections grossly outweigh the benefits.

Outcome

The prognosis in infants requiring resuscitation at birth is determined by the in-tensity and duration of the asphyxial process and by the presence of other condi-tions. The Apgar scores at 1 minute have little predictive values (Drage and Kennedy 1966). The majority of resuscitated infants have a relatively uneventful neonatal course and can look to a normal neurological development. Those in whom the Apgar score at 5 minutes was < 2 or < 4 after 10 minutes or those who had seizures or prolonged hypotonia have a high incidence of late sequelae or mortality (Scott 1976; Nelson 1977, 1979, 1981; Ergander and Erikson 1983).

Transport to the nursery

Transport should commence only after abnormalities in colour, heart rate, ventila-tion, perfusion and body temperature have been corrected. The resuscitating team must accompany the baby and continue providing assistance during transport. Re-suscitation is only the first step in the management of an asphyxiated or otherwise compromised infant. Very often the benefits obtained during resuscitation are lost because of failure to recognise that the infant needs continued assistance during transport and in the nursery.

Management of high risk infants

Maternal medical disease or obstetric complications

These may predispose the baby to early problems such as hypothermia, hypogly-cemia, respiratory distress, inability to suck, septicemia and seizures, all of which are generally preventable by careful neonatal management in the first few hours after birth. The babies should therefore be transferred immediately after birth to a special care nursery. In the absence of pediatricians the obstetric team is obliged to initiate this early monitoring and treatment.

Diabetes mellitus (DM)   When DM is poorly controlled and is associated with macrosomia, the risk in the neonate of hypoglycemia and subsequent CNS damage and the possibility of cardiomyopathy and immature lungs, warrant the provision of special monitoring for about 48 hours even if the baby is initially well. Blood glucose levels are likely to reach a nadir at about an hour to two of age. False low values will be obtained when sampling occurs in the presence of hypothermia, poor peripheral perfusion and polycythemia.

Thyrotoxicosis   The maternal late acting thyroid stimulating (LATS) anti-bodies are capable of producing thyrotoxicosis in the fetus. If the mother is not treated, the baby will be symptomatic from birth; when the mother has been treated but if the disease is still immunologically active, neonatal thyrotoxicosis may manifest in the latter part of the first week. Suppressed TSH levels at birth and at 2 weeks should identify the baby at risk of symptomatic thyrotoxicosis.

Chorioamnionitis   Early congenital bacterial infections tend to remain asymp-tomatic for a period and then suddenly present as early as 12 hours of age in shock. Institution of treatment before the disease becomes symptomatic is a prerequisite for decreasing mortality and morbidity. When chorioamnionitis is suspected, it is advisable for the baby to be investigated (blood counts, surface swabs and deep cultures) and for broad spectrum antibiotics (penicillin and aminoglycoside) to be started soon after birth on the presumption of infection. The antibiotics are with-drawn usually by about the third day if clinical behaviour and investigations are not suggestive of infection.

Other conditions   If the mother is a Hepatitis B carrier with e Ag positivity, then the baby will require not just the vaccine, but also 0.5 ml of Hepatitis B immunoglobulin within 12 hours of birth. Chicken pox infection with the rashes erupting in the mother in the five days before delivery markedly increases the chances and morbidity of neonatal chicken pox. Such babies need early passive immunisation with 125 units of varicella zoster immunoglobulin (VZIG). VZIG increases the incubation period, does not reduce the attack rate but reduces the intensity of symptoms. Babies of mothers with untreated tuberculosis need to be isolated from their mothers. Babies of mothers addicted to narcotics, alcohol and other recreational drugs also need to be watched for withdrawal symptoms. The various alpha thalassemia states are easily distinguishable and diagnosable in the newborn period because of their distinctly differing concentrations of Bart's hemoglobin as determined by hemoglobin electrophoresis in cord blood. If the mother has not been screened for syphilis, the child must be screened with a VDRL or RPR test.

Antenatal diagnosis of fetal abnormality

Congenital heart disease   As early medical and surgical intervention are criti-cal in a significant number, it is preferable that parents be guided depending on the lesion (especially duct dependent lesions), to having the delivery in a setting where the appropriate level of general medical, cardiac and surgical care can be provided, rather than being forced after birth to initiate urgent, emotionally devastating and often prognosis worsening transports.

A word of caution: antenatal diagnosis of cardiac lesions even in experienced hands is associated with mistakes because of restricted viewing windows; thus lesions considered to be poorly amenable to treatment may on assessment in the newborn period be found to be anatomically different and have a better prognosis. The reverse is also being documented. Antenatal prognostication should thus always be conditional to postnatal cardiac anatomy definition and equally important, detection of abnormalities in other organs. Accurate cardiac, brain and renal anatomy definitions are being regularly attained postnatally by experienced hands with just two dimensional (2D) and colour Doppler studies.

Thus in the absence of an inhouse 2D echo facility, it is better for the child to be transported to the appropriate centre for a good 2D echo study than to be subjected to an inhouse cardiac catheterisation.

Renal Abnormalities   Except for the very obvious and severe abnormalities like renal agenesis or dysplasia, polycystic disease or urethral obstructions, a good prognosis can be given and child enrolled in an extended programme of non-invasive evaluation; immediate surgery is only very rarely needed.

Early manifestation of disease in the newborn

Birth injuries   These with functional consequences like brachial plexus injury, facial nerve palsy, subaponeurotic hematoma, and bone fractures are all recognisable at birth; the first examination after birth at the delivery suite must aim to pick them up. Though most babies do not need any immediate intervention, the parents must be informed of the injury, its cause, prognosis and the intervention needed.

Cosmetic abnormalities   These are a source of intense distress to parents. Since most of them do not produce any sickness in the child and are also amenable to treatment, immediate counselling of parents is necessary.

Genital abnormalities   Genital abnormalities are very anxiety provoking, particularly when there is ambiguity of the sexual phenotype. In counselling, the emphasis is to point out that genital development is incomplete and therefore sexual identification is not readily possible by inspection. Parents should also be told that the child is not half male and half female. Examination of the buccal smear for chromatin bodies cannot be depended on. Chromosomal analysis is needed for genotype identification and the result can be available within 48 hours of receiving the specimen. Sex identification can thus be quick; the gender of assignment however is generally made on the basis of external anatomy. In general, if the phallus is less than 2 cm in length, it would be best to raise the child as a female irrespective of the chromosomal or gonadal sex. The rare exception is in 5 alpha reductase deficiency or pituitary deficiency with concomitant growth hormone deficiency.

Mildly preterm infant   Mildly preterm (> 34 weeks gestation) infants who have not been compromised prior to delivery have a relatively uneventful postnatal period provided the first few minutes are stress free and hypothermia and hypoglycemia have been prevented. They can easily be handled in any Level 1 nursery. The need to be nursed in higher level nurseries arises only if rare complications develop. As these infants are prone to hyperbilirubinemia it is advisable that discharge be delayed till after the fourth day when a further rise in bilirubin level is unlikely. Those having to stay in hospital for whatever reason are susceptible to nosocomial infections. Strict hand washing by all categories of staff before handling babies, assuring sterile milk supplies and minimising invasive procedures are more important in preventing infections than wearing gowns, changing footwear, or denying access to parents into the nursery.

Moderately preterm infant   If between 32 and 34 weeks, these babies will suffer unnecessarily in the absence of dedicated facilities and staff. They should preferably be delivered in such centres; if this is not possible, they must be electively transferred. Studies have demonstrated that the high mortality and morbidity that such babies experience occur only when they are transferred after complications set in (Paneth et al 1982).

As respiratory disease may set in early and progress rapidly, they must be transferred under trained medical supervision with provision for maintaining body temperature, blood glucose levels and cardiorespiratory function.

Severely preterm infant   The prognosis for intact survival in those born between 28 and 32 weeks has improved over the last decade (Saigal et al 1982; Yu et al 1982; Ho 1985; Biswas et al 1995). The majority however will need sustained intensive care and a long hospital stay (Loke et al 1993). Their prognosis easily becomes poor if the care during labour, delivery and after birth is not anticipatory and proactive. Heroic care after a dismal start is a sure prescription for death or significant neurological sequelae.

Though the Apgar scores may not be very low, these infants are nevertheless unable to maintain adequate respiratory efforts and will therefore need to be intubated even in the absence of bradycardia or apnoea.

The advent of the artificial surfactant is likely to create a false sense of security and suggest that the problems of birth in a low care setting can be nullified by the administration of surfactant and an immediate transfer.

In spite of the ability to offer an optimistic note in general, the outcome in each particular baby can be quite unpredictable. It is imperative to provide hope to the parents; nevertheless, neither undue optimism nor pessimism is appropriate in the early days of life.

Preterm of doubtful viability   These are babies born below 28 weeks of gestation and in most parts of the world they do not survive. About half of them may survive with intensive and prolonged care (Yu et al 1986; Ho and Lim 1995). The approach to these babies is heavily influenced by the national health policy, funding sources, the expectations of society, parental opinions, and resources available. In view of the heavy utilisation of nursing staff and equipment, a prolonged hospital stay, the unpredictability of the outcome, and costs involved it seems appropriat that an informed decision whether to continue with care should be taken by the parents (Joseph 1989). If in doubt, there must be no delay in initiating care in the labour ward. Intervention can always be discontinued later.

Management of the healthy term infant

Many mothers continue to deliver without having received any antenatal care or without antenatal screening of their fetuses for congenital abnormalities. Healthy term infants are therefore also at risk, albeit a much lower risk, for morbidity and mortality in the first few days after birth. There is the onus to ensure screening for diseases that can be diagnosed before they produce irreversible morbidity.

Population screening at birth

Congenital dislocation of the hip (CDH), G6PD deficiency and congenital hypo-thyroidism are the three diseases for which every newborn should be screened. They all have the essential characteristics of a disease that merits screening. The morbidity that these diseases can produce when unrecognised is significant. There are simple procedures for screening and confirming the diagnosis and treatment is equally simple.

Congenital dislocation of the hip   This has been shown in our population to occur with an incidence of about 1 in 1,000 births. The newborn female, or one who was presenting with the breech or who has a history in the sib of CDH is at higher risk. The majority have developed stable hips with the simple intervention of a hip plaster cast for about 3 months. Screening is easily done by performing the Barlow procedure which dislocates the femoral head followed by the demon-stration of the Ortolani sign indicating reduction.

G6PD deficiency   This is present in about 4% of Chinese males, and 1% of Chinese females and Malay males. Among Indian males in Singapore, the incidence is about 0.5% (Wong 1964). In an Indian community in a malaria endemic area a 7.8% incidence with no male preponderance has been reported (Ramadevi et al 1994). Even in the absence of a hemolytic crisis, the incidence (20%) of severe neonatal hyperbilirubinaemia (serum bilirubin > 256 umol/L) is about double that in the non G6PD deficient newborn (Tan 1981). Such babies therefore benefit from early diagnosis, protection from triggers and close observation in the hospital at least in the first four days of life and can then be discharged with advice on potential triggers and the mode of inheritance.

   With the high gene frequency particularly in Asia and the rising frequency of inter-racial marriage, the need to screen all babies becomes obvious. The disease can easily be screened by determining the enzyme activity in an anticoagulated specimen of cord blood using the semi-quantitative modified Bernstein's technique (Brown and Wong 1968). Results are available within a few hours, well before the mother is ready to go home.

Congenital hypothyroidism   Twenty years of newborn screening of many mil-lions of infants have confirmed the highly asymptomatic nature of congenital hypothyroidism, an incidence of about 1 in 3,500 births and the almost complete prevention of intellectual deficits when treatment is started within the first month of life.

   Since most mothers in Asia go home fairly soon after delivery, we advocate and have been practising for the last ten years, primary cord serum TSH screening for congenital hypothyroidism (Joseph et al 1992). Those with a TSH greater than the 99th centile (about 25 mU/L) are recalled for further evaluation. The current generation of highly sensitive and automated non-radioimmunoassays are easily incorporated into any laboratory service and results can be available within 12 hours of receipt of the specimen enabling the first evaluation to be done before discharge from hospital. If found to be elevated a repeat assay is performed. With this only 1 per 1,000 of those screened will be detected to have persistent elevation of TSH levels and will need a subsequent evaluation in the first week after discharge. About 1 in 3 in this group can be expected to have hypothyroidism.

Check list of screening symptoms

Most healthy term infants will remain in the care of the obstetrician. The following checklist of symptoms will help considerably to identify infants with potential problems: infrequent or delay in stooling, vomiting of feeds, inability to suck, early jaundice, cyanosis on crying, poor urinary stream and/or abdominal distension. If by 48–72 hours of birth, these symptoms and signs are absent, it is extremely unlikely that there is an ongoing subclinical pathology and it should therefore be safe for discharge to be effected.

Although most babies do not need much attention at birth, there are a few who do. This attention is in the form of examination and investigation to detect abnormalities, treatment to facilitate cardio-respiratory adaptation to extrauterine life, triage to determine the level of care needed and finally communication with their parents. All these must be readily available in every birthing centre; their complete provision will not always prevent death or illness but will go a long way in ensuring a satisfactory end to a pregnancy.

References

Biswas A, Chew S, Joseph R, Arulkumaran S, Anandakumar C, Ratnam SS 1995. Towards improved perinatal care - Perinatal audit. *Ann Acad Med Sing* 24:211-217.

Brown WR, Wong HB 1968. Hyperbilirubinemia and kernicterus in glucose-6-phosphate dehydrogenase deficient infants in Singapore. *Pediatrics* 41:1055-62.

Drage JS and Kennedy C 1966. The Apgar scores as an index of infant morbidity. *Develop Med Child Neurol* 8:141-148.

Ergander V and Erikson M 1983. Severe neonatal asphyxia. *Acta Paediatr Scand* 72:321-325.

Ho LY 1985. Growth and early developmental outcome of the VLBW infants at Alexandra Hospital, Singapore 1978-1982. *Ann Acad Med Sing* 14:546-54.

Ho LY 1988. Predictability of perinatal risk factors on the need for resuscitation at birth. Handbook of Abstracts. 22nd Singapore-Malaysia Congress of Medicine, Singapore, p 111.

Ho NK, Lim S B,1995. Outcome of infants weighing 500-999 grams at birth in a Singapore hospital (1990-1993). *Sin Med J* 36:185-188.

Jain L, Ferre C, Vidyasagar D, Nath S, Sheftel D 1991. Cardiopulmonary resuscitation of apparently stillborn infants: survival and long-term outcome. *J Pediatr* 118:778-782.

Joseph R 1989. Intensive care of extremely premature newborns. *Sing J Obstet Gynecol* 20:45-47.

Joseph R 1990. Resuscitation at birth. *Sing Med J* 31:166-170

Joseph R, Ho LY, Gomez JM et al 1992. Non isotopic cord serum screening for congenital hypothyroidism in Singapore - The TSH and T4 strategy. In: Wilcken B and Webster D, eds. Neonatal screening in the Nineties. Manly Vale NSW, pp 69-70.

Loke HL, Mui PR, Tan KW 1993. Outcome of a cohort of 2 year old very low birthweight survivors managed in Singapore during 1988 and 1989. *J Sing Paed Soc* 35:154-160.

Paneth N, Kiely JL, Wallenstein S, Marcus M, Pakter J, Susser M 1982. Newborn intensive care and neonatal mortality in low birthweight infants - a population study. *N Engl J Med* 307:149-155.

Ramadevi R, Savithiri HS, Devi AP, Bittles AH, Rao NA 1994. An unusual distribution of glucose-6-phosphate dehydrogenase deficiency of South Indian population. *Ind J Biochem-Biophys* 31:358-60.

Saigal S, Rosenbaum P, Stoskopf B, Milner R 1982. Follow up of infants 501 to 1,500 g birthweight delivered to residents of a geographically defined region with perinatal intensive care facilities. *J Pediatr* 100:606-624.

Scott H 1976. Outcome of very severe birth asphyxia. *Arch Dis Child* 51:712-6.

Simmons MA and Bowes WA 1978. Apgar scores in infants less than 1,500 grams. *Pediatr Res* 12(abst):534.

Tan KL 1981. Glucose-6-phosphate dehydrogenase status and neonatal jaundice. *Arch Dis Child* 56:874-877.

Wong HB 1964. Neonatal hyperbilirubinemia. *Bull Kandang Kerbau Hosp,* Singapore.3:1

Yu VYH, Zhao SM, Bajuk B 1982. Results of intensive care for 375 very low birthweight infants. *Aust Paed J* 18:188-192.

Yu VYH, Loke HL, Bajuk B, Szymonowicz W, Orgill AA, Astbury J 1986. Prognosis for infants born at 23 to 28 weeks gestation. *BMJ* 293:1200-1203.

24

Postpartum Psychiatric Disorders

Pamela Chan Siew Ling

It does seem rather incongruous that pregnancy, delivery and motherhood can be associated with psychiatric morbidity and even mortality (Robin 1962). Birth is after all considered to be a happy event and is celebrated in a myriad of rituals across many different cultures. However, pregnancy and delivery are also considered major life events. In the Chinese culture this is marked by many superstitions, beliefs, taboos and practices that have been handed down many generations. Modern mothers of this generation often struggle with the dilemma of whether to play safe and follow these rules or to dismiss these quaint customs as being so much archaic nonsense. One custom that still appears to persist is the Chinese 'confinement month' in the immediate postnatal period. This custom recognises the new mother's need for additional care and close surveillance in the puerperium. In this month, the new mother is confined to the house and forbidden to bathe, eat anything other than specially cooked nourishing food or be exposed to 'wind'. Household chores and cooking are all undertaken by a female relative or a hired confinement nanny specially trained for these tasks. It really serves a culturally sanctioned protective function enabling the early recognition of any postnatal mental illness and gives the necessary support to any afflicted mother and her child.

Pitt in 1968 postulated that postnatal depression was a disorder specific to the puerperium and distinguishable from classical depressive illness.

The types of postnatal psychiatric disorders considered here include:

a. postnatal or maternity blues

b. postnatal depression

c. postnatal psychosis

d. preexisting psychiatric disorders in pregnancy.

The prevalence of postnatal blues has been estimated in different western studies to be anywhere from 50 to 70% (Kumar and Robinson 1984; Paffenbarger 1964). Postnatal depression is somewhat less common at 10%. Postnatal psychosis is rare and estimated to occur in about 2 per 1,000 births.

In Singapore, Kok et al (1994), studied 200 postnatal women for depressive symptoms for six months using the Edinburgh postnatal depression scale (Cox et al 1983). No cases of psychosis were detected. In the study, high levels of mild depressive symptoms were found in 80% of the women over the entire study period with a peak at the third month. These findings were comparable to that found in another similar study (Kendell et al 1984).

Aetiology

a) Biological factors

Biological factors have been implicated in the genesis of puerperal mental illness because of the frequency of the emotional change and the timing of the onset. Oestrogen and progesterone both increase greatly during late pregnancy and fall precipitously after childbirth. Changes also occur in the corticosteroids and corticosteroid-binding globulin levels.

Other researchers have noted a link between premenstrual syndrome complaints and the subsequent development of a puerperal mental illness. Some report that the development of a mood change when on oral contraceptives is another risk factor.

Although the actual etiological factor for puerperal disorders is unknown, the current state of research seems to suggest that the dramatic hormonal changes may act in concert with other stressors to induce mental illness in vulnerable, predisposed women (Kendell 1985).

b) Psychological factors

Psychodynamic factors implicated in the etiology of puerperal mental illness usually point to the woman's ambivalence about motherhood or the feminine role (Brockington and Kumar 1982). Her attitude to the pregnancy is often shaped by the attitudes of others, for example, her husband, other children and in-laws. Lack of social support, adverse socioeconomic status and the legitimacy of the pregnancy are other risk factors.

Marital conflicts are known to precipitate such disorders. Some couples use the pregnancy as an attempt to cement an already shaky relationship. Others struggle with the 'death' of the relationship between the couple as they are 'invaded' by another person, the infant.

The woman herself has to struggle with major changes in body image both during the pregnancy and delivery as well as in the puerperium (Fervers-Schorre 1991). Dramatic physical changes in her body occur during these phases in response to hormonal shifts.

In late pregnancy, the changes are most dramatic as her girth enlarges to incorporate the growing fetus. At this time, severe fatigability often forces the woman to rethink her priorities. She may have to decide on how to balance her roles as mother and career person. If she decides to stop work, there is a loss of income and status, the additional expense of the new baby and the added stress on the new father, now the sole breadwinner.

Women particularly at risk of developing puerperal psychiatric morbidity are:
* primigravida
* those with a poor marital relationship
* those who lack a confiding relationship
* those whose social and economic circumstances are at risk
* those with a family or a personal history of mental illness

CLINICAL FEATURES

Postpartum blues

- ❑ Benign onset in first three days postdelivery
- ❑ Adjustment reaction to puerperium
- ❑ Transient
- ❑ Resolves in two weeks with no treatment
- ❑ Depression and anxiety
- ❑ Poor concentration
- ❑ Lability of mood
- ❑ Sleep disturbance

Postpartum depression

- ❑ Lasts more than two weeks
- ❑ Depressed mood
- ❑ Anxiety
- ❑ Tiredness
- ❑ Psychomotor retardation or agitation
- ❑ Depressive cognitions (e.g. guilt, self blame)
- ❑ Poor concentration
- ❑ Indecisiveness
- ❑ Suicidal thoughts
- ❑ Insomnia or hypersomnia

Postpartum psychosis

- ❑ All features present in Postpartum depression (above) and
- ❑ Suspiciousness
- ❑ Incoherence or confusion
- ❑ Irrational statements
- ❑ Obsessive concern about baby's health/welfare
- ❑ Thoughts of harming self/baby
- ❑ Delusions that baby is not normal
- ❑ Hallucinations of voices telling her to harm baby

Differential diagnosis

In the postnatal period it is prudent to do a careful physical examination and relevant investigations to exclude possible organic causes that may give rise to a deranged mental state. Anemia, infection, urinary problems or thrombosis should be treated if present.

It is sometimes quite difficult to differentiate between a true puerperal mental illness and other mental disorders like schizophrenia or affective disorder. Only with hindsight can it be ascertained if the episode of illness was puerperal or actually the first onset of manic depressive psychosis or schizophrenia with the delivery being the precipitating stressor (Good 1991).

Physical examination and investigations

A careful physical examination should be conducted to exclude organic causes after which routine investigations that should be done include a full blood count, erythrocyte sedimentation rate, renal, liver and thyroid functions.

If confusion and incoherence are marked, the clinician may proceed to a computer tomographic scan of the brain and an electroencephalogram to exclude intracranial causes like infarct or hemorrhage.

Social investigations

A detailed enquiry about the social circumstances will allow the doctor to assess the possible contributory stressors in the patient's background It will also allow an understanding of the extent of social support available and which should be provided to the patient and new baby.

Treatment

In the first instance, the doctor must assess the extent of suicide risk and risk to the new baby in each case of postnatal mental illness. This should be balanced against the degree of social support available.

Admission to an inpatient mother and baby unit where mentally ill mothers are nursed with their babies by nursing staff trained both in psychiatry and neonatology would be ideal. Unfortunately this is not currently available in many centres. Mothers who require admission have now to be separated from their babies and families.

In *postnatal blues,* usually no specific treatment is needed. The doctor needs to ensure adequate support for the mother and baby at home by enlisting the help of relatives. Reassurance and education should be given to the mother. The condition is self limiting and resolves spontaneously in two weeks.

In *postnatal depression* or *psychoses,* specific intervention is often required. If at risk, the patient should be admitted and closely supervised.

In mild to moderate cases, medication in the form of antidepressants (for example, prothiaden) or antipsychotics (for example, haloperidol, chlorpromazine) should be prescribed. In more severe cases, electroconvulsive therapy is the treatment of choice as it has been proven to be effective and rapidly enables the mother to resume the care of her new baby, enhancing the mother–child bond. Breastfeeding is contraindicated because of its stressful nature and because all psychotropic drugs are excreted in the breast milk.

In mothers with *preexisting psychiatric illness* like schizophrenia, major affective disorder or substance abuse, a close liaison should be maintained between the managing obstetrician and psychiatrist the moment the pregnancy is confirmed (Robinson and Steward 1993). Often patients conceive while still on psychotropic medication despite medical advice to the contrary. They need to be monitored for fetal abnormalities and given clear, sound and consistent advice on the risks of these abnormalities and the option of termination. If they decide to continue the pregnancy, the managing psychiatrist should wean the patient on to the lowest possible dose of medication that enables adequate control of the symptoms. The stress of the advancing pregnancy, delivery and motherhood carry the risk of precipitating a relapse of the patient's illness. If such a relapse occurs, the psychiatrist must balance the wellbeing of the mother against that of the developing fetus. Often this means restarting medication and a very close antenatal follow up jointly by both the obstetrician and psychiatrist.

Management of labour

When patients at risk can be identified before the onset of labour, the managing staff can exercise extra vigilance during delivery.

Labour ward staff should be briefed on the patient's psychological problems on admission. A list of current medications and last dose consumed should be recorded. Drugs should not be routinely omitted just because the patient is in labour. Antenatal and psychiatric notes should contain instructions on the continuation of medication in labour or the psychiatrist's contact number where he can be consulted on this matter. It is reassuring for both patient and staff if the patient's usual obstetrician and psychiatrist are available for consultation.

Pain relief in labour should have been discussed antenatally and a decision already made. In general, unless there is an obstetric contraindication, adequate obstetric analgesia should be offered early. The patient should be accompanied by a relative and closely supervised throughout labour by the midwife, who should be instructed to be sensitive to the woman's mental state. If instrumental delivery is required, this must be discussed clearly and unhurriedly with both the patient and the relative who is present.

It is prudent to have a neonatologist on standby at delivery to check the newborn.

Post delivery, these patients should be observed in the postnatal ward for a week to ten days. A psychiatric review should be done from the third to the fifth day, or sooner if the ward staff note any changes in mood. Transfer to a psychiatric ward or a mother and baby unit may become necessary if the patient is disturbed or distressed.

Prognosis

Most patients recover fully from a puerperal mental illness and the prognosis is excellent if the illness is diagnosed early and treated adequately.

In *postnatal blues,* almost all cases resolve spontaneously with reassurance, emotional support and advice. The recurrence rate in subsequent pregnancies is up to 20%.

In *postnatal depression,* which is similar to a major affective disorder, and *postnatal psychosis,* the response to drug treatment or electroconvulsive therapy is good. There is a real risk of infanticide or suicide. Historically, English common law has recognised that the mother is criminally insane if she injures her child during this illness (Inwood 1989). Again, the recurrence rate in subsequent pregnancies is up to 20% and couples should be counselled about this risk before embarking on the next pregnancy so that adequate supervision can be arranged (Davidson and Robertson 1985).

Women who have a preexisting personal or family history of schizophrenia have up to a 25% chance of developing a schizophrenic psychosis in the puerperium. Those with a history of bipolar affective disorder have up to a 50% risk of relapse in the puerperium (McNeill 1988; Inwood 1989).

A case history

CBL was apparently healthy and functioning well as an orthopaedic staff nurse in a restructured hospital until the delivery of her third son about eight months before initially consulting me. After an uneventful vaginal delivery she stayed only two days in the postnatal ward and was discharged well. She said that she began to feel very low in mood on the fifth postnatal day. Once at home she was full of fears and worried about coping with her third child. She slept badly, waking up frequently and had a poor appetite. She also thought that her baby had brought the household bad luck and started to regret having had the child. She took no pleasure in her new baby and avoided holding him. At the same time she experienced guilt at having these thoughts and felt upset that the baby appeared to prefer the company of the family's Filipino maid.

CBL gradually became unable to cope with the household and the care of the children. She persuaded her husband to move the whole family to her mother's apartment where she felt more secure. The husband did so reluctantly as they were then preparing to move into their own new upgraded flat.

CBL appeared to improve slightly in the six months that she lived with her mother. She returned to work after two months of maternity leave. Her mother helped her with cooking and household chores. However she found that she was forgetful at work and could not perform her duties with her usual efficiency. She found the job meaningless and mechanical and took no enthusiasm or pride in her duties unlike previously.

After six months in her mother's house, her husband continued to be puzzled by his wife's change in behaviour. He could not accept her apparent regressive behaviour and over-dependency on mother. He then insisted that they take possesion of their new house. After the move, the patient's condition began to deteriorate. She was negative about her new neighbourhood and anxious about being alone in the house. She looked markedly dejected in appearance. She admitted to morbid thoughts about death and said that life was meaningless. She had no plans to commit suicide but hoped the whole family might be killed suddenly in an accident so she could be 'put out of her misery'. She experienced no enjoyment in any aspect of her life and found it difficult to cope with work and family. She had depressing thoughts about being a bad wife and mother and an incompetent nurse. She felt that she was a burden to the family and to her colleagues and that she did not deserve their concern and support.

It was only after suffering these symptoms for eight months that she decided to consult the staff doctor to be referred for a psychiatric opinion. As a staff nurse, she feared the stigma of a psychiatric diagnosis and worried about the implications on her employment in the hospital.

CBL responded to an outpatient course of antidepressants after three weeks of treatment. She managed to resume her work after two months' leave and described a complete reversal of all her depressive symptoms.

In her own words, she said, 'As a nurse, I should have known better and got treated earlier. I was so afraid of psychiatrists and mental illness. I really suffered for eight months and it was a completely unnecessary torture for myself and my family.'

The failure to recognise and treat psychiatric disorders in the puerperium can have far-reaching effects on the patient, the newborn, the family and society. There may be a permanent disruption of the mother–child bonding process that has long term effects on the child's intellectual and emotional adjustment (Murray and Stein 1989). Cox (1988) found that 13% of women with depression had difficulty coping with their babies. More acutely there is a small but significant risk of suicide and infanticide in severely depressed or psychotic new mothers.

Obstetricians, midwives and community nurses are ideally placed to detect psychological changes in new mothers. They can be taught to be more sensitive to early features of the illness and to recognise those at risk even in the antenatal period. Raising awareness of these disorders in antenatal or 'parentcraft' classes among parents-to-be would also be a good preventive measure. Services available for treatment should also be publicised.

Postnatal mental illness is highly amenable to treatment. Early recognition and appropriate intervention are the most effective measures to reduce the psychiatric morbidity and mortality associated with these disorders.

References

Brockington IF, Kumar R, eds 1982. Motherhood and mental illness. London, UK: Academic Press.

Cox JL, Connor, YM, Henderson I, Mcquire RJ, Kendell RE 1983. Prospective study of the psychiatric disorders of childbirth by self report questionnaire. *J Affective Disord* 5:1-7.

Cox JL 1988. The life event of childbirth: sociocultural aspects of postnatal depression. In: Kumar R, Brockington IF, eds. Motherhood and Mental Illness Vol II. London: Wright, pp 64-7.

Davidson J, Robertson E 1985. A follow-up study of postpartum illness 1946-1978. *Acta Psychiatr Scand* 71:451-459.

Fervers-Schorre B 1991. Change of body image after childbirth. In: Richter D et al, eds. Advanced Psychosomatic Research in Obstetrics and Gynecology. Berlin, Heidelberg: Springer-Verlag.

Good RS 1991. Postpartum psychiatric admissions. In: Richter D et al, eds. Advanced Psychosomatic Research in Obstetrics and Gynecology. Berlin, Heidelberg: Springer-Verlag.

Inwood DG 1989. Postpartum psychotic disorders. In: Kaplan HI, Sadock BJ, eds. Comprehensive Textbook of Psychiatry. Vol 1, 5th edn. Williams and Wilkins.

Kendell RE, Mackenzie WE, West C, Mcquire Cox JL 1984. Day to day mood changes after childbirth: further data. *Br J Psychiatry* 145:620-5.

Kendell RE 1985. Emotional and physical factors in the genesis of puerperal mental disorders. *J Psychosom Res* 29:3-11.

Kok LP, Chan P, Ratnam SS 1994. Postnatal depression in Singapore women. *Singapore Med J* 35:33-5.

Kumar R, Robinson K 1984. A prospective study of emotional disorders in childbearing women. *Br J Psychiatry* 144:35-47.

McNeil TF 1988. A prospective study of postpartum psychoses in a high-risk group: 3) relationship to mental health characteristics during pregnancy. *Acta Psychiatr Scand* 77: 604-610.

Murray L, Stein A 1989. Effects of postnatal depressions on the infant. *Baillieres Clin Obstet Gynecol* 3:921-31.

Murray D, Cox JL 1990. Screening for depression during pregnancy with the Edinburgh

Depression Scale. *J Reprod Infant Psychiatry* 8:99-107.

Paffenbarger RS 1964. Epidemiological aspects of postpartum mental illness. *Br J Prev Soc Med* 18:189-95.

Pitt B 1968. Atypical depression following childbirth. *Br J Psychiatry* 114:1325-35.

Robin A 1962. Psychological changes in normal parturition. *Psychiatr Q* 36: 129-50.

Robinson GE, Steward DE 1993. Postpartum disorders. In: Stewart DE, Stotland NL, eds. Psychological aspects of women's health care: The interface between psychiatry and obstetrics and gynaecology. Washington, DC: American Psychiatric Press, Inc.

Steward DE, Klompenhouwer JL, Kendell RE, Van Hulst. AM 1991. Prophylactic lithium in postpartum affective psychosis - 3 centres' experience. *Br J Psychiatry* 158:393-398.

Index

myometrial contractility 3, 269
  regulation of 2, 3
myometrial contractions 1, 12
myometrial receptors 7
myometrial sensitivity 4
myometrium 1–4, 12, 15
  structure and function of 2
myopathy
  congenital 349
myosin 3

nalbuphine 46
naloxone 27, 345, 348
naproxen 271
nausea 45, 110, 126, 267, 270
necrosis
  cortical 164, 340
  tubular 188, 340
neonatal
  acidemia 101
  death 288, 330
  jaundice 147, 224, 287
  immediate problems
    management of 344
  resuscitation 158, 344
nerve block
  pudendal 49, 143
neurotransmitter
  adrenergic 4
  cholinergic 4
  peptide 4
  release of, in sensory fibres 44
nifedipine 265, 272, 341
  sublingual 341
nitrazine paper test 231
nitric oxide
  donors 265, 273, 274
nitrofurazone 237
nitroglycerine 273
  patch 274
nitrous oxide 27, 47, 153
nomograms 29
  of cervical dilatation 22
nonstress test (NST) 290
noradrenaline 180
normovolemia 180
norpethidine 45
nulliparae
  failed induction in 286
non-steroidal anti-inflammatory drugs
(NSAIDs) 199

obesity
  maternal 147
oesophageal atresia 350
oestradiol 5–8, 217
oestriol 7
oestrogen 1, 2, 4, 6–8, 15, 70, 261
  receptor 6, 8
oestrone 8
oligohydramnios 232, 233, 237, 239, 241–244,
  247, 248, 252, 272, 291, 296
oliguria 110, 114, 179, 181, 184, 244, 340
operative delivery 132, 252
opiates 44, 45
orciprenaline 265
Ortolani sign 356
oxygen 43, 52, 53, 57, 58, 87, 89, 90, 100
129, 177, 180, 334, 339, 346, 347
  saturation 67
  tension 57
  use of 99
oxytocin 1, 3-6, 8-13, 15, 16, 30, 33, 34,
36-38, 70, 82, 97, 109, 113, 114, 123, 141,
144, 146, 171, 173, 177, 185-187, 200, 216,
217, 221, 222, 234-237, 261, 322–324
  analogues 273
  augmentation 24, 32, 37, 190, 302, 303,
  328
  antagonist 10, 13
  dosage 34–36, 80, 83, 110, 219, 220,
  303
  infusion 30, 35, 79, 83, 100, 109, 110,
  122, 142, 152, 153, 162, 190, 191,
  214, 220–224, 234-237, 239, 240,
  252, 285, 303
  radioimmunoassay of 35
  receptors 1, 3, 9, 10, 12, 13, 15
  receptor antagonist 15
  regime for induction of 111
  role of 9, 261
  time increment schedules 34, 35
  titration 35, 36, 78–80, 220
  treatment 141, 144, 149
  use of 27, 82, 109, 219, 224, 236, 286,
  322, 323
oxytocic 163, 171, 172, 176–179, 181,
187, 193, 194
  administration of 83, 176, 177
  agents 15
  augmentation 37, 78, 323
  drugs 28, 50, 87, 104, 171, 172
  induction of labour 7
  titration 252
  use of 82, 83, 166, 171, 175, 177,
  186, 235

ventilation
   intermittent 342
   over 348
ventricular failure
   left 338
VLBW baby 309, 310, 313
verapamil 272
vernix 230
vesical calculus 306
vocal chord spasm 352

volume expanders 345
vomiting 110, 187, 267, 273, 357
Vulsalva manoeuvre 231
vulval varicosities 167

washout phenomenon 339

Zavanelli manoeuvre 148